Epilepsy 101

The New Patient and Family Guide
to Living Well

Ruben Kuzniecky, MD

Cover image: Ya no hay pecho que resista by Fernando Toledo © 2000

To order copies, please visit www.medicuspress.com or write to:

Medicus Press
P.O. Box 284
Leonia, NJ 07605

www.MedicusPress.com

ISBN: 978-0-9787727-4-1

To the Memory of my mentor and friend

Fred Andermann, MD, FRCP
1930–2019

Contents

Acknowledgments

This book is the end result of many people's efforts directly or indirectly. I am very appreciative to many of my collaborators who wrote chapters, book sections, made comments and critiques, provided art and figures, etc. If this book is better, it is because of all of them.

I am especially thankful to my close collaborators and friends—Steve Pacia, Souhel Najjar, Derek Chong, Howard Weiner, Andy Kanner, Jackie French, Werner Doyle, Robert Goodman, Carmen Baez, Sam Berkovic, Graeme Jackson and Heath Pardoe. All are superb physicians, surgeons, and scientists who have taught me so much through the years. Special thanks to my dear friend and colleague, Dan Lowenstein, MD, a real mench, super scientist, physician, and teacher. To my wife, Yvonne, and family who have never ceased to support and encourage me. I remain ever thankful.

I dedicate this book to the memory of my mentor, Dr. Fred Andermann who passed away as this book was being completed. Everything I will ever know about epilepsy and how to take care of patients came down from Fred. He had an immense intellect, a prodigious memory, enormous skills, unlimited energy, and empathy for others. He was mentor-in-chief to possibly dozens, if not hundreds, of neurologists around the world. He was an incredible clinician, teacher, and researcher. Above all, he continued to be our mentor and friend for many years, guiding us through our private and professional lives.

Finally, I am thankful to our patients and families that have given me an opportunity to be better. It is a daily privilege to care for them.

Editor and Contributors

Editor

Ruben Kuzniecky, MD, FAAN, FANA
Professor and Vice Chair
Department of Neurology
Zucker School of Medicine
New York

Contributors

Bassel Abou-Khalil, MD
Department of Neurology
Vanderbilt University Medical
Center
Nashville, Tenessee

G. Barkley, MD
Department of Neurology
Henry Ford Health System
Detroit, Michigan

Jorgeo G. Burneo, MD, MSPH
Department of Neurosciences
University of Western Ontario
London, Ontario

Gregory Cascino, MD
Department of Neurology
Mayo Clinic
Rochester, Minnesota

Edward Faught, MD
Department of Neurology
Emory Healthcare
Atlanta, Georgia

Jacqueline French, MD
Department of Neurology
NYU Langone Health
New York, New York

Daniel Friedman, MD
Department of Neurology
NYU Langone Health
New York, New York

Frank Gilliam, MD
Department of Neurology
Kentucky Neuroscience Institute
Lexington, Kentucky

Andres Kanner, MD
Department of Neurology
University of Miami Health System
Miami, Florida

Shefali Karkare, MD
Pediatric Neurology
Zucker School of Medicine
Northwell Health
New York, New York

Sanjeev Kothare, MD
Pediatric Neurology
Zucker School of Medicine
Northwell Health
New York, New York

Daniel Lowenstein, MD
Department of Neurology
UCSF Medical Center
University of California
San Francisco, California

Kimford Meador, MD
Department of Neurology and
   Neurosciences
Stanford University
Palo Alto, California

Foram Mehta
Editoral Assistance
San Francisco, California

Anne Marie Morse, DO
Pediatric Neurology
Geisinger Medical Center
Danville, Pennsylvania

Steven Pacia, MD
Department of Neurology
Zucker School of Medicine
Northwell Health
New York, New York

Alison Pack, MD
Department of Neurology
Columbia University Medical
   Center
New York, New York

Page Pennell, MD
Department of Neurology
Brigham and Women's Hospital
Harvard Medical School
Boston, Massachusetts

**Courtney Schnabel Glick,
   MS, RD, CDN**
Department of Neurology
NYU Langone Health
New York, New York

David Vossler, MD
Valley Medical Center
Neuroscience Institute
Renton, Washington

Introduction

Epilepsy, seizures, convulsions, attacks, events, spells, and falls; these are some of the most common terms we hear people use when dealing with epilepsy. Centuries of misunderstanding, demonization, and discrimination caused those with seizures and epilepsy to hide their burden in the closet. Fortunately, over the past 30 years, we have seen the gradual disappearance of these attitudes to the great benefit of patients and families affected by epilepsy and seizures.

The world *epilepsy* is a general term that cannot be considered a disease or a diagnosis. To say that a person has epilepsy has no specific meaning, and it should not be considered a final diagnosis. While the term may give a general indication of the nature of a problem, it is so unspecific as to be almost meaningless in many ways. Epilepsy includes a large number of conditions that can manifest in many ways. Although this may seem complicated, a good way to gain a better understanding is to think about epilepsy in the same way we think about anemia (low blood count). Neither epilepsy nor anemia is a disease. Anemia can be caused by low blood iron, lack of vitamins, loss of blood, and many other causes. Similarly, epilepsy can result from abnormal genes, a malformation of the brain, trauma to the brain, a brain infection, a brain tumor, and so forth. A seizure or epilepsy is simply a manifestation of abnormal brain function (see Chapter 1).

One has to remember that the brain is the most complex and marvelous organ of the human body and, thus, is very sensitive to minor changes in function. If something goes wrong, the problem manifests itself in abnormal functioning within the various systems of the body, such as problems with vision, hearing, language, memory, behavior, and so forth. In simpler terms, abnormal brain function can be exposed by either a loss of function or excess of activity, due mostly to an imbalance between the affected systems. For example, a stroke will destroy an area of brain tissue, resulting in a loss of function in that area. The most common case in point is a stroke victim who has lost the ability to use their arm and hand due to paralysis. On the other hand, seizures or epilepsy can also arise from too much abnormal activity in a brain region. The following section explores all aspects of seizures and epilepsy in more detail.

Historical Background

In the earliest of writings, it was believed that epilepsy, also known as the "sacred disease," was caused by the possession of evil spirits or gods. The word *epilepsy* is derived from the Greek verb *epilamvanein,* which means "to be seized" and is associated with possession by evil spirits. Treatment, therefore, involved the use of religious, occult, and magical powers, and some less than pleasant experiences. The Mesopotamia, Hebrew, and Egyptian civilizations knew of the disease for centuries. The symptoms are mentioned in the Bible. The Greek physicians of the Hippocrates school mentioned epilepsy as the sacred disease, despite the fact that the Greek's rejected the idea that epilepsy was a form of punishment inflicted by the gods. On the contrary, they believed that something in the brain was its cause. Even though they attempted to refute its connection to the supernatural, epilepsy remained attached to charlatans, superstition, and magic powers for many centuries.

In the middle ages, fear of epilepsy and seizures became even more radical. People with epilepsy were accused as possessed by evil spirits and were targeted for death, which wrought much destruction on many people, particularly women. If patients continued to have seizures—despite exorcism—they were frequently put to death. Even at the end of the nineteenth century, a reputable medical practitioner specializing in the treatment of epilepsy might advocate in a lecture in New York that various forms of mutilation, including castration, were appropriate for the treatment of epilepsy. This was because convulsions were known to originate in the testes and masturbation was known to exacerbate epileptic seizures.

The modern view of epilepsy is generally considered to have originated with the studies and work of Dr. John Hughlings Jackson, an English physician born in Yorkshire. At the age of 27, Jackson was appointed as assistant physician in the National Hospital for the Relief and Cure of the Paralyzed and Epileptic (now the National Hospital for Neurology and Neurosurgery), Queen Square, London, in 1862. As in many cases in medicine, Jackson had a close relationship with epilepsy, as his wife had developed motor seizures following a stroke. During the attacks, her hand began jerking, then her leg, and then her face. This type of epilepsy, with its typical march of symptoms, became known as Jacksonian epilepsy, as he himself described the seizures in his wife. Since Dr. Jackson was puzzled by brain function, he used his observations to develop a view of neurology that related where functions were located in the brain. In 1873, Dr. Jackson presented his classic definition of epileptic seizures as "occasional sudden excessive, rapid, and local discharges of gray matter." This view established focal seizures as being truly epileptic in origin. The combination of scientific research and clinical findings enabled Dr. Jackson's ideas to be confirmed by other scientists performing experiments in animals. As a result, the first step of the modern area of epilepsy began (see Chapter 1).

The Modern Era

In 1934, Dr. Wilder Penfield, who founded the Montreal Neurologic Institute at McGill University in Montreal, became the lead figure in furthering the development of the surgical treatment for epilepsy and the localization of brain function. In common with Dr. Jackson, his extensive writings, coupled with a clear, detailed, and objective skill in observation, provided a wealth of information, which remains important to this day.

In 1929, Dr. Hans Berger, a German psychiatrist published the technique of EEG and showed for the first time that electrical activity of the brain could be recorded. Although Dr. Berger was disappointed that the EEG was of limited use in psychiatric patients, he showed that abnormal waves could be recorded in patients with seizures. Soon after his findings were confirmed, many centers around the world began using the EEG to study and treat patients with seizures. This important technology was further developed by many researchers to provide a means whereby the seizure origin in the brain could be localized. This was an exciting time in neurology because, for the first time ever, physicians had a real test that could be used not only to find the area in the brain that caused seizures, but also to separate different seizure types. In 1934, in Boston, Dr. Frederick Gibbs showed the spike and wave EEG of "petite mal" for the first time. A few years later, Dr. Herbert Jasper worked with Dr. Wilder Penfield in Montreal to use the EEG to help in the surgical treatment. The EEG technology developed to the point that in 1951, Dr. Percival Bailey, a neurosurgeon in Chicago, published a paper documenting a series of patients who had temporal lobe surgery based *only* on EEG alone. The results were encouraging and helped established the EEG as the prime method to study seizures. Over the next 30 years, the study of epilepsy was dominated by the technical development and understanding of the information obtained from the EEG. During this period, surgery—as a treatment of epilepsy—also gained considerable ground.

A More Modern View of Epilepsy and Seizures

As we enter the twenty-first century, we have gained much knowledge about epilepsy and seizures. No longer are patients hidden from society because we now know and understand that epilepsy is not an "untouchable" disorder. Additionally, we have many new diagnostic tests, medications, and better surgical techniques. In particular, modern imaging techniques, such as MRI, have had an impact as large as that of EEG more than 70 years ago. In this day and age, we are now entering the genetic era of epilepsy as we try to solve the puzzles of why, what, and how epilepsy occurs. What has become clear over time, though, is that no single mechanism or cause underlies all epilepsies. Therefore, treatment of seizures and epilepsy is likely to change in the years to come.

CHAPTER 1

Epilepsy and Seizures: An Overview

- A *seizure* is what happens when the brain has abnormal, uncontrolled electrical activity.
- *Epilepsy* describes a condition in which a person has a tendency for recurrent seizures.
- About 10 billion neurons are in the human brain.
- Focal seizures come from a discrete *focus* in the brain.
- An aura can occur as a stand-alone event, but it often progresses into a complex focal seizure.
- The tonic-clonic (or *grand mal*) seizure is probably the most commonly recognized seizure type.
- *Myoclonic seizures* refer to extremely brief, jerking movements.
- The most common example of a symptomatic, localization-related epilepsy occurs in *temporal lobe epilepsy.*
- Epilepsy is widely thought as a disorder of childhood, but it is common at any age.

Defining Some Basic Terms

Before getting into a description of what goes on in the brain when a person has a seizure, it is important to first be clear about the definitions of words such as "seizure" and "epilepsy." A *seizure* is what happens when the brain has abnormal, uncontrolled electrical activity leading to a sudden change in a person's behavior. (Technically, a seizure can occur without any obvious change in behavior and even without the person being aware of it, but we will cover this later.) So, you should think of a seizure as a single event. On the other hand, the term *epilepsy* is used to describe a condition in which a person has a tendency for recurrent seizures. Thus, rather than being a single event, epilepsy generally refers to a chronic condition. This definition means that a person who has had only one seizure does not have epilepsy. In fact, even two or three seizures might not mean a person has epilepsy, as long as the reason for the seizures can be fixed and there is no "tendency" or high likelihood for recurrences.

What Goes On in the Brain During a Seizure?

To understand what is going on in the brain during a seizure, you need to have a general idea of the brain structure. Everyone knows that the brain is a mass of gelatinous material that sits inside the skull and is responsible for our ability to think, speak, move our body, and sense the world, to name just a few of its amazing functions. Exactly how does the brain do these things? Neuroscientists have been working on this question for years now, and we are only beginning to get an idea of exactly how the brain accomplishes these tasks. However, we do know that one main cell type in the brain— the neuron—is a key player in brain function Figure 1.1. About 10 billion neurons are in the human brain, and each neuron makes numerous connections with other neurons, forming an incredibly complex and intricate network. Some scientists have estimated that each neuron makes an average of 100,000 connections with other neurons, which means that the brain's neuronal network has a total of 1,000 trillion connections! Nature designed

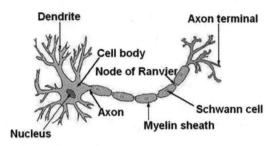

FIGURE 1.1 A typical neuron and its parts.
The dendrite connects the neuron with other cells.

neurons to accomplish one main task—to communicate with one another by generating electrical impulses that can travel along the length of the cell and create a signal that influences the ability of other neurons to generate electrical impulses. Thus, *neurons* are miniature signaling devices that can detect incoming electrical impulses and, depending on the circumstances, relay the information to other cells in the form of electrical signals.

If it were possible to "listen" to the firing of electrical impulses by a large group of neurons during normal brain activity (for example, what your brain is doing right now as you read these words), you would hear many neurons firing away, but the overall sound would not make much sense. That is, the overall signaling occurring in the brain is so complex that the sum total of the firing by a large number of neurons would sound like chaotic noise. This chaotic, seemingly random activity is actually similar to what you can see with an electroencephalograph (EEG), a device that measures the overall electrical activity of neurons during normal brain function in a conscious person.

Now, here is the *key concept* in understanding what is going on in the brain when a person is having a seizure. During a seizure, large groups of neurons are out of control—they fire excessively—and they synchronize their firing with one another. Thus, if you were listening in on a group of neurons involved in a seizure, you would hear loud, high-speed bursts of activity coming from many neurons at the same time. This is dramatically different from the relatively quiet and seemingly random background noise that you would hear normally.

A good way to visualize what is happening during a seizure is to imagine standing at the entrance of a large, busy restaurant and listening to the sounds of all the people talking at once. There are presumably meaningful conversations taking place at each table—whether it is the couple at a table for two or a large party of ten or twelve. However, the sound from where you are standing is just chaotic noise. If you think of each person in the restaurant as a neuron, you are hearing what the brain normally "sounds" like during normal activity. Now, imagine that suddenly a line of waiters and waitresses emerges from the kitchen. At the head of the line is a waiter carrying a birthday cake, and they are headed toward a table in the distance, which is obviously the scene of a birthday celebration. As soon as the birthday cake comes into sight, the raucous group at the table begins singing "Happy Birthday" very loudly. Their loud singing represents the high-amplitude, super-synchronized activity that occurs in a group of neurons during a seizure. And, you, standing at the doorway some distance from the singing, can detect this "abnormal" synchronized activity in much the same way that an EEG can detect seizure activity in the brain.

Believe it or not, this is a fairly accurate analogy of what is going on in the brain during a seizure. As you learn next, a variety of different seizure types exist, with the main distinguishing feature being whether the seizure activity stays restricted to just one part of the brain or whether the seizure involves the entire brain. When a seizure stays restricted to one part of the brain, it is just like the song is being sung by only the people at the birthday table. However, sometimes a seizure "focus" can spread to other regions of the brain, to the point at which the entire brain is undergoing a seizure—a so-called "generalized" seizure. This is analogous to people at neighboring tables joining in and singing the birthday song, to the point where every person in the restaurant is singing (loudly and synchronized!).

More On the Different Types of Seizures

As previously mentioned, a variety of seizure types exist, depending on where the abnormal neuronal activity is occurring. In fact, an internationally recognized seizure classification system is used by epilepsy doctors to try to make the most accurate diagnosis of a patient's problem and to provide a guide to the best therapy.

The basic classification system is shown in Table 1.1 and explains each group in some detail.

TABLE 1.1   Classification of Seizures

1. **Focal Onset** (Can be further described as having intact or impaired awareness, motor, or nonmotor onset, or evolve from focal to bilateral tonic-clonic)

2. **Generalized Onset**
  a. Motor
    • Tonic-clonic
    • Other motor (e.g., atonic, myoclonic)
  b. Nonmotor (absence)

3. **Unknown Onset** (Can be further described as motor or nonmotor, or unclassified)

Focal Onset Seizures

Note that the first main category is seizures having a "focal onset." Focal onset seizures come from a discrete *focus* in the brain. That is to say the abnormal firing of neurons start and stay restricted to one brain region. To confuse matters, previous classification systems have used the term "partial" synonymously with "focal." Many people misinterpret the term "partial" to mean that a seizure is partial or incomplete, but that is not the case. Just substitute the word "focal" every time you hear "partial."

To understand the different types of focal seizures, you need to have a general appreciation for how the brain is organized. You can see in Figure 1.2 that each half of the brain is composed of four major regions or "lobes," and, as a general rule, each one of these lobes has a distinctive set of functions. The *occipital lobe* at the back of the brain analyzes the signals coming from the eye, and it enables us to see. The *parietal lobe,* just in front of the occipital lobe, interprets information coming from sensory receptors throughout the body—it is responsible for our ability to feel skin sensa-

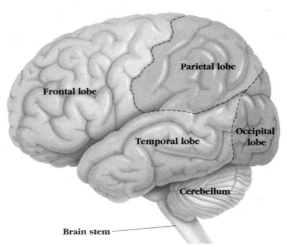

FIGURE 1.2 The human brain with the different lobes. This is a view of the left hemisphere.

tions, including things like light touch, temperature, pain, and the position of our limbs. The *temporal lobe* sits below the parietal lobe and allows us to form memories, experience, emotions and, along with the frontal lobe, to use language. (Actually, language typically resides on one side of the brain or the other; in the majority of people this is on the left half of the brain.) Finally, the *frontal lobe*, at the front of the brain, is responsible for many of the higher-level functions that are the most distinctive of human traits, such as judgment, planning, personality, planning, and abstract reasoning. Also, a very important function of the frontal lobe (coming from the backmost part right next to the border with the parietal lobe) is the control of motor movements.

Now, back to the question of the various types of focal seizures. Since different parts of the brain do different things, the nature of the seizure, or the behavior you might observe in a person during a seizure, depends on which part of the brain is undergoing seizure activity. Suppose, for example, we could create a seizure focus precisely in the part of the frontal lobe responsible for motor movement. Since the seizure focus creates uncontrolled activity in a group of neurons, the seizure the person experiences may be uncontrolled shaking movements of the arm, the leg, the face, or a combination of these, depending on the extent of the region involved. This would, therefore, be a *focal onset* seizure. Importantly, when we describe or classify a seizure, we also consider whether there is any abnormality of awareness or consciousness in the person, so in this case, we would say the seizure is *focal onset with intact awareness.*

If we created a seizure focus slightly farther back in the brain—in the parietal lobe—the person might experience odd sensations, since the parietal lobe is responsible for (among other things) detecting sensations in the skin. But there would not be any abnormal movements or behavior. In this case, we would describe the seizure as *focal onset, nonmotor with intact awareness.*

What happens when the seizure focus is located in the temporal or frontal lobe? Now things get a bit more complicated because most functions of these two parts of the brain are more complex than the regions just described (refer to Figure 1.2). For example, let's place the seizure focus in the left temporal lobe. In this case, the seizure activity would disrupt the normal function of the brain dealing with memory, emotions, and possibly language. Try to imagine what you would feel like if you suddenly were unable to remember anything (such as recognizing the faces of people around you), you became anxious (because your emotions were difficult to control), and you were unable to speak or understand the words other people were saying. This interruption of your normal thinking would cause you to have an abnormal level of consciousness. To an outside observer, you might appear confused (e.g., with a dazed, "far off" look), perhaps afraid, and unable to communicate with others. For reasons we don't fully understand, seizures of this type can also cause repetitive, automatic-like behaviors, such as lip smacking or picking movements of the hands, which are called *automatisms.* As you can see, this type of focal seizure has much more complex behaviors associated with it, compared with the pure motor seizure and pure sensory seizure described earlier. We would classify this as a focal seizure with automatisms and impaired awareness.

A somewhat similar situation happens when the seizure occurs in the frontal lobe. Again, the abnormal neuronal activity would disrupt functions of the brain, such as judgment and abstract reasoning, so you can see how the person with a frontal lobe seizure might have an interruption of their normal consciousness. We would, therefore, also classify this seizure as being focal with impaired awareness.

Not surprisingly, focal seizures can cross the boundaries of the various lobes of the brain or involve multiple functions. So, for example, a focal seizure of the frontal lobe might not only cause a change in a person's awareness, but it could also cause abnormal motor movements due to the involvement of the region of the frontal lobe responsible for the control of movement.

We want to review one last point before moving on to the other main categories of seizures. A seizure that comes from the temporal lobe or frontal lobe can cause an odd awareness that something is not quite right, such as a feeling of rushed thoughts, déjà vu (feeling as though you have already experienced what is happening around you), sudden emotions (e.g., fear), or sensing unusual odors or sounds. These seizures are similar to what may be experienced during focal seizures, but no actual impairment of awareness occurs. That is, the person is awake and aware of what is going on, and can describe it to others. Since awareness is not impaired, this is classified as a *focal nonmotor seizure*. Also, these particular experiences are usually what is meant when a person says he is having an *aura*. An aura can occur as a stand-alone event, but it often progresses into a focal seizure with impaired awareness. People with epilepsy quickly learn that an aura is a warning sign that a larger seizure may be coming. (In fact, the word "aura" comes from the Greek word meaning "breeze," as if the breeze is a signal that a storm may soon follow.)

Generalized Onset Seizures

Generalized seizures are, not surprisingly, quite different from focal seizures, because the abnormal neuronal firing seems to occur in most of the brain all at once. Purists might say that a seizure cannot possibly start precisely all over the brain at exactly the same time—it must start somewhere! And they are right. However, in practical terms, a generalized seizure takes over the brain so quickly, it is impossible (using current methods) to detect where the first electrical discharge begins. Generalized onset seizures are further classified into motor and nonmotor types.

The most commonly recognized seizure type of all is the tonic-clonic (or grand mal) seizure. The seizure activity rapidly spreads over both sides of the brain, leading to a loss of consciousness. Since the part of the brain controlling motor movement is affected on both sides of the brain, the person usually has stiffening of the arms and legs on both sides of the body, which causes them to fall if standing. The stiffening is referred to as the *tonic phase*. Depending on when the seizure begins during the breathing cycle, the sudden contraction of the muscles of the diaphragm and the voice box may cause the person to let out an unusual cry. After a short while, the constant stiffening is replaced by cycles of stiffening and relaxation of the muscles, which leads to shaking movements (the *clonic phase*). Finally, once the seizure passes, the person becomes limp and remains unconscious until the brain recovers sufficiently to allow them to wake again. The duration of tonic-clonic seizures can vary a great deal, but the tonic and clonic phases usually last about a minute or two. It usually takes at least 15 to 30 minutes (and often longer) for a person to begin to return to normal.

A more unusual generalized seizure is an atonic seizure. *Atonic* refers to a loss of tone, so you can imagine what happens when a seizure of this type suddenly occurs while a person is upright. The person abruptly becomes limp and collapses to the ground. Many individuals with this form of seizure must wear a protective helmet to prevent a serious head injury from falling. It might be a bit difficult to understand how hyperexcitable, super-synchronized neurons could lead to a *loss* of tone, rather than increased tone. However, researchers have learned that the overall output of certain networks of activated neurons can be inhibitory, rather than excitatory; it is thought this is the basis for atonic seizures.

Myoclonic seizures refer to extremely brief, jerking movements. For example, the movements are the same as the very sudden movement that can occur when a normal person is falling asleep in a classroom. A myoclonic seizure can be a single jerking movement lasting a fraction of a second, or repetitive jerking movements lasting seconds or minutes (and rarely longer). These are frequently seen in people who have other types of generalized seizures.

Absence (also called *petit mal*) seizures are a form of generalized onset nonmotor seizures in which a sudden abnormality occurs in the circuitry that connects the surface of the brain with a deeper structure called the *thalamus*. Interestingly, these are the same pathways that enable us to transition from being awake and being asleep, and some parallels exist between the behavior of a person having an absence seizure and being asleep. During the seizure, which usually starts abruptly and without warning, the person just goes blank for a few seconds. There may be a small amount of facial movements, such as fluttering of the eyelids or movements of the mouth, but the patient otherwise maintains their posture or position, and the seizure stops as abruptly as it began. People are usually able to maintain their posture during the seizure, for example, they can remain standing. These seizures tend to occur in children, and the EEG shows a characteristic wave pattern known as "3-per-second spike-and-wave" that emanates from the so-called *thalamo-cortical* circuitry.

Focal Seizures that Evolve to Generalized Tonic-Clonic Seizures

If you have a good idea of what is happening in a focal seizure versus what is happening in a generalized seizure, then this additional type of seizure, in which a focal seizure evolves into a generalized seizure, should not be too difficult to understand. Imagine a focal seizure beginning in the part of the frontal lobe controlling motor movements. As previously discussed, this leads to shaking movements of the arm, leg, or face. But now imagine that the overall state of the brain is such that the brain tissue surrounding the seizure focus is relatively susceptible to abnormal excitation and, under certain conditions, can be "recruited" to join in to the seizure focus. In this case, the seizure focus begins to grow and spread, and it can rather quickly take over the entire brain. Thus, the person who was initially having shaking movements in one part of the body will become unconscious (and fall to the ground if upright) and have the other manifestations of a generalized seizure. It is important to try to discriminate between a pure, generalized seizure and a focal seizure that evolves into a generalized seizure because the causes of these two types of seizures can be quite different.

Unknown Onset Seizures

The last category in the seizure classification system includes seizures in which we cannot determine whether the onset is focal or generalized. In these situations, we do our best to describe what we observe (e.g., whether the seizure has motor manifestations).

Epileptic Syndromes

In addition to classifying seizures, experts in the field have developed a separate classification system for the different epilepsies or epileptic syndromes. Classifying epilepsy by seizure type alone creates problems when an individual has more than one seizure type. In addition, it leaves out other critical information that may be important in understanding each individual's condition. When doctors classify an individual as having a specific epilepsy syndrome, they take into account a number of characteristics including seizure type, EEG recordings, age of onset of the seizures, family history, precipitating features, and accompanying neurologic symptoms or problems. Making a diagnosis of a specific epileptic syndrome often allows the physician to provide more accurate information about the expected response to treatment and better counseling regarding the possibility that the epilepsy may be inherited. An understanding of the epilepsy syndrome may also affect what treatment the doctor chooses for the seizures.

Table 1.2 provides a simple outline for the classification scheme for the epilepsies and epileptic syndromes. It is based on an international classification scheme that is much more complex and beyond the focus of this discussion. Just as with the classification of seizures, the classification of the epileptic syndromes is divided into those with focal-onset seizures (*localization-related or focal epilepsies*) or generalized seizures (*the generalized epilepsies*). Within both the localized and generalized groups are additional subdivisions into *idiopathic* (unknown cause, often determined to be genetic), *symptomatic* (identified cause), and *cryptogenic* (hidden cause).

Under the heading of localization-related epilepsies, most of the syndromes are defined by where in the brain the seizures originate, such as in the temporal, frontal, parietal, or occipital lobes. For example, in frontal lobe epilepsy, there are examples of idiopathic, symptomatic, and cryptogenic subtypes. An example of an idiopathic frontal lobe epilepsy is the syndrome of *autosomal dominant nocturnal frontal lobe epilepsy*. This syndrome initially had no identified cause, but it was recognized to occur in families. Eventually, it led to the identification of a specific gene for a particular chemical receptor that caused the syndrome. In many cases, the use of the term "idiopathic" implies that the cause of the epilepsy is thought to be genetic. Frontal lobe epilepsy may also arise from a structural lesion in the frontal lobe that can be seen on magnetic resonance imaging (MRI). When we are able to identify an abnormality in the frontal lobe that is the cause of the seizures (such as a tumor or blood vessel abnormality), the syndrome is classified as *symptomatic frontal lobe epilepsy*. Similarly, many

TABLE 1.2 Simplified Classification of Epilepsies and Epileptic Syndromes

I.	Localization-related (involves one or more distinct areas of the brain)
II.	Generalized (involves both sides of the brain at the same time)
III.	Undetermined whether localized or generalized
IV.	Special syndromes

individuals diagnosed with frontal lobe epilepsy have no identified cause (even after exhaustive testing); they are labeled as having *cryptogenic epilepsy*. Here, the doctors believe that a scar or brain abnormality is present, but it is too small to discover with our present tools.

The most common example of a symptomatic, localization-related epilepsy occurs in temporal lobe epilepsy. The temporal lobe, an area of the brain that sits on each side of the head just above the ear, is the most common site for the onset of epileptic seizures. Individuals with temporal lobe epilepsy frequently have a history of brain insult in infancy, such as a prolonged fever-related seizure (complex febrile seizure) or brain infection (bacterial meningitis). Many years later, complex partial seizures develop that are often difficult to control with medicines. The EEG shows abnormal epileptiform or spike activity over one or both temporal lobes. The MRI, particularly when special images are done through the temporal lobe, reveals scaring or shrinkage of the hippocampus. The *hippocampus* is a structure deep within the temporal lobe that is primarily involved in memory but, for unclear reasons, is also very likely to give rise to seizures. **Many patients with temporal lobe epilepsy are not controlled with antiepileptic drug treatment**. These individuals with uncontrolled *mesial temporal lobe epilepsy* are often treated with surgery to remove the scarred hippocampus, and this surgery has an excellent chance of stopping the seizures.

The second category of epilepsy syndromes, the generalized epileptic syndromes, centers on individuals with predominantly generalized seizures. This category includes many of the most common epileptic syndromes, such as *juvenile myoclonic epilepsy, childhood absence epilepsy, infantile spasms*, and *Lennox-Gastaut syndrome*. All these syndromes will be discussed in subsequent chapters.

A few uncommon epileptic syndromes appear to have features of both generalized and localization-related seizures. They are classified in a third and separate category in Table 1.2. An example of this type is the *Landau-Kleffner syndrome* (LKS), which is also called acquired *epileptic aphasia*. LKS is a syndrome characterized by two major symptoms: the development of aphasia or language impairment and a profoundly abnormal EEG with epileptiform activity occurring over the temporal regions and/or in a generalized distribution. It usually has its onset between the ages of 3 and 8 years. Seizures do occur, but they are much less of a problem than the cognitive and language impairments.

The fourth category of epileptic syndromes is called *special syndromes.* These are often syndromes that are clearly defined but are so different that they do not fit comfortably into any of the other three categories. Two examples include *febrile seizures* and *reflex epilepsy.* **A febrile seizure is a specific syndrome that involves generalized seizures occurring with a fever**. Not all experts consider this a true form of epilepsy, but it does appear in the international classification. Febrile seizures occur in 3 percent to 4 percent of children, usually between the ages of 6 months to 5 years of age, with the peak at approximately 18 months of age. Children with febrile seizures are usually not treated because the seizures occur infrequently and the medicines are of questionable effectiveness. Most children simply outgrow the tendency to have seizures with fever and never have problems with seizures again. However, approximately 5 percent of children with febrile seizures will develop focal or localization-related epilepsy later in life, particularly if the febrile seizures were very long or had other complicated features. Reflex epilepsy is an uncommon but fascinating group of disorders, which is also considered under the heading of special syndromes. *Reflex epilepsy* is the name given to seizures that are triggered by sensitivity to sensory stimulation in the environment. The most common form is *photosensitive epilepsy*, in which seizures are precipitated by exposure to intense or fluctuating levels of light, such as those given off by a strobe light. The condition usually begins in childhood and is generally outgrown by adulthood. Other rare triggers for reflex epilepsy include certain sounds, reading, immersion in hot water, and even eating.

Causes of Epilepsy

When a person is told that they have epilepsy, many questions immediately come to mind. Usually the first question is "Why me?" Understandably, you want to know what is causing your seizure disorder. Despite the development of sensitive tests such as MRI, doctors still are unable to identify the cause of epilepsy in about half of individuals with the new onset of epilepsy. When doctors are able to identify a cause for epilepsy, the likely cause varies depending on the age when seizures begin. Newborn infants very frequently have seizures due to problems surrounding their birth, discussed further in Chapter 8. In young children, common causes of epilepsy include abnormalities in the brain present at birth and infections in the central nervous system. These nervous system infections include *meningitis* (an infection of the covering of the brain and spinal cord) or *encephalitis* (an infection of the brain itself). When epilepsy begins in a school-age child, genetics often plays a prominent role. The specific genetic pattern of inheritance is often complex, but it is clear that many seizure disorders, particularly those discussed under generalized epileptic seizures (see Table 1.2) are due to a genetic predisposition. In adolescents and young adults, head trauma (particularly if associated with loss of consciousness or accompanied by bleeding in or around the brain) often leads to the development of epilepsy. When adults develop epilepsy, the first concern usually is "Do I have a brain tumor?" Although brain tumors of all sorts are a possible cause of epilepsy throughout adulthood, they represent only a small percentage of all cases of new-onset epilepsy. A much more common cause of epilepsy is stroke. A *stroke* is an injury to the brain that occurs when the blood supply to an area of the brain is cut off. Strokes happen much more frequently in the elderly and, as a result, epilepsy is surprisingly common in older individuals. Epilepsy is widely thought to be a disorder of childhood, but it is common at any age, and the largest number of new-onset cases of epilepsy is actually in people over the age of 65.

Factors That May Provoke Seizures

Even in people without epilepsy, seizures can be provoked if enough bio-logic stresses are present. In fact, about 10 percent of people will have a sei-zure sometime in their life, but only about 1 percent will go on to have epi-lepsy (meaning recurrent unprovoked seizures). Some have seizures with a high fever as an infant or child (febrile seizures, as previously mentioned). Others will have a seizure due to the effect of a medical illness (kidney failure) or drugs (both street drugs and prescription drugs). Everybody has a certain threshold, or propensity, to have seizures. The difference in an individual with epilepsy is that the *threshold* (or "hurdle") is lower, and it is easier to "get over" the threshold and go on to have a seizure. The use of antiepileptic drugs helps raise that seizure threshold, making it less likely a seizure will occur.

However, many things that happen in your daily life may lower that seizure threshold and, as a result, make having a seizure more likely. The two most common lifestyle factors that provoke seizures are sleep-depri-vation and alcohol. *Sleep deprivation* can be due to staying up all night for only one night, such as when trying to finish a school or work project, or it can be due to being short on sleep over several days or weeks due to work or social demands. The bottom line is that getting adequate rest is important for anyone with a seizure disorder. Alcoholic beverages are also a common cause of breakthrough seizures. Having several alcoholic drinks clearly lowers your seizure threshold and makes seizures more likely. It is less clear whether a single alcoholic drink helps bring on seizures, but avoiding alcohol altogether is commonly recommended for anyone with epilepsy. Other stresses that may push you toward having seizures are listed in Table 1.3.

Table 1.3 lists drugs, both recreational and medical, that are known to lower the seizure threshold. Of the recreational or street drugs, stimulants (such as cocaine) and hallucinogens (PCP) seem to be the drugs that most commonly cause seizures. Several over-the-counter (OTC) or prescription medicines can also bring on seizures. Sedating antihistamines (which are

TABLE 1.3 Factors That Lower Seizure Threshold

Common	Occasional
Sleep deprivation	Hyperventilation
Alcohol	Flashing lights
Infection (fever)	Stress (physical, emotional)
Recreational drugs (cocaine, stimulants)	Medications (sedating antihistamines, some antibiotics)
Menstruation	

found in many multisymptom cold or allergy remedies) are the OTC medicines that seem most commonly to precipitate breakthrough seizures. A few prescribed medications (such as the antibiotic ciprofloxacin [Cipro]) also are reported to increase the risk of seizures.

Many people with epilepsy attempt to identify factors in their daily life that seem to bring on seizures. Diet is often examined as a possible cause, but most evidence suggests that diet (specific foods or missed meals) is rarely a significant contributor to seizure risk. Many women identify an increase in seizures with their menstrual cycle, which is supported in the scientific literature. An increase in seizures is commonly seen just at the onset of menstrual flow or during mid-cycle (at the time of ovulation).

The Risks or Dangers Associated with Having Seizures

Do Seizures Cause Brain Injury?

Up until about 20 years ago, the answer to this question was easy and simple: No, a single isolated seizures whether partial or generalized, does not cause injury to brain cells. Only if the seizure activity was prolonged (lasting less than 30 minutes) did doctors begin to worry about the possibility of permanent brain injury due to seizure activity. However, over the last two decades, evidence has accumulated in animal studies (as well as some evidence in human studies) that even recurrent isolated seizures can lead to further brain injury. In real life, though, the majority of people with epilepsy, even after years of active problems with seizures, still have no evidence of additional brain injury or brain function impairment. So, while complete seizure control is obviously everyone's goal, recurrent seizure activity, unless it is excessive, is rarely identified to cause additional injury to the brain.

Risks of Injury During a Seizure

A major concern for many people with epilepsy is the possibility of injury during a seizure. During a tonic-clonic seizure, an intense and unnatural muscle contraction occurs beyond what anyone can carry out voluntarily. This results in the muscle soreness that frequently is noted in the days after a convulsive seizure. Often the tongue may be bitten as the jaw muscles clamp down. This can be extremely painful, but, unfortunately, it cannot be prevented because the contraction usually occurs too quickly for any intervention. The intense muscle contraction can also sometimes result in shoulder dislocations or compression fractures of the spine. Shoulder dislocations are painful but can be *reduced* or put back in place in the emergency department. A *compression fracture* of the spine is probably more common and occurs when the muscles surrounding the vertebrae in your spine contract so strongly that they compress or partially collapse one of the bones that makes up your spinal column. This does not lead to injury to the spinal cord, but it does result in significant pain over the area of the compression.

With tonic-clonic seizures, abrupt loss of consciousness **usually occurs,** so that falls from a standing position are common. Individuals with active seizure problems are counseled to avoid dangerous activities (working at heights, operating large machinery, swimming alone) in which they would be at a markedly increased risk if they suffered a seizure. In a fall from a standing position, any number of injuries can occur: head trauma, broken bones, cuts, and bruises. Significant head trauma is the most worrisome for fear of concussions, brain contusions, and bleeding inside the skull. This is why some people with extremely uncontrolled epilepsy, particularly with frequent tonic, atonic, or tonic-clonic seizures, may be required to wear a helmet to avoid serious brain injury.

FREQUENTLY ASKED QUESTIONS

Q **My doctor says he doesn't know the cause of my seizures, so why do I have them?**

The two terms doctors use to describe your epilepsy, if there is no evident cause, are cryptogenic or idiopathic. *Cryptogenic* comes from the Greek words meaning "obscure or unknown origin." And, *idiopathic* comes from the Greek words meaning "one's own private suffering." In either case, these terms are a fancy way of saying that the cause of your epilepsy remains unknown to the doctor. In most cases of cryptogenic epilepsy, it is likely that a small brain abnormality is present that is too small to be discovered by any of our tests. This small area of abnormality cannot be seen on the MRI, but it still is able to cause the abnormal electrical activity that leads to your seizure. When doctors use the term idiopathic epilepsy, it has come to imply that the cause is likely genetic. Even in idiopathic epilepsy, it is common not to have a clear family history, but the clinical suspicion focuses on an inherited trait that may have predisposed you to developing epilepsy.

Q **I'm told my seizures are coming from a scar on my brain that occurred during an auto accident 10 years ago. Why did it take so long for my seizures to show up?**

To have a delay of months or even years after a brain injury before the development of epilepsy is common. Exactly what is going on in the brain during this interval is unknown. Scientists continue to explore the changes happening to the brain cells during this time, but the answer as to why epilepsy develops after this delay is not completely known. The hope is that with better understanding of this process, doctors may be able to intervene during the "lull in the action" and prevent the subsequent development of epilepsy. Unfortunately, no medicine or treatment has been identified that can interrupt this process in humans.

Q   How can I tell what type of seizures I have?

Your doctor combines the information from your history (age of onset, description of your seizure behavior, risk factors for epilepsy) and medical tests (EEG, MRI) to determine the type of seizures that you have. If your seizures began before the age of 15, about half will be focal onset and half will be generalized in onset. The presence of an abnormality on your MRI or focal epilepsy-type changes on your EEG, would make the diagnosis of a focal epilepsy likely. If the EEG showed a generalized pattern, a generalized epilepsy would likely be the diagnosis. This information is then combined with the clinical history, including a description of the seizures themselves, to make the diagnosis or determination. The doctor uses your description of your seizures and combines it with what observers say about your seizures to get as clear a picture as possible about the type of seizures that you are experiencing. However, sometimes the tests are all normal, and the description of the seizure is not conclusive enough to allow a diagnosis of a specific seizure type. In older individuals, say over 30 or 35 years old, it is much easier. Almost everybody presenting with new-onset seizures in this age group will have focal epilepsy.

Q   Can I die from having a seizure?

The biggest danger from a seizure comes from what the individual is doing when a seizure occurs. Obviously, if you are driving a car, there is a real risk of serious injury to yourself and others. So, creating lifestyle restrictions (such as not driving, not swimming alone, not working at heights) is the first step to assuring the safety of someone with uncontrolled seizures. Once seizures are brought under control with treatment, however, it's safe to resume these activities. It should be noted that the extent of the activity heavily depends on the unique situation of each person with epilepsy. For example, in some cases, there may be legal restrictions to keep in mind. In Chapter 14, we review important tips for how to live an independent life with epilepsy, including what you should know about obtaining a driver's license in your state. As discussed in this chapter, there are also risks from falls during the seizure or from confusion after the seizure. However, the seizure itself, although often terrifying to observe, is not immediately life threatening. Rarely, individuals with epilepsy can suffer an unexpected sudden death. These episodes usually are unwitnessed and occur more commonly in poorly controlled epilepsy. The exact cause or causes remain unknown. Thankfully, sudden unexpected death in epilepsy (SUDEP) is rare, especially in people who have their seizures fully controlled.

Q   When should I call for emergency help?

When someone witnesses a tonic-clonic seizure for the first time, emergency help will almost always be summoned due to the frightening nature of the seizure and the fear that the person is dying or seriously ill. However, in someone with an established diagnosis of epilepsy, emergency help does not need to be summoned for each seizure. Proper "seizure first-aid" should be carried out (see the Appendix) and the person observed until they achieve a normal degree of alertness. However, there are situations in which it is appropriate to summon emergency help, even for someone who has an established diagnosis of epilepsy. Three main situations exist in which summoning emergency assistance is appropriate:

1. If the seizure duration (active motor jerking) lasts more than 5 minutes (as timed by a clock).
2. If the person has a second seizure before regaining a normal degree of alertness.
3. If the person has injured themselves significantly during the seizure (such as a head injury due to a fall).

These are general guidelines and are not meant to replace your doctor's advice and instructions. Please discuss and consult with your physician about the details of your particular form of epilepsy.

CHAPTER 2

Diagnosis of Seizures and Epilepsy

- Approximately 90 percent of the new-onset cases in adults have focal or partial ("part" of the brain is involved in seizure onset) epilepsy.
- With the occurrence of a first seizure or a recurrence of a first seizure, it is important to seek an explanation or a cause.
- The *electroencephalogram* (EEG) is the only test that can prove someone has epilepsy.
- Patients with seizure disorders, even drug-resistant epilepsy, may have repetitive "normal" EEG studies.
- Video-EEG monitoring is predominantly used by most physicians for diagnostic classification.
- MRI is the best imaging technique we have to find the cause of seizures.
- It is not uncommon for patients with nonepileptic behavioral events or psychogenic spells to have many normal EEG recordings.

As discussed in Chapter 1, epilepsy is a chronic medical condition characterized by recurrent and unprovoked seizures that afflicts close to 4 million people in the United States. Epilepsy is one of the most common neurologic disorders. One in 25 Americans will develop a seizure disorder during their lifetime. Approximately 90 percent of the new-onset cases in adults have focal or partial ("part" of the brain is involved with seizure onset) epilepsy. Nearly 70 percent of focal seizures are associated with temporal lobe epilepsy, a form of epilepsy in which seizures arise from the temporal lobe in the brain.

As you will see, the abnormal behavior or symptoms associated with seizures and the area of the brain involved with the seizure onset are used to understand and classify the seizure activity (Tables 2.1 through 2.3). As explained in Chapter 1, the generalized seizures (involving both the right and left side of the brain at onset) include *tonic-clonic* (grand mal or convulsions), *absence* (petit mal), *myoclonic, atonic* (drop attacks), and *tonic* (increased tone in the arms and legs). Focal seizures include *focal seizures with impaired awareness* (behavioral arrest and staring), *focal seizures with the patient aware* (patient remains awake), or *focal seizure evolving into tonic-clonic* (part of the brain initiates a tonic-clonic seizure). It is important to remember that the majority of "convulsions" (tonic-clonic seizures) are *focal* in onset with secondary generalization (see Table 1.3). The distinction between the two types of focal seizures depends on the presence of impairment in consciousness or *awareness* during the seizure; making this distinction can be challenging.

Establishing a Diagnosis of Seizures and Epilepsy

With the occurrence of a first seizure or a recurrence of a first seizure, it is important to seek an explanation or a cause. Almost 10 percent of individuals will experience one or more seizures during their lifetime. Over 150,000 people in the United States will experience an unprovoked first seizure each year. Adults with an unprovoked seizure are at greatest risk of a recurrent seizure within the first 2 years (21 percent to 45 percent). The diagnostic evaluation of the patient with a first seizure may be useful to determine the cause of the seizure and any indication for antiepileptic drug therapy. A medical doctor (MD) or physician should be consulted. As in any other field of medicine, there are specialists who are trained in the diagnosis and treatment of seizures. For those 18 years and older, a neurologist will be the most appropriate physician; for children, a pediatric neurologist should be consulted. Some neurologists specialize in epilepsy (epileptologist), and those may be particularly appropriate when seizures are difficult to control or when other treatments are needed.

Several steps are taken in the neurologic consultation and investigation of patients with seizures or epilepsy. These steps are:

1. Clinical evaluation
2. Laboratory testing
3. Neurophysiologic testing
4. Neuroimaging
5. Other special tests

Clinical Evaluation

The clinical evaluation takes place when a patient walks into the neurologist's office or when the neurologist sees the patient in the hospital. The visit is first directed at establishing the details of the seizure and the patient's medical history. This is one of the most important aspects of the evaluation. The physician tries to establish whether the seizure was indeed a seizure or if it was something that looked like a seizure, but may have been something else (Table 2.1). This part of the evaluation is called the *differential diagnosis,* and it is very important since a number of conditions can look like epileptic seizures.

Let's suppose that the initial interview suggests a seizure. The physician will try to establish whether the seizure's features are consistent with the typical expected manifestations. For example, was there an aura? Did

TABLE 2.1 Differential Diagnoses in Patients with Possible Epilepsy

1. Nonepileptic disorders may present a diagnostic challenge in the individual with epilepsy. Many individuals with nonepileptic paroxysmal disorders do not have a determined *etiology* or cause for their spells, despite an extensive evaluation. Most of these patients have either nonepileptic behavioral events (*pseudoseizures*) or indeterminate spells.
2. The physiologic causes of these spells include: a. Cardiac syncope b. Vasodepressor syncope c. Simple faint d. Migraine e. Movement disorder f. Hyperventilation g. Cerebrovascular disease h. Autonomic disorder i. Drug toxicity j. Vertigo and dizziness k. Sleep disorders
3. The psychological causes include: a. Panic attacks b. Mood disorder c. Behavioral events (*pseudoseizures*) d. Psychotic episodes e. Anxiety disorder

the patient lose consciousness? Did any motor activity occur? Were vision changes experienced? Was the tongue bitten? Because the patient may have lost consciousness during the seizure, it is a good idea to have someone who witnessed the event accompany the patient, or at least have them be available to answer the doctor's questions.

Once the patient's history, including any other medical issues in addition to the seizure event, has been obtained, the physician performs a physical and neurologic examination. The physical examination may uncover clues to the cause of the seizure. For example, certain skin lesions are associated with a brain disorder called *tuberous sclerosis*, which can present with epilepsy (see Chapter 6). Other physical changes the neurologist will look for may include weakness or sensory changes in one part of the body, visual field loss, or other symptoms. Once the history and physical examination have been completed, the neurologist will establish an impression and design a plan of action.

General Laboratory Testing

In the context of a first seizure, it is often necessary to run some routine tests that may explain the cause of the seizure. A number of changes in the normal blood composition can induce a seizure. The most common changes are reductions in sodium (salt) or glucose (sugar). The presence of drugs, both legal and illegal, may be the cause of a seizure. Some antipsychotics, asthma medications, stimulants, and antidepressants can also cause seizures. Similarly, cocaine, heroin, and other illegal drugs can induce seizures. For that reason, a *drug screen* is often done the first time a seizure takes place in certain patients. An electrocardiogram (EKG) is also done to check for potential heart problems that may present like a seizure. For some patients with recurrent seizures associated with other conditions, specialized laboratory testing is done, but this is much less commonly needed.

Neurophysiologic Studies

Routine Electroencephalography

The electroencephalogram (EEG) is the only test that can prove someone has epilepsy. The brain produces electrical activity that may be analyzed using an EEG machine. A routine EEG in the office or hospital is typically collected for 30 to 60 minutes by the application of metal electrodes placed on the scalp with a conducting paste. (Figure 2.1) The electrodes are attached to wires that connect to the input box of the EEG machine. The EEG machine displays the electrical activity on a computer screen or paper (Figure 2.2). The outpatient scalp-recorded EEG predominantly observes *interictal* (brain activity between seizures) EEG changes, and may be altered by the presence of antiepileptic medications and other factors.

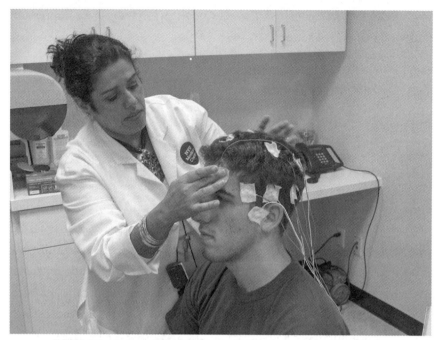

FIGURE 2.1   Patient being prepared with electrodes for an EEG study.

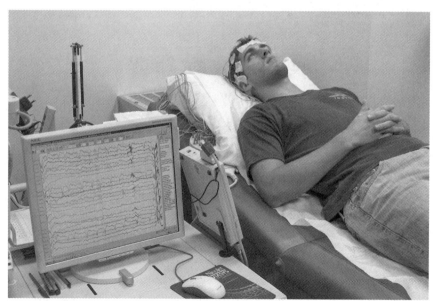

FIGURE 2.2   Computer screen showing the collection of an EEG study.

The human brain has fairly predictable electrical activity that varies with its location within the brain and whether the person being recorded is awake or asleep (Figure 2.3). In people with epilepsy, the EEG shows evidence of irritability, reported as either a spike or a sharp wave. These abnormal waves are a hallmark of epilepsy, and they occur even when a person with epilepsy is not experiencing a seizure. Spikes and sharp waves may occur in one location, multiple locations, or throughout the entire brain at once (Figures 2.4 and 2.5). The type and localization of the epilepsy you have can sometimes be diagnosed when these discharges are recorded with an EEG. Spikes and sharp waves may be provoked by sleep, deep breathing (hyperventilation), or flashing lights (photic stimulation).

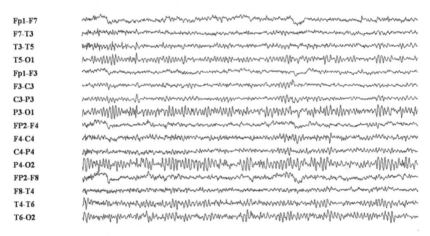

FIGURE 2.3   Normal, adult, awake EEG showing the effect of eye opening on the posterior alpha activity.

Although the EEG may tell your neurologist if you have epilepsy, it may not tell him what type of epilepsy you have. EEG studies are not always reliable indicators of the classification of seizure type. The routine EEG may be insensitive to (it may fail to identify) *epileptiform discharges*, which are abnormalities associated with an increased risk of seizure activity, or it may yield nonspecific findings. EEG alterations may rarely be identified in a patient with nonepileptic behavioral events. Patients with seizure dis-

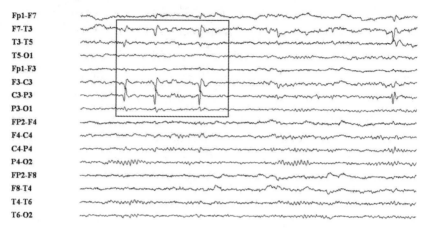

FIGURE 2.4   EEG showing focal spikes (interictal EEG) in a patient with left centro-temporal lobe epilepsy.

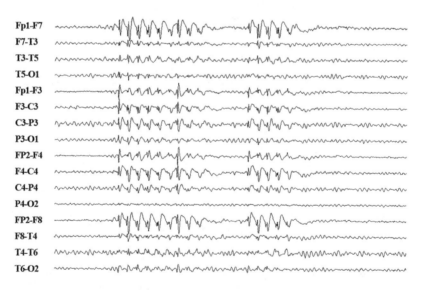

FIGURE 2.5   Generalized spike and wave abnormality (interictal EEG) in an awake patient with primary generalized epilepsy.

orders, even medically intractable epilepsy, may have repetitive "normal" EEG studies.

If a laboratory or office EEG does not detect an abnormality, the physician may order a *sleep-deprived EEG*, during which the patient is kept awake all night and an EEG is obtained while he is awake, and then asleep. If the EEG is still inconclusive or unrevealing, your doctor may order an *outpatient ambulatory EEG*, or he may want to hospitalize you for *video-EEG monitoring*.

Ambulatory Electroencephalography

An ambulatory EEG uses basically the same technology as a regular in-office EEG, but instead of recording activity for 30 to 60 minutes, it records the patient's brain activity for days at a time. The patient carries a small pouch or device on his belt, while the electrodes are attached to their head (Figure 2.6). The ambulatory EEG device runs on batteries and has memory cards that can store EEG data for several days. Most ambulatory EEG studies are run for 24 to 72 hours. The advantage of ambulatory EEG is that it can record your EEG for one or more days, and it might detect infrequent abnormal discharges. The other major advantage is that it may record actual seizures, which seldom can be recorded on the routine EEG (Figure 2.7). In those cases, the electrical activity can be analyzed, and sometimes an opinion can be formed regarding where in the brain seizures might be starting. Newer devices may permit video monitoring during the ambulatory EEG recording. Disadvantages of ambulatory EEG is degradation of the EEG quality due to electrodes poor contact, and so forth.

Video-Electroencephalographic Monitoring

If the routine EEG and/or the ambulatory EEG are negative or do not provide a definite answer on the diagnosis, your doctor may refer you for video-EEG monitoring. This is typically done in the setting of a specialized

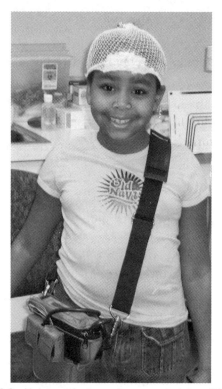

FIGURE 2.6   Young patient carrying an ambulatory EEG pack.

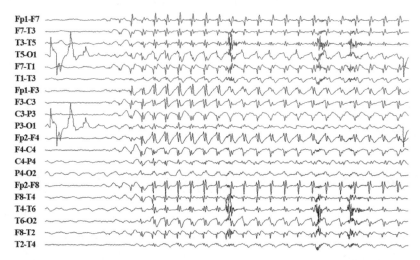

FIGURE 2.7   EEG pattern during an absence seizure in a child with staring spells.

epilepsy monitoring unit in a hospital. The technology is similar to a routine EEG or ambulatory EEG, except that a video camera is running during the EEG recording (Figure 2.8). The main advantage of video-EEG is that the neurologist can observe seizures and correlate the EEG with the seizure behavior. Trained nurses or EEG technologists can also perform testing during the seizure. Because seizures may occur relatively infrequently in some people, antiepileptic medication can be reduced or stopped to induce seizures.

Additional body changes that can be evaluated during video-EEG monitoring include heart rhythm (using an EKG), and changes in blood pressure, heart rate, and breathing. These assessments may be necessary in differentiating a seizure from other medical events, such as passing out from a drop in blood pressure. In addition, seizure-inducing maneuvers can also be done, such as sleep deprivation. People may be admitted to the hospital for a few days or up to a week, depending on how often their seizures occur and how many need to be studied. In some patients, video-EEG monitoring may be essential in the care and management of their seizure disorder.

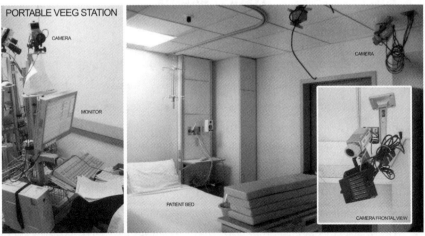

FIGURE 2.8 Video EEG set up in a patient's room with the camera installed on the ceiling (*right*) and a portable video EEG station (*left*).

Video-EEG monitoring is predominantly used by most physicians for diagnostic classification; that is, to determine epileptic from nonepileptic events, to classify the seizure type and syndrome, and sometimes to count the number of seizures and to evaluate whether a patient is a good candidate for epilepsy surgery (see Chapter 6). The high value of video-EEG monitoring in children and adult patients with recurrent and unprovoked spells has been confirmed by many studies and by many years of experience. Recognition of a seizure's EEG pattern is extremely important in making the diagnosis of epilepsy in selected patients. Scalp-recorded interictal EEG study, neurologic history and examination, and brain imaging procedures (discussed next) may not always permit clear event classification. The potential disadvantages of video-EEG recordings include the cost of the study and hospitalization, as well as the need for special resources and personnel. The EEG patterns may also be difficult to interpret because of artifacts related to movement and eye blinking. Finally, patients may not have a typical clinical event during video-EEG monitoring. However, in the majority of patients, the video-EEG study is helpful, and it may be the definitive test for most patients.

Neuroimaging

Magnetic Resonance Imaging

Magnetic resonance imaging (MRI) is the structural imaging procedure of choice for people with seizures and epilepsy. Nearly all patients being evaluated for unprovoked first seizure or epilepsy require an MRI. An MRI machine uses a big magnet that, through a complicated set of changes, can make beautiful pictures of the body. The patient usually has to lie still inside a large tube or tunnel while the magnet scans their body (Figure 2.9). Most studies of the brain last about 30 to 40 minutes. The MRI machine can be quite noisy while it is scanning.

The MRI supplies detailed information about the structure or anatomy of the brain. It is highly sensitive for localizing strokes, tumors, birth

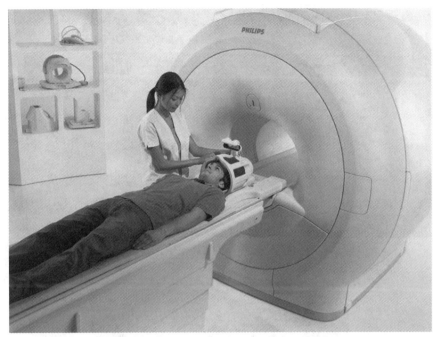

FIGURE 2.9   An MRI unit is shown with a patient being prepared for scanning.

defects, scar tissue from traumatic injury, and other abnormalities associated with seizures. In temporal lobe epilepsy, which is the most common type of epilepsy treated with surgery, shrinkage of a deep part of the temporal lobe (the *hippocampus*) can be seen. Sometimes, a contrast agent, *gadolinium*, is injected during the MRI as well. This contrast agent allows the neurologist to see certain details of the brain more clearly.

Because many studies have shown that MRI is the best technique we have to find the cause of seizures, it is the imaging procedure of choice in patients with epilepsy (Figure 2.10). MRI is very good at revealing common physical disturbances within the brain, such as head trauma, vascular malformations, and tumors (Figure 2.11). MRI is better and more specific than X-ray computed tomography (CT or CAT scan) in patients with seizure disorders. The MRI has an important role in identifying potential patients for *epilepsy surgery* and in planning the operation for the surgeon. The negative aspects of MRI include patient claustrophobia (fear of small

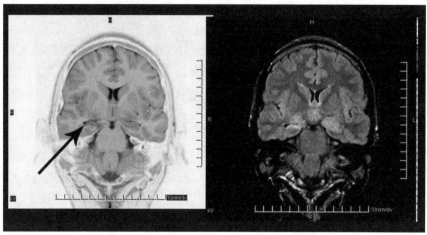

FIGURE 2.10 MRI of a normal patient.

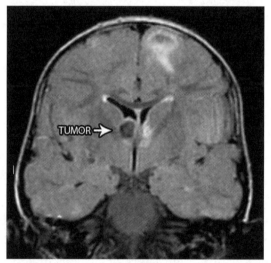

FIGURE 2.11 MRI that shows medial temporal lobe atrophy in a patient
with temporal lobe epilepsy (*arrow*).

spaces), excess body size, and the presence of some foreign metallic objects
(such as cardiac pacemakers and certain heart valves or aneurysm clips).
The latter may not permit the MRI study. Dental work and minor surgical
procedures (like suturing of scalp lacerations or paranasal sinus surgery)
usually have little effect on the quality of an MRI.

MRI is a painless technique, although it may be uncomfortable for people who suffer from claustrophobia. Claustrophobia can usually be managed through sedation or the use of an "open" MRI scanner that does not require the patient to be placed entirely within the MRI machine. Patients who are excessively large (both by body weight and shoulder width) may not fit into the tunnel of the typical MRI scanner. These patients may also be candidates for an open MRI scan. Unfortunately, open MRIs have lower resolution and may be less likely to find something wrong than the traditional tunnel-type scanner. Young children and adults with mental retardation may require general anesthesia to safely complete an MRI study. MRI has no known harmful side effects if the patients imaged do not have the contraindications noted earlier (metallic implants, and so forth). MRI does not involve any radioactive substances. The benefits of MRI must be weighed against any potential risks in pregnant women.

Positron Emission Tomography

Positron emission tomography (PET) is a nuclear medicine imaging study that may be useful in identifying a localized abnormality in patients with partial epilepsy. This may assist the surgical planning in individuals being considered for epilepsy surgery. This test is not routine, and it should be used only if epilepsy surgery is a consideration. PET studies are typically performed "in between" the patient's clinical seizures when they are not experiencing seizure activity. Further information on PET is provided in Chapter 6 (see Figure 2.12).

Single Photon Emission Computed Tomography

Single photon emission computed tomography (SPECT) is another nuclear medicine imaging study used in patients being considered for epilepsy surgery. SPECT identifies a focal blood flow alteration that may indicate the location of the epileptic brain tissue. An advantage of SPECT is the capability to perform imaging studies during the clinical seizure. The nuclear medicine isotope is injected when the patient is having a seizure in an epilepsy monitoring unit and subsequently is brought for the SPECT scan. This may label the site of seizure onset in the individual with focal epilepsy. SPECT is more available than PET, but it is reserved mainly for patients who are considering surgery; it is discussed further in Chapter 6 (see Figure 2.13).

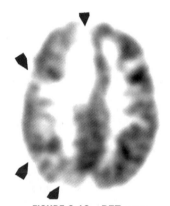

FIGURE 2.12   PET scan.

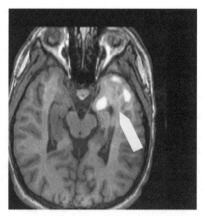

FIGURE 2.13   SISCOM subtraction ictal SPECT co-registered to MRI reveals a left frontal lobe blood flow change.

Clinical Applications of Diagnostic Studies

Recurrent Spells

Patients may be referred for the evaluation, as well as for treatment of recurrent and unprovoked clinical spells. An estimated 20 percent of patients referred to comprehensive epilepsy programs for medically refractory "seizures" do not have epilepsy (Table 2.1). The issues to be considered in caring for these patients include diagnostic classification, potential causes, and treatment options. The neurologic history and examination, and routine EEG, indicate the classification of the seizure type and allow selection of an appropriate antiepileptic medication in about half the patients.

Common events that are referred for diagnosis include potential psychological and physiologic nonepileptic disorders that involve sudden changes in behavior. Patients with an underlying psychiatric disease, such as depression, anxiety, or psychosis, may experience recurrent events that look like seizures. Nonepileptic behavioral events also known as *psychogenic spells* or *pseudoseizures* may be present in the absence of a major psychiatric disorder. It is not uncommon for patients with nonepileptic behavioral events to have many normal EEG recordings, a remote history of emotional or sexual abuse, an unusual response to medication (increase in spells with the use of antiepileptic drugs), coexistent chronic pain syndromes such as disabling headache or fibromyalgia, and unusual symptoms suggesting a behavioral or "functional" disorder. The spells may be prolonged in duration and associated with headache, generalized pain, or crying. Importantly, the clinical features alone may be unclear in differentiating nonepileptic behavioral events from seizures. For that reason, video-EEG evaluation is needed for many of these patients.

Other nonepileptic events with episodic behavioral changes include cardiac disease, syncope, tremor, chemical dysfunction, and medication toxicity. These can be differentiated from psychogenic spells through the use of laboratory testing and video-EEG.

Seizure Type Classification

A very important indication for video-EEG monitoring in patients with epilepsy is seizure classification (type). Classifying the seizure type in a patient with epilepsy is important for choosing the correct drug treatment (Table 2.2). The routine EEG study and neurologic history may not always be able to determine the seizure type(s). One potential clinical problem is the patient with frequent "convulsions" (generalized tonic-clonic seizures) who may have either generalized or focal epilepsy. Classification of the exact epileptic condition will be used to determine what other tests are needed and the best medication to control the seizures. Some patients with periods of blank behavior may have absence, atypical absence (petit mal), or focal seizures with impaired awareness (see Chapter 1). The introduction of so many new antiepileptic drugs has made diagnostic classification more important now than ever. (Over 90 percent of new-onset cases of epilepsy in adults are focal seizure disorders, whereas in children it may be close to 60 percent.)

TABLE 2.2   Summary of the International Classification of Epileptic Seizures

I. Focal seizures
A. Focal seizures (without impaired awareness) With motor symptoms With somatosensory or special sensory symptoms With autonomic symptoms With psychic symptoms
B. Focal seizures (with impaired awareness)
B.1. Beginning as focal seizures without impaired awareness and progressing to impairment of consciousness With no other features With features as in I.A With automatisms
B.2. With impairment of consciousness at onset With no other features With features as in I.A With automatisms
C. Focal seizures evolving into tonic-clonic seizures

| II. **Generalized seizures (convulsive or nonconvulsive)** |
| Absence seizures |
| Myoclonic seizures |
| Clonic seizures |
| Tonic seizures |
| Tonic-clonic seizures |
| Atonic seizures |
| III. **Unclassified epileptic seizures** |
| IV. **Status epilepticus and provoked seizures** |

Source: Commission on Classification, 1981

FREQUENTLY ASKED QUESTIONS

Q   Do I have epilepsy when I experience a single seizure?

The diagnosis of epilepsy is confirmed when a patient experiences two or more unprovoked seizures. Many individuals with a single seizure will not experience seizure recurrence. Approximately 10 percent of individuals will experience one or more seizures during their lifetime. However, there is now evidence that selected patients with a first unprovoked seizure may be appropriate candidates for antiepileptic drug therapy if they are at increased risk of recurrence. The risk of recurrent seizures is greatest in patients with a history of a previous significant neurologic disorder (like a brain tumor), an abnormal MRI head study, an abnormal EEG that shows epileptiform activity, an abnormal neurologic examination that suggests a localized structural alteration in the brain, and a positive family history of epilepsy. One or more of these factors may increase the risk of seizure recurrence. Patients with a normal neurologic evaluation may be at lower risk of a second seizure. Patients who experience a single seizure should undergo an appropriate medical and neurologic evaluation. In the adult patient, this almost invariably means an MRI head and EEG study will be performed. A cerebrospinal fluid examination may be indicated if the patient is thought to be at risk of *meningitis* (an infection in the spinal fluid and lining of the brain). The rationale for the use of antiepileptic medication is to lower the risk of seizure recurrence. There are conflicting findings regarding the use of antiepileptic drug therapy in patients who experience only a single seizure or very few seizures. The potential disadvantages include the potential for drug side effects, interaction with other medications, pregnancy-related complications, and the cost and expense associated both with the prescription and need for laboratory studies. Not uncommonly, the physician will individualize the need for antiepileptic drug therapy at the end of the diagnostic evaluation. The prevailing evidence suggests that many individuals who experience a single seizure do not require long-term antiepileptic medication.

Q   If my EEG is normal, do I not have epilepsy?

Patients may have a single normal wake–sleep EEG and still have a seizure disorder. Approximately 50 percent to 90 percent of patients with epilepsy will have an abnormal EEG if multiple EEG recordings are performed. The yield of the routine EEG recording depends on multiple factors, including the type of seizure activity, location of seizure onset, age of the patient, frequency of seizures, and presence of antiepileptic medication. The timing of the last seizure may affect the sensitivity of the EEG recording. The closer the EEG is done in relation to a seizure, the more likely the study will be abnormal. Use of additional scalp electrodes, a prolonged period for an EEG recording, and activation procedures (like hyperventilation and photic stimulation) may enhance the likelihood of recording a specific abnormality that indicates a seizure disorder. Selected individuals may have repetitively "normal" EEG recordings and still have a seizure disorder. The diagnosis of epilepsy requires the appropriate clinical history with supporting evaluation. In some instances, admission to an epilepsy monitoring unit for long-term EEG recordings may be necessary to confirm the diagnosis and initiate therapy.

Q **If the EEG and MRI are normal, should I not receive antiepileptic medication for my seizure disorder?**

Patients with epilepsy may have normal routine EEG results *and* MRI scans. The decision regarding the use of medication in these patients depends on the clinical history and additional information. The diagnosis of epilepsy does not necessarily require an abnormal routine EEG and MRI. As discussed in Question 2, the EEG may be unremarkable, especially with only a single recording. MRI may demonstrate a structural abnormality associated with a partial seizure disorder. However, in a significant number of patients with partial or generalized epilepsy, the MRI does not reveal a specific alteration. The technique used for the MRI study is important. Your doctor should personally review the MRI to make certain the study has been done appropriately, and to see if, in the context of your particular history, a subtle abnormality is present. The decision regarding medical therapy in patients with normal EEG and MRI studies depends on the seizure type, the likely "mechanism" of seizure activity, and potential underlying cause(s). Subsequent EEG and MRI studies in selected patients may reveal abnormalities that may provide indispensable information concerning the cause of epilepsy, type of seizure disorder, and likely site of seizure onset.

Q **What happens if I am admitted to the epilepsy monitoring unit for seizure classification and I do not have a seizure?**

Patients are admitted to an epilepsy monitoring for two important reasons. The first is to classify seizure type. The second may be to localize the site of seizure onset prior to possible epilepsy surgery. To increase the likelihood of recording a seizure or spell, your antiepileptic medication may be discontinued or reduced. Other seizure-precipitating factors that may be used include sleep deprivation, photic stimulation, hyperventilation, and exercise using a treadmill or bicycle. The average duration for epilepsy monitoring is variable and depends on a number of factors, including the frequency of seizure activity. Prolonged EEG recordings made between the clinical spells (*interictal* EEG patterns) may be useful for diagnostic classification. Approximately 80 percent of individuals with drug-resistant epilepsy admitted to an epilepsy monitoring unit 3 days or longer will have recorded epileptiform discharges in the absence of seizure activity. The convergence of diagnostic studies (routine EEG, MRI) and the neurologic history-examination may also permit a presumptive diagnosis of epilepsy, despite the fact that you do not have a typical spell. Often this information may allow your doctor to determine the most likely effective antiepileptic drug therapy. Finally, in selected patients, further inpatient monitoring may need to be performed at another time to try to record seizure activity if the initial evaluation is nondiagnostic.

> **Q** **How can the doctor localize the site of seizure onset if the MRI is normal?**

Localization of seizure onset is particularly important in patients with medically refractory or drug-resistant focal seizures being considered for surgical treatment. The EEG is the appropriate study to determine the site of region or zone associated with the initial onset and spread of focal seizure activity. MRI may demonstrate a structural lesion or abnormality that may indicate the cause of the seizure disorder and indirectly suggest the localization of the epileptic brain tissue. Video-EEG monitoring has been the "gold standard" to determine the classification of seizure type and the area of the brain involved in the seizure activity. The *ictal* EEG pattern (the pattern present during the habitual seizures) is pivotal to select candidates for the surgical treatment of intractable epilepsy. Most operative procedures (referred to commonly as *epilepsy surgery*) involve *resection* or removal of the epileptic brain tissue. In selected candidates, EEG recordings may be performed in the operating room (directly from the brain and not the scalp; this is referred to as *electrocorticography*). Not uncommonly, scalp-electrode EEG monitoring does not permit the exact localization of the site of seizure onset to determine the most effective operative procedure. *Chronic intracranial EEG monitoring* (placement of electrodes on the brain surface or in regions of the brain) is performed to record the habitual seizures and better localize the epileptic brain tissue. This requires a neurosurgical procedure to place the electrodes, and it is only performed after a comprehensive noninvasive evaluation. Other imaging studies are commonly performed in patients with a normal MRI when there is concern regarding the site of seizure onset in potential surgical candidates. PET, SPECT, or magnetic resonance spectroscopy (MRS) may be useful in guiding the presurgical evaluation.

CHAPTER 3

Epilepsy Treatment: General Considerations

■ A single seizure may occur in any person under certain extreme provocations.

■ It is important to prevent recurrent seizures because seizures can be associated with various injuries.

■ Diagnosing the seizure type is important when choosing the best medication to prevent seizures.

■ When a medication is started, it should be started at a low dose, and then increased in small, slow steps, unless it is urgent to move faster.

■ Some medications have to be titrated, or adjusted, slowly for safety reasons.

■ Studies show that approximately two-thirds of people who just started having seizures will stop having seizures with drug treatment.

■ Certain forms of epilepsy are more likely to respond to treatment.

As we now understand, epilepsy is a condition characterized by recurrent unprovoked seizures, or at least one seizure, in addition to a persistent tendency to develop additional seizures. This chapter focuses on the treatment of epilepsy to prevent recurrent seizures. Since most seizures stop by themselves, there is usually no need to treat individual seizures, unless they continue beyond 5 minutes. At present, no medication can eliminate the tendency for seizures altogether, unless the seizures are caused by an underlying treatable infectious or inflammatory condition. Discovering treatments to cure epilepsy, however, is a strong focus of research. If a treatment is found that can permanently reverse the seizure tendency in patients (in the same way that an antibiotic can cure pneumonia), such a treatment could become very important.

This chapter discusses treatment decisions, beginning with the first seizure. It also discusses the duration of successful treatment, the management of recurrent seizures that do not respond to initial medications, and other various aspects of treatment.

Single Seizures

Provoked Seizures

A single seizure may occur in any person when subjected to certain extreme provocations. For example, anyone may develop a seizure if exposed to certain toxic substances or if an extreme change in the mineral composition of their blood occurs. Single seizures may also occur in individuals who drink alcohol heavily on a regular basis, and then suddenly stop drinking. In this setting, the tendency to have seizures is short-lasting. The seizures occur typically within 2 days of the last drink. A similar pattern may occur in individuals who suddenly stop taking certain sleeping pills or "nerve" medications. Although there could be a series of seizures, the tendency does not persist and, after the seizures have stopped, they do not keep coming back.

Provoked Seizures and Long-term Treatment

In the setting of a single seizure clearly provoked by a drug or a change in blood composition, correcting the underlying problem can eliminate the seizure tendency. Long-term treatment is only for the prevention of recurrent seizures. This is not usually necessary for provoked seizures, unless the underlying provoking factor cannot be easily corrected. In one study, the risk of an unprovoked seizure was only 13 percent after a short provoked seizure. However, if the first seizure was very long (known as *status epilepticus*), then the risk of an unprovoked seizure increased to about 41 percent.

Reasons for Treatment to Prevent Recurrent Seizures

It is important to prevent recurrent seizures because seizures can be associated with various injuries. Because of the risk of injury, recurrent seizures result in certain lifestyle restrictions, specifically restrictions on driving, on working in environments that could result in an injury in the event of a seizure, and on working at a job in which a seizure can be disruptive.

Recurrent seizures may also result in loss of brain cells if allowed to continue uncontrolled. Seizures may occasionally become more severe. For example, it is possible that after a mild focal seizure, the second seizure could be a more severe seizure that evolves to become bilateral tonic-clonic.

Uncontrolled seizures may interfere with functioning. In particular, people with uncontrolled seizures frequently report difficulties with memory because seizures often involve parts of the brain (the temporal lobes) important for memory.

There is a small but definite risk of sudden unexpected death during seizures, but it has been demonstrated that this increased risk is largely eliminated if seizures are well controlled.

The risk of brain injury with recurrent seizures does not apply to every seizure type. It is well known that generalized absence seizures (frequently called *petit mal seizures*) do not cause cell loss in the brain. However, they do interfere with reaction time; people with generalized absence seizures will be restricted from driving and engaging in other potentially risky activities.

Risk of Recurrence and Treatment for a Single Unprovoked Seizure

When the first seizure is unprovoked or is related only to a trigger (such as sleep deprivation) that does not generally result in seizures in most individuals, and then treatment may be considered. Studies indicate that a second seizure occurs in only 40 percent to 50 percent of people overall. If everyone with a single unprovoked seizure were to be treated, then a lot of people would be treated unnecessarily. As a result, doctors look into factors that can help predict who will have a second seizure.

Medical Tests Before Treatment of a First Unprovoked Seizure

In most instances, when a decision has to be made about treatment, the neurologist needs a very good description of the seizure. This requires talking to a witness who has seen the seizure. Based on this description, the neurologist will decide if the seizure was indeed epileptic. Many conditions can imitate epileptic seizures (see Chapters 1 and 2). If it is decided that the seizure was indeed epileptic, the neurologist should explore past diseases or injuries that may have affected the brain and produced a tendency for seizures. Tests that the neurologist will obtain are described in Chapter 2.

Factors That Predict Recurrent Seizures

Individuals who are more likely to have recurrent seizures include people who have a structural abnormality in the brain (for example, an old injury such as scar, a tumor, or other *lesion*), people who have other members of their family with epilepsy, and people who have an abnormal EEG (Table 3.1). People with a single seizure who have none of these factors

TABLE 3.1   Factors Predicting a Higher Risk of Another Seizure After a Single Seizure

Cause of epilepsy—Abnormal brain structure or brain function as a cause of seizure (e.g., cerebral palsy, intellectual disability)
Abnormal electroencephalogram (EEG)
Seizure type—Focal seizures predict greater likelihood of recurrence than generalized seizures (but this is not consistently found)
Other factors found in some studies: • Seizure while asleep • Prior seizures with high fever • Weakness on one side of the body after the seizure

are much less likely to have another seizure, with odds of another seizure as low as one in four or one in three. However, the decision to start a new medication or not must involve the patient and take into consideration the patient's personal situation. Certain personal factors may make it wise to treat an individual with a low risk of another seizure, while other factors may make it worthwhile to withhold treatment in someone who has a high risk of another seizure. For example, a working adult may be at risk of job loss in the event of another seizure. Treatment may then be recommended for such an individual, even though the risk of recurrence is not high. On the other hand, treatment may be withheld in a child who is not working or driving, if the family is very concerned about the risk of side effects from medication or the effect that a medication may have on learning.

Risk of Seizure Recurrence After Two or More Seizures

If a second seizure occurs, then the risk that a third seizure will occur is almost three out of four. Once three seizures have occurred, approximately 81 percent of people will experience another seizure. The majority of recurrences will occur within the first year. Because of these statistics, treatment is almost always recommended after two or more seizures. However, some circumstances could make the decision to treat not so straightforward. For instance, if the seizures are several years apart, it may be hard to justify taking daily medications to prevent another seizure that may not happen for several years.

These case studies are real examples of the problems facing patients and doctors when decisions regarding treatment must be made.

EXAMPLE 1. Single seizure during sleep.   A 13-year-old boy had a single seizure in sleep. His parents heard a noise and walked into his room to find him jerking all extremities and producing a snorting noise. The next day, his pediatrician finds him completely normal. The neurologist also finds a completely normal neurologic examination. MRI of the brain and EEG are normal. The advantages and disadvantages of starting a seizure medication are discussed with the family. In this case, the risk of another seizure is probably around 30 percent. The child is not yet of driving age, and the risk of another seizure does not seem to be major. In addition, the family is concerned that medications may affect learning in school. All these factors tilt the balance toward not treating, but just observing the child for the possibility of another seizure.

EXAMPLE 2. Single seizure in working adult.   A 35-year-old nurse has a seizure at work characterized by staring, lip smacking, and unresponsiveness for about 2 minutes. During that time, she picks repeatedly at the bed sheets of a patient. Testing shows that she has a normal MRI and a normal EEG. Neurologic examination is completely normal. There are no definite risk factors for epilepsy. The advantages and disadvantages of treatment are discussed with the patient. She feels that her job is at risk, and that another seizure may cause her to lose her job. Even though the risk of another seizure is low, the consequences seem to be too great, and the patient decides to start a medication.

EXAMPLE 3. Adult with a single seizure and abnormal neurological status.   A 40-year-old man awakens his wife at night with jerking of all extremities for about 1 minute, after which he is limp and unresponsive, with loud respirations. He goes back to sleep and has no memory of the event the next day. He had a severe head injury 5 years previously, resulting in weakness on the left side of the body ever since that injury. MRI shows a scar in the right brain with evidence of old injury. The EEG shows abnormal waves in the right frontal region of the brain. In this case, the risk that a second seizure will occur is greater than 50 percent. It seems quite advisable to start treatment.

Medication Choices After First Unprovoked Seizure

Many seizure medications are available for us to choose from. Some of the available medications have been compared with each other to see how effective they are and how well a patient can tolerate them. For example, the older medications such as carbamazepine (Tegretol/Carbatrol), phenytoin (Dilantin), primidone (Mysoline), and phenobarbital were compared in patients with focal seizures. It was clear that primidone and phenobarbital were less well tolerated than the other medications, therefore, these are no longer recommended as first-line drugs. Among the new medications, those that have been tested for initial use include gabapentin (Neurontin), lamotrigine (Lamictal), topiramate (Topamax), oxcarbazepine (Trileptal), levetiracetam (Keppra), zonisamide (Zonegran), lacosamide (Vimpat), and eslicarbazepine acetate (Aptiom). The U.S. Food and Drug Administration (FDA) previously had strict criteria for approving a drug to be used alone (monotherapy) as first treatment. More recently, the FDA relaxed its rules, adopting an extrapolation policy, granting monotherapy approval for drugs found effective in adjunctive use. Nevertheless, when treating newly diagnosed epilepsy, neurologists are more likely to prescribe drugs that have undergone testing as initial monotherapy.

Influence of Seizure Type on Choice of Medication

Diagnosing the seizure type is important when choosing the best medication to prevent seizures because not all seizure types respond to the same medications. For example, generalized absence seizures respond to ethosuximide (Zarontin) and divalproex sodium (Depakote), but not to phenytoin (Dilantin), carbamazepine (Tegretol/Carbatrol), or phenobarbital, which are effective against focal seizures and generalized tonic–clonic seizures. As a result, it is important to diagnose the seizure type and the form of epilepsy before choosing the most appropriate drug.

Considerations in Choosing the First Drug

Choosing the most appropriate drug takes into account many considerations. These considerations include age, gender, potential for becoming pregnant, other medical illnesses, other medications being used, and other factors. For example, several recent studies compared immediate-release carbamazepine (Tegretol) and lamotrigine (Lamictal) in seniors with new-onset seizures and found that lamotrigine (Lamictal) was better tolerated in this age group. It is now established that exposure during pregnancy to divalproex (Depakote) is associated with an increased risk of birth defects, lower IQ, and increased risk of autism; therefore, this drug may not be appropriate as a first choice in a woman who may get pregnant. Many people with new-onset seizures have migraine headaches. Using one medication to treat both migraine and seizures is an attractive possibility that would certainly influence the choice of medication. Medication side effects also affect the choice. For example, in a person with a strong family history of kidney stones, topiramate (Topamax) and zonisamide (Zonegran) may not be good choices because they are associated with an increased risk of kidney stones. In a person who has a history of severe skin reaction, lamotrigine (Lamictal) may be avoided because it has a higher risk of serious skin rash.

Guidelines to Starting the First Medication

Once a medication is started, it should be started at a low dose and increased in small, slow steps. The principle "start low and go slow" is almost always wise, unless there is a rush to reach an effective level because the first seizure was particularly severe, or because several seizures have occurred within a short time. After a single seizure, it is hard to know how much medication is needed to prevent subsequent seizures. It may, therefore, be wise to increase the dose to an amount known to be effective from experience with other individuals. In people who have had frequent repeated seizures, this may not be the case: As the dose is slowly increased, the seizures may stop, even if the dose is smaller than what is well known to be generally effective.

If there is a need to reach a protective dose very rapidly, some medications are not a good choice. For example, lamotrigine (Lamictal) cannot be started and increased rapidly because we know this increases the risk of allergic rash. Topiramate (Topamax) cannot be increased rapidly because that can result in difficulty concentrating.

Monitoring and Optimizing Treatment

Monitoring Treatment with Blood Tests

Two forms of blood tests are used to monitor people taking seizure medications. One measures the level of the medication in the blood—the *drug level*. The other test measures blood count, liver enzymes, and mineral blood composition because these may rarely be affected by treatment. It is generally felt that measuring the level of medication in the blood is not essential, although it is helpful as a reference point once the target dose is reached. This may help show a doctor how much leeway there is with increasing the dose. In addition, should seizures recur or side effects appear during the course of treatment, the drug level can be obtained and compared with the earlier level when seizures were controlled and there were no side effects. This comparison could help explain what caused the seizures to recur or what caused side effects to appear.

It is usually a mistake to make adjustments based on the blood level of a medication alone. Enough variability exists between people that a blood level effective for one person may be ineffective for another, or a blood level that is well-tolerated by one person can be toxic for another. For most medications, the blood-level test does not need to be repeated at set periods. For most seizure medications, the change in blood level is proportional to the change in dose. For example, if the dose is increased by 25 percent, one expects the level of drug in the blood to increase by about 25 percent. However, there is one important exception to this rule, which is the drug phenytoin (Dilantin), which was one of the most frequently used medications for seizures. Neurologists must be very careful about how fast they increase the dose of phenytoin (Dilantin) because it builds up rapidly in the bloodstream. A doctor may use very small dose increases of phenytoin (Dilantin) when it is close to the range that is most often effective.

For the older medications, such as phenytoin (Dilantin), carbamazepine (Tegretol or Carbatrol), divalproex sodium (Depakote), and phenobarbital, we have a fairly good idea of the effective blood-level range. For the newer medications, the effective range is generally not well established, except for lamotrigine (Lamictal). When a new medication level is obtained, the laboratory provides a comparison with the usual range seen on doses that were used in research studies (rather than the known most effective range). However, lamotrigine (Lamictal) has a general range defined; above this range, it is likely that side effects will appear. Birth control pills and pregnancy markedly reduce the level of lamotrigine (Lamictal) in the blood. Therefore, it is indicated to check the blood level of lamotrigine (Lamictal) after starting birth control pills and periodically throughout pregnancy for appropriate adjustments in the dose.

Checking and Monitoring Blood Count and Liver Enzymes

Some seizure medications (particularly the older ones) have been associated with occasional changes in liver enzymes or blood count. Other medications may reduce sodium level. When starting these medications, it may be reasonable to check these levels at baseline, and then once or twice after treatment is initiated. For individuals in whom these values do not change, it is unnecessary to continue these blood tests.

Optimizing Treatment and Determining That a Drug Has Failed

If the diagnosis of epileptic seizures is very clearly established and an appropriate medication has been started, but seizures continue to occur, certain steps should be considered before concluding that the medication has failed. The possibility should be considered that the medication dose has not been pushed to an optimal level. So much variation exists among individuals that a dose effective for one person may be ineffective for another. This could be because the medication was less well absorbed or because of rapid breakdown of the medication in the patient's system. Thus, if no side effects are present, it is usually appropriate to continue increasing the dose as long as seizures are not yet controlled. A blood level can help determine how much room there is to increase the dose. However, this is true only for some medications. For individuals who are clearly resistant to the maximum tolerated dose of an appropriately chosen medication, a change in treatment must be considered. Once at least two drugs have failed in this manner, and if the diagnosis and the classification of epilepsy are identified beyond doubt, then the possibility of surgical treatment should be considered for patients who have focal epilepsy. If a well-defined lesion or *hippocampal sclerosis* (a condition with cell loss and scarring affecting the hippocampus, a structure in the temporal lobe that is a common source of seizures) is present, then surgical treatment can be highly effective and should be considered early.

EXAMPLE 4. Optimizing treatment with a new drug.   A young man is taking 600 mg per day of lamotrigine (Lamictal) and still having one seizure every 2 months. He is not experiencing any side effects. His physician is worried that these seizures continue despite a dose of Lamictal that is higher than he normally prescribes. He obtains a blood level, which is 4 micrograms per milliliter (mcg/mL). Studies suggest that some people can continue to derive benefit from Lamictal up to a level of 20 mcg/mL. A level of 4 mcg/mL is an indication that there is a lot of leeway for increasing the dose. The appropriate step is to increase the dose of lamotrigine. This may not need a blood level, and the dose could be increased as long as no adverse experiences occur. However, the blood level helps increase confidence in the appropriateness of increasing the medication dose.

Determining Effectiveness of Treatment

Studies show that approximately two-thirds of the people who just started having seizures will stop having seizures with drug treatment. Thus, approximately one-third of the people may continue to have seizures and would thus be considered as having *drug-resistant epilepsy*.

Defining Good Seizure Control

Only the complete absence of seizures can be considered a good end-point of treatment. Even though some individuals may be pleased to have only one seizure every 2 months when they used to have seizures every day, this is not satisfactory seizure control. *Any* persistent seizures are associated with the risks and restrictions listed earlier.

Reversible Causes of Treatment Failure

When seizures continue, it is essential to search for factors that may explain why treatment is failing. Some of these factors can be easily reversed. For example, sleep deprivation may be a cause of seizures not responding to treatment. This is particularly true in a form of epilepsy called *juvenile myoclonic epilepsy*. Evidence suggests that *sleep apnea*, which is a very common condition, particularly in overweight men, may cause poor quality sleep, and therefore may imitate the effect of sleep deprivation. This can cause seizures to be resistant to treatment. Treatment may also fail because of the use of some recreational drugs or certain medications that can trigger seizures. In some individuals, an excessive intake of caffeine can result in breakthrough seizures. The effective treatment of epilepsy requires taking seizure medications regularly. Missing doses can reduce the medication blood level to the point at which the medication is not sufficient to protect from seizures. It is also possible that the drug has not been given a fair chance. Before a medication trial is considered to have failed, the dose may need to be pushed to the maximum amount tolerated, although this may not be necessary if it is clear that no benefit has been gained from repeatedly increasing the dose. The dose necessary to stop seizures may be higher for some than for others. In the case of a medication like phenytoin (Dilantin), it is easy to totally skip the effective dose by making dose increases that are too large. Therefore, it is important to use small steps while exploring the dose that will control seizures eventually. It is also possible that the medication chosen is not appropriate. This is why it is essential to have a clear idea of the type of seizures present before starting treatment. Finally, it is also possible that the seizures are not epileptic, or that the patient has both epileptic and nonepileptic seizures; nonepileptic seizures will usually not respond to seizure medications. Even after accounting for these factors, approximately one-third of patients will continue to have seizures despite the best medical treatment.

Predicting Response to Treatment

Certain forms of epilepsy are more likely to respond to treatment, and others are more likely to be resistant to treatment. For example, patients with genetic epilepsies (who had no neurologic problem other than epilepsy) are more likely to be seizure-free with treatment. Patients with hippocampal scarring are less likely to be seizure-free. Because epilepsy with hippocampal sclerosis is very effectively treated with surgery, this should be considered early in these patients (see Chapter 6).

Likelihood of Complete Seizure Control with First and Subsequent Medications

One important study showed that approximately one-half of patients stopped having seizures with the first drug tried, but only 13 percent stopped with the second drug. If the first drug failed because of side effects rather than lack of efficacy, then the chance of the second drug being effective is no different from the chance of the first drug. However, if the first drug failed because of lack of efficacy, then the chance of the next drug being effective is less. In the same study, after failing the first and second drug, only 1 percent of patients became seizure free with a third drug and 3 percent became seizure-free by combining two drugs. Therefore, failing two drugs seems to indicate a high chance of drug-resistant epilepsy. This is true only if the drugs have failed despite using an adequate dose and without causing unacceptable side effects. When the drugs fail because of bad side effects only, the chances are better that another drug without side effects will work.

Managing Recurrent Seizures and Drug-Resistant Epilepsy

Once two drugs have failed, it becomes likely that the epilepsy is going to be difficult to control. At this stage, it is important to reevaluate the condition. Before deciding that treatment has failed, it is important to consider all the possible explanations listed earlier. If the drug has been appropriately pushed to the maximum dose tolerated, and if lifestyle factors (such as sleep deprivation, poor-quality sleep, recreational drugs, other medications, alcohol abuse, and excess caffeine) are excluded, the possibility should be considered that the drugs failed because the seizures are nonepileptic. If that is a possibility, then it becomes important to perform long-term video and EEG (V-EEG) monitoring. This test is designed to record seizures and analyze them for definitive diagnosis.

Adding a Second Drug Versus Switching to Another Drug

Most neurologists will try another drug before combining two drugs. (The use of one medication at a time is referred to as *monotherapy*. The use of two or more drugs in combination is referred to as *polytherapy*.) However, no evidence suggests that monotherapy is more effective than polytherapy. If the first drug failed because of complete lack of efficacy, then it is most appropriate to switch to another. However, if the first drug was effective, but not completely, then adding a second drug may be quite appropriate. Some drugs have not been sufficiently tested as stand-alone treatments and are best used in combination with another drug (even though the new FDA policy allows extrapolation from adjunctive therapy to monotherapy). It should be noted that if the decision is made to switch to another monotherapy (single drug), the switch usually involves adding the second drug before removing the first. If, in the process, the patient becomes seizure-free while still on both drugs, the neurologist may hesitate to remove the first drug, and *dual* or *polytherapy* may then result.

Many factors must be considered in the choice of the next monotherapy drug. If the previous drug failed because of side effects, the doctor may want to consider a drug that does not share the same side effects as the first. If the previous drug failed because of lack of efficacy, then doctors may consider another drug with a different mechanism of action.

Advantages of Monotherapy Versus Polytherapy

It is the rule that many medications for epilepsy are best tolerated when used alone. Using drugs in combination increases the chance of extra side effects and increases the chance of interaction between drugs. Early on in the treatment of drug-resistant epilepsy, most neurologists will try to stick with one drug. However, if the drug currently used has produced an excellent but incomplete benefit, the possibility could be considered of adding another drug, rather than completely replacing the existing drug. Studies that compared these two approaches did not clearly identify one approach as superior to the other. However, when using two drugs in combination, the selection of the add-on drug must be made carefully. In addition, it may be wise to avoid adding a drug that has a similar mechanism of action because this may increase the chances of extra side effects. For example, it is well known that using two drugs that block the sodium channel (for example, lamotrigine [Lamictal] and carbamazepine [Tegretol]) together can increase the risk of blurred vision, double vision, or dizziness.

Occasionally, however, the interaction of two medications could be favorable, such that they complement each other's action. For example, studies suggested that combining lamotrigine (Lamictal) and divalproex (Depakote) might produce an incremental benefit that is greater than the benefit of each of the two drugs taken separately. This is an appealing concept, but one that has not been clearly proven in practice for other combinations.

It is usually desirable not to exceed two medications at the same time. However, there are instances where the epilepsy is so resistant that the doctor is forced to add a third medication. In these instances, the neurologist may consider removing one of the previous two medications, but this is not always possible. The interactions of these medications should be always taken into consideration.

After two or three failed medication trials, it is important to consider if epilepsy surgery is a good option (Figure 3.1). For that purpose, special testing will be needed (see Chapter 6).

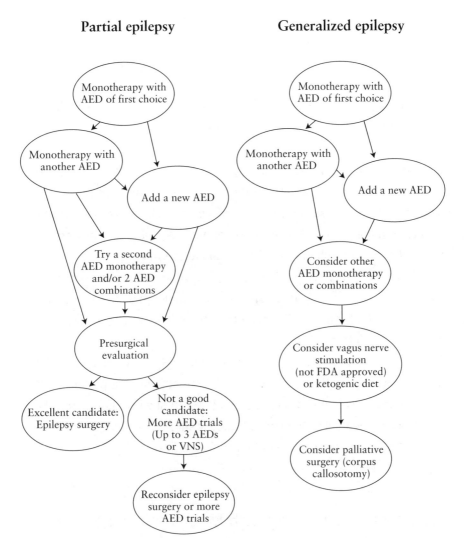

FIGURE 3.1 General guidelines for treatment steps. Vertical position generally reflects the order in which options are considered (higher position considered first). In this algorithm, it is assumed that the diagnosis is secure. The diagnosis must be confirmed with V-EEG early on, after the failure of no more than two drugs.

AED, antiepileptic drug; VNS, vagus nerve stimulation; RNS, responsive neurostimulation; FDA, Food and Drug Administration

Example 5. Managing drug-resistant epilepsy. A 24-year-old man started having seizures at age 19. These begin with a butterfly sensation in the pit of the stomach that rises to the throat, at which point he loses awareness and is noted to have lip smacking and picking movements with his right hand. After the seizure, he is tired for several minutes. He was started on one seizure medication that controlled his seizures completely for 2 years. Then, seizures started again and did not respond to increasing the dose of his medication. The dose was increased to the point at which he developed dizziness and excessive sleepiness. He wants to know what he should do next. His EEG shows abnormal sharp waves in the right temporal lobe. His MRI shows right hippocampal scarring.

This patient most probably needs a change in treatment. He can be switched to a different drug, or another drug could be added to his current regime. Early on, at this stage of treatment, most neurologists would probably switch to another drug.

If the second drug does not work, even though it was pushed to high levels, this patient should consider surgical treatment. The pattern of the seizures and the results of the EEG and the MRI suggest that he may be an excellent candidate for surgery. Epilepsy surgery will give him a 70 percent to 80 percent chance of being seizure-free.

Avoiding and Dealing with Medication Side Effects

Every medication has a potential for side effects that may affect a variable proportion of patients taking that medication. It is important for the patient and the physician to discuss the most common side effects of every medication before starting it. Some individuals are particularly susceptible to developing certain side effects. For example, people who have a tremor before starting treatment should know that some medications, for example divalproex (Depakote) or lamotrigine (Lamictal), might increase the tremor. Similarly, people who have problems with finding words may need to avoid topiramate (Topamax), which can cause speech difficulties.

Certain types of side effects can be managed without changing medications. For example, an inability to sleep that develops with lamotrigine (Lamictal) may be managed by changing the timing of the doses. Instead of taking the last dose at bedtime, it may be taken with supper or even as early as lunch. Some side effects occur 1 or 2 hours after taking a dose and last for only 30 minutes to 2 hours, linked to the timing of the medication dose. This is probably related to the medication level peaking in the blood. Such a side effect may be managed by splitting the dose in two or by taking the medication with food, which usually evens out the blood level peak. Because of this phenomenon, it may be advantageous to give the largest dose at bedtime (provided the medication does not interfere with sleep). Several medications are available in extended-release preparation. Such a preparation may help smooth out the blood level fluctuations and provide both reduced side effects and greater efficacy throughout the day. Some side effects tend to disappear with the passage of time. This is particularly true of side effects that are mild to start with. One example is mild drowsiness.

Other side effects may be treated with supplements or medications. This is usually not a good idea unless the medication has produced excellent seizure control. For example, hair loss seen with divalproex (Depakote) may be helped by supplementing the diet with zinc and selenium. The excessive tiredness sometimes encountered with divalproex (Depakote) has been helped in some cases by the addition of L-carnitine. There is also anecdotal evidence that the mood swings sometimes encountered with levetiracetam (Keppra) can at times be helped by the addition of vitamin B_6 (also called pyridoxine).

In many instances, reducing the dose of the medication may take care of the side effects without losing seizure control. If seizures recur with dose reduction, the dose can be reduced for a while, and then another attempt can be made at increasing it. Some side effects require stopping the medication, if the side effects are severe and are not helped by reducing the dose. This is particularly true if the medication also did not control the seizures.

Predicting and Preventing Serious Complications from Medications

Several seizure medications also have the potential for rare, serious complications. These rare complications are difficult to predict. Sometimes, it is possible to identify people who are at risk for these adverse reactions. For example, people of Asian descent are at greater risk of serious skin reaction from carbamazepine (Tegretol, Carbatrol) if they possess a genetic marker called HLA-B1502. The drug felbamate (Felbatol) is associated with a risk of bone marrow failure (aplastic anemia), which is often lethal. It is known that people who have baseline immune conditions, such as lupus, are at increased risk of developing this complication, and these individuals should not be started on this drug.

Discontinuing Medications

The treatment of epilepsy is not necessarily lifelong. Some forms of epilepsy are known to recover spontaneously, and it is therefore quite appropriate to consider removing treatment after seizures have been controlled for a period of time. In children, the waiting period before considering stopping seizure medications is usually 2 years. In adults, most neurologists wait longer before stopping seizure medications.

Reasons to Consider Stopping Medications

In some individuals, some medications may reduce concentration and learning, cause sleepiness or tiredness, or cause other bothersome side effects. Some patients also report changes in sexual function. In addition, some medications may have long-term effects, such as weight gain or reduced bone density. Because of these possible effects, a neurologist may favor removing medications if they are no longer necessary. However, it may be difficult to tell if or when the medication is no longer necessary.

Risk of Seizure Return After Stopping Medication

The risk always remains that seizures may come back after stopping seizure medications. Estimates of the risk of seizure recurrence after stopping seizure medications have varied. It is estimated that about 30 percent of patients will have seizure recurrence within 2 years of stopping medications. However, this depends on many factors.

A recurrence of seizures is more likely in people whose seizures are due to brain injury (Table 3.2). It is also more likely that seizures will come back if they started in adolescence, as opposed to childhood. In addition, an abnormal EEG at the time of stopping medications makes it more likely that seizures will come back. We can now predict that certain forms of epilepsy are unlikely to disappear.

The decision to stop medications depends on more than just the calculated risk of seizure recurrence. The doctor and patient should discuss

TABLE 3.2 Factors That Predict a Higher Risk of Another Seizure After Stopping Seizure Medications

Cause of epilepsy—Abnormal brain structure or brain function as a cause of epilepsy (e.g., intellectual disability or cerebral palsy)
Abnormal electroencephalogram (EEG)
Epilepsy starting in adolescence or adulthood has a greater risk than epilepsy starting in childhood.
Juvenile myoclonic epilepsy has a high risk of seizures after stopping medications.
Other factors found in some studies: • History of status epilepticus (continuous seizure activity) • Seizures that were frequent before they were controlled • History of epilepsy in other members of the family

the potential impact of a seizure on work and life in general. For example, a mother who has to drive her children to school every day should probably not plan on coming off seizure medications any time soon. The same would be true of a man whose job necessarily involves operating a forklift. If a patient decides to go ahead with medication withdrawal, it is best to plan for a time when driving can be avoided. Most neurologists will suggest not driving for 3 to 6 months in association with medication withdrawal. Medication withdrawal is much easier to consider in children who are not driving yet.

Duration of Medication Withdrawal

It is the usual practice to stop a medication very gradually, usually over 3 to 6 months. However, one study showed no difference in outcome between *tapering* the medication over 6 weeks or over 9 months. If the patient is taking two medications, one medication should be slowly removed first, before the second medication is tapered.

The majority of individuals whose seizures return with removal of seizure medications will become seizure-free again after medications are restarted. However, some patients will continue to have seizures that can no longer be controlled. It is not totally clear if this was going to happen anyway, or if this is the result of stopping the medications.

Example 6. Deciding to stop seizure medications.   A 16-year-old boy had seizures starting at the age of 12 in which he lost consciousness first, and then had jerking of all extremities. These seizures came quickly under control with one seizure medication, and he has been seizure-free for 2 years. He is eager to start driving as soon as possible, and hates to take his medication. In fact, he often misses his morning dose, and has not had any problems with that. His MRI is normal. His first EEG showed epileptic discharges in one frontal lobe, but his EEG at age 16 was normal.

This may be the ideal situation to consider medication withdrawal. This should probably be done before the patient starts driving. There is a suggestion that the epileptic condition may have resolved, since the EEG has become normal and no seizures occur when he misses his medication. It is probably best not to start driving until at least 3 months after coming off the medication.

FREQUENTLY ASKED QUESTIONS

Q   I have had one seizure. Should I be treated?

At present, the purpose of medication treatment is to prevent more seizures from happening. If the seizure was clearly provoked by a cause that is no longer present, then treatment is not necessary. For example, if the seizure is due to a very low sodium level, which is now corrected, treatment is not necessary. If the seizure occurred without provocation, then treatment could be advisable, and the pros and cons of treatment should be discussed with your neurologist. Overall, a second seizure occurs in only 40 percent to 50 percent of patients. People who have a normal neurologic examination, normal MRI scan of the brain, and normal EEG have a lower risk of seizure recurrence. They may consider not receiving any treatment. However, the decision may also depend on personal factors. For example, if there is a serious risk of job loss in the event of another seizure, this may affect the decision to treat.

Q   Why is it important to prevent repeated seizures?

It is important to prevent seizures if a high risk exists that another seizure may occur. The reasons include the following:

- Recurrent seizures could become more severe.
- Direct or indirect physical injury may result from a seizure.

- Loss of brain cells may occur from repeated severe seizures.
- Sudden death may occur rarely with severe seizures.
- Seizures can be associated with injury.
- Seizures result in legal restrictions on driving.

Q **Now that I have been seizure-free for 6 months, I would like to come off seizure medications. Can I?**

It is recommended that treatment for seizures should continue for at least 2 years. Evidence suggests that the risk of seizure recurrence may be higher if medication is stopped earlier than that. Even after 2 years of no seizures on treatment, the risk is always present that seizures will come back after treatment is stopped, with approximately one-third of people having seizure recurrence. The risk of seizure recurrence can be predicted to some extent by the type and cause of epilepsy, the neurologic examination, and the result of EEG testing. For example, the risk of seizure recurrence in people with juvenile myoclonic epilepsy is very high, such that only a minority of affected individuals can come off medications in the long-term. When seizures start in later life, for example after age 60, the risk of recurrence after stopping medications is also high, and medication treatment may need to be lifelong.

Q **Should I have blood tests every 3 months because I take a seizure medication?**

Routine blood testing is usually not necessary, except for some specific medications. Drug levels are usually not useful as a routine test. Drug levels can be useful if they answer a specific question. A drug level is useful:

- For future reference in a patient who is seizure-free
- To help explain lack of response at a high medication dose, and explore how much leeway there is for increasing the dose
- To help explain side effects at a low dose

■ To monitor a known interaction for dose adjustment (for example, lamotrigine (Lamictal) dose changes may be needed after a birth control pill is added)

Q   **I am still having seizures! Why is the drug not working?**

Not all patients with epilepsy become seizure-free with treatment. Approximately one-third continue to have seizures despite the best treatment. After failing one medication, there is a fair chance that a second medication will work. However, when two medications have not worked, the chance of complete seizure cessation with a third medication becomes much smaller. When seizures are resistant to treatment, it is most important to verify that the attacks being treated are indeed epileptic seizures. It is also important to verify that the seizure type and form of epilepsy have been correctly diagnosed and treated with the most appropriate drug. Inpatient V-EEG monitoring is generally essential for answering these questions. If the seizures are indeed epileptic and are correctly diagnosed and treated, factors such as sleep deprivation, substance abuse, or the use of another medication that can trigger seizures must be explored and corrected.

CHAPTER 4

Antiepileptic Drugs

- The goal of medication is to achieve the best seizure control possible, with few to no side effects.
- So far, no medication can cure epilepsy; AEDs work instead by suppressing seizure activity.
- The dose of a medication needed to control seizures varies considerably among people. Some people need only a small dose, while some need a larger dose.
- All medications have the potential of causing adverse side effects, and each drug comes with a long list of potential problems.
- Sometimes several medications need to be tried to find the one that best controls seizures with the fewest side effects.

Antiepileptic drugs (AEDs) are the mainstay of treatment of epilepsy. Even people who have had successful surgical treatment for their seizures usually continue to take at least some medication. When a firm diagnosis of epilepsy is made, treatment using antiepileptic medication is usually started either immediately or within days. Your doctor will prescribe a medication based on multiple factors, such as epilepsy and seizure type, age, gender, significant medical history, the side-effect profile of each medication, as well as the cost of the drug. The goal of medication is to achieve the best seizure control possible, with few to no *side effects* (unwanted, bad effects).

The majority of people with epilepsy, over 50 percent, will achieve this goal. But, for others, seizure control will be more difficult and may require multiple medication trials or the use of more than one medication at the same time. Some 20 percent to 30 percent of people with epilepsy will experience only partial control of seizures with medication, while another 20 percent will remain *refractory* (resistant) to medication.

About 20 antiepileptic medications currently are available, with more being developed and tested every day. This gives an individual and their doctor more options and a better chance at controlling epilepsy today, as compared to 10 or 15 years ago.

When a new drug is started, your doctor will provide a schedule to follow, as well as information about the possible side effects or problems that could occur with the medicine. Most drugs must be started gradually, increasing the dose a little at a time. Other drugs can be started more quickly. Slowly increasing a dose, which is called titration, usually gives your system a chance to get used to the medicine. This leads to fewer side effects. Therefore, it's important to make sure that your doctor's instructions are clear and that you can follow them exactly.

Many AEDs can produce side effects such as sleepiness or dizziness. In most cases, these side effects are mild and go away as you get used to the medication. Sometimes slowing the rate of dose increase is helpful. However, sometimes side effects are unusually troublesome or do not go away even at low doses, and a different medication must be tried.

Unlike some other types of medicines, there is no standard dose of AEDs. In some cases, a relatively small dose is enough to stop seizures completely. In other people, larger doses are needed. Your doctor will often increase the dose of your medication gradually until the seizures either come under control or until it is clear that the medication is not working. You cannot compare milligram doses between medications — this refers only to the size of the pill or capsule. Thus, 10 mg of one medication may be stronger than 1000 mg of another medication.

What Is the Most Effective Drug?

Most of the available AEDs are about equally effective when used at proper doses for the seizure types for which they are indicated. The choice of drug depends more upon other factors, such as ease of use, possible side effects, cost, and age and sex of the patient.

Thus there is no "best" or most effective drug for epilepsy.

Continued Treatment

Doctors typically use one medication to treat seizures. Using one drug alone is called *monotherapy*. If a medication fails, either because it failed to control seizures or because it caused side effects, a second medication may be added. The use of one medication is often preferable for multiple reasons: it's cheaper, easier for increased adherence (taking the correct medicine at the scheduled time), and produces fewer side effects and interactions between medicines. While most people with epilepsy do best using a single medication, patients with difficult-to-control seizures may require two or more medications (known as *polytherapy*). AEDs must be taken every day. Skipping doses increases the chance of seizures. Some people think that because they did not have a seizure every time they missed a dose, that regular dosing may not be important. However, because seizures are unpredictable, this is not a safe practice. Although it is difficult to take medication every day for months or years, that is essential to protection against seizures. You should ask your doctor what to do if you happen to miss a dose. For some medications, it may be possible to "catch up" by adding an extra dose, but for other medications, this can cause unpleasant side effects.

How Antiepileptic Drugs Work

Some AEDs are listed in Table 4.1. The *mechanism of action*, or how these medicines work to stop seizures, is often not known completely. Most medications work by preventing epileptic cells from firing abnormally, while leaving the normal firing of brain cells unchanged. Because seizures are thought to be a sign of brain-cell overexcitation, some medications increase *inhibitory pathways*, by increasing a normally occurring brain chemical called *gamma-amino butyric acid* (GABA). Other medications decrease *excitatory pathways* through systems that use the excitatory chemical *glutamate*. Other AEDs work in more than one way.

TABLE 4.1   List of Antiepileptic Drugs (USA)

Brivaracetam (Briviact)	Gabapentin (Neurontin)
Carbamazepine (Tegretol, Tegretol XR, Carbatrol)	Perampanel (Fycompa)
Clobazam (Onfi)	Pregabalin (Lyrica)
Phenobarbital (Luminal)	Oxcarbazepine (Trileptal)
Phenytoin (Dilantin)	Eslicarbazepine (Aptiom)
Primidone (Mysoline)	Rufinamide (Banzel)
Valproate (Depakote, Depakene)	Tiagabine (Gabitril)
Lamotrigine (Lamictal)	Topiramate (Topamax)
Levetiracetam (Keppra)	Vigabatrin (Sabril)
Felbamate (Felbatol)	Zonisamide (Zonegran)
Ethosuximide (Zarontin)	Cenobamate (Xcopri)

So far, no medication can cure epilepsy. AEDs work instead by suppressing seizure activity. That means they have to be constantly present in the brain. After a medication is taken by mouth, it is passed through the stomach and absorbed by the small intestine, and then transported to the bloodstream. Eventually it reaches the brain. Some medicines leave the body when they are broken down (*metabolized*) by the liver. Others are not metabolized by the liver, but are cleared from the body by the kidneys, through the urine.

Drug Interactions

Many combinations of two or more drugs can interfere with one another by reducing each other's effectiveness, or less often, they make the effect of each other stronger. These are called *drug interactions*. Some interactions are simply additions of expected effects, for example, if you take two drugs, both of which make you sleepy, you could be twice as sleepy. Other interactions, however, affect the actual amount of drug reaching your brain. This is especially true of combinations that include drugs processed by the liver, such as phenytoin and carbamazepine.

It important for your doctor to know about all of the drugs you are taking, including nonprescription drugs and dietary supplements, so that unwanted drug interactions can be avoided. We have listed some of the more common interactions in the descriptions of the following individual drugs. However, because literally thousands of possible interactions exist, we cannot provide a complete list. Computer programs that are now in many doctor's offices and pharmacies may be able to provide a warning of possible drug interactions.

Blood Levels and Blood Testing

After a medication is ingested, it reaches a maximum level in the bloodstream within a certain amount of time, usually between 30 minutes and 6 hours. After that, the amount of medication in the bloodstream gradually drops, as does the amount reaching the brain. If the level of medication in the brain drops too far, it may no longer be able to protect against a seizure. The amount of time it takes for the medication level to drop to half the amount of the peak level is called its *half-life*. The half-life of a medication can be short, intermediate, or long. A medication with a short half-life must be taken more frequently to maintain a constant level in the bloodstream and brain, while a medication with a long half-life can be dosed at less frequent intervals. Most AEDs are taken once or twice a day. For some drugs, a blood test can measure the amount of medication in the bloodstream. This is called a *drug level*.

Routine measurement of drug levels is not necessary for most AEDs, especially for more modern drugs. The proper dose is determined by gradual increases in the dose until seizures stop completely or until unacceptable side effects, such as dizziness, occur.

However, drug levels are useful for some medications in certain circumstances. Long experience has shown that certain drug levels of phenytoin, carbamazepine, valproate, and lamotrigine usually produce the best seizure control with the fewest side effects in most people. These are called *therapeutic levels*. However, they should be used as general guides only. Some people are free of seizures at lower blood levels and some people need blood levels above the usual range. A "low" blood level may not need action if seizures are completely controlled, and a "high" blood level may not need action if there are no side effects. For some drugs, blood levels do not match up well with the effect of the drug on the brain. For these drugs, blood level testing is less useful. Examples are levetiracetam (Keppra) and gabapentin (Neurontin)

Routine blood testing for drug side effects is also unnecessary for most drugs. Drugs that are processed by the liver, such as phenytoin, carbamazepine, valproate, and phenobarbital, may cause slight increases in blood levels of some liver enzymes. This is not harmful. In rare cases, more abnormal liver tests may require stopping the drug.

Persons taking carbamazepine, oxcarbazepine, or eslicarbazepine may need to have blood sodium (salt) levels measured a few weeks after starting the drug because a low sodium level may occur, especially in older persons or those taking diuretics.

Valproate can sometimes lower blood platelets and cause bruising or bleeding, especially at higher doses. Felbamate is the only AED for which regular blood testing is strongly recommended because it can affect blood or liver function. Although not considered a typical anti-epileptic drug, liver monitoring is needed in patients using CBD at least during the initial phase.

Medication Side Effects

All medications have the potential of causing unwanted side effects, and each drug will come with a long list of potential problems. Your doctor will tell you the most commonly expected side effects of the drug prescribed, but they cannot provide a complete list of everything possible. There are more complete listings on the Internet or in the pamphlets that you receive from your doctor or pharmacist, but it is important to understand that most of these side effects are uncommon or not serious. It is helpful to divide side effects into categories:

1. **Starting dose side effects.** These are common side effects that many people experience when they first start a drug. Most are not serious and may go away in days or weeks. Examples of such effects seen with many AEDs are sleepiness or dizziness. Unless these are severe, you do not need to notify your physician.

2. **Dose-related side effects.** These are side effects that typically appear with higher doses of a drug. Often they are the same as the starting dose side effects, but they may not go away and may require lowering the dose. Unless they are mild and temporary, your doctor should be consulted if they should occur.

3. **Rare serious side effects.** These are sometimes called *idiosyn-cratic* side effects because they are unpredictable, not related closely to the drug dose, and probably affect only people with certain genetic makeups. The most common of these is a rash. If you should develop a rash, especially a red, widespread rash within the first three months of starting a new drug, you should notify your doctor *immediately*—certainly within 24 hours. If it is determined that the drug is the likely cause, it will be necessary to change drugs. However, do not stop taking the drug abruptly without your doctor's advice. Stopping an AED abruptly can cause a dangerous condition called *status epilepticus* (one seizure after another).

   Rashes usually go away quickly when the drug is stopped, but they can be a part of more dangerous allergic reactions. AEDs are relatively safe drugs, but no drug is completely safe. About one out of 1000 to 25,000 people will have a very severe allergic reaction to a drug, with or without a rash, which may result in hospitalization or death. This may involve damage to the liver, blood, or other organs. This is true of all AEDs and, in fact, of all other drugs, including those available without a prescription. These reactions cannot be foreseen, but you should tell your doctor if you have had allergies to any previous drugs. Some of the side effects that should prompt you to call your physician are rash, fever, skin blisters, unusual bleeding or bruising, severe stomach pain, vomiting, change in skin color, or generally feeling ill. If you are in doubt, it is best to discuss the problem with your doctor.

   It is also important to understand that in almost all cases uncontrolled seizures, especially convulsions, are far more dangerous than taking any medication.

4. **Long-term use side effects.** These are cumulative side effects that may appear after months or years of drug use. These side effects are not directly life-threatening, but they can affect health

or quality of life. Some older drugs, including phenytoin, phenobarbital, carbamazepine, and possibly valproate can cause *osteoporosis* (thinning of bones) over time. Peripheral nerve and joint
problems occasionally occur. Endocrine effects of some drugs can
affect sexual function.

5. **Birth defects (teratogenicity).** Pregnant mothers with epilepsy
    are often worried about the effects of their AEDs on their unborn
    babies. However, there is good evidence that seizures during
    pregnancy, at least tonic-clonic seizures (convulsions), are much
    more likely to harm mother or baby than taking any AED. For
    this reason, pregnant women should never stop taking an AED
    without their doctor's advice.

    Some AEDs do carry a higher risk of causing birth defects.
    Phenobarbital has been reported to carry a risk of 6.5 percent and
    valproate to carry a risk of 10.7 percent. Newer drugs are proba-
    bly safer, but women should discuss their AED therapy with their
    doctors well before a chance of pregnancy exists.

Brand-Name and Generic Drugs

Every drug has a chemical (*generic*) name as well as one or several brand
names (given in parentheses in this book), which are specific to the company that markets the drug. A drug may also have different *formulations*,
such as liquid, solid, sprinkle, immediate-release, or long-acting. Generic
drugs are usually much less expensive than the original brand name drug
and work perfectly well for most people. There are occasional people who
do better with a particular brand. In that case, the doctor will need to spec-
ify the brand and often provide information to the insurance company
about why this is necessary.

We've listed the most common drugs for epilepsy here in alphabetical
order and described them in detail. Included are the seizure types the drug
is commonly prescribed for, as well as common dose-related and rare seri-

ous side effects, and common drug interactions to look out for. This list is not meant to be exhaustive. Each drug should be discussed with your doctor before starting it. We have also described less-commonly used AEDs briefly at the end of this section.

Carbamazepine (Tegretol, Carbatrol)

- ■ Used for focal seizures and generalized tonic-clonic seizures. May cause absence, atypical absence, and myoclonic seizures to worsen.
- ■ Common side effects:
  - ● Double vision, headache, nausea, incoordination, drowsiness, difficulty concentrating, and dizziness are the most frequently reported side effects at the start of treatment. These side effects usually improve as the body adjusts to the medication or the dose is lowered.
- ■ Rare less serious side effects, which may or may not require discontinuation:
  - ● *Hyponatremia* (low sodium level), *leukopenia* (decrease of white blood cells).
- ■ Rare serious side effects that usually require discontinuation:
  - ● Liver failure, bone marrow failure, drug-related rash, and hypersensitivity.
- ■ Potential long-term effects:
  - ● Carbamazepine has an effect on the liver (*enzyme induction*) that speeds the metabolism of other substances. This may increase the metabolism of vitamin D, which can contribute to *osteopenia* (a mild thinning of bone mass) and *osteoporosis* (a loss of normal bone density that leads to fragile bones and an increased risk of bone fracture). People who are on carbamazepine often have slight increases in liver enzymes measured on blood tests; these are not harmful. However,

higher elevations, or elevations that continue to rise, may be a sign of liver injury.

- Drug–drug interactions:
  - Cimetidine, diltiazem, erythromycin, clarithromycin, fluoxetine, omeprazole, propoxyphene, and verapamil can increase carbamazepine levels. Antipsychotics, lamotrigine, narcotics, oral contraceptives, theophylline, topiramate, valproate, and warfarin can be affected by carbamazepine, causing a decrease in their effectiveness.
  - Carbamazepine can lower the effectiveness of oral contraceptives (birth control pills).

Cenobamate (Xcopri)

- Used for focal seizures.
- Common side effects:
  - Dizziness, sleepiness, headaches, fatigue, blurred vision.
- Serious rare side effects:
  - Skin rash or significant allergic reaction. The chance of allergic reaction is higher with increasing the medication too fast.
- Drug–drug interactions:
  - Xcopri reduces levels of lamotrigine and carbamazepine and increases levels of phenobarbital and phenytoin in the blood.

Ethosuximide (Zarontin)

- Used for absence (*petit mal*) seizures. No effect on other seizure types.
- Common side effects:
  - Gastrointestinal distress, drowsiness, irritability, dizziness.
- Rare side effects:
  - Skin rash, blood disorders, psychosis.

- Drug–drug interactions:
  - Carbamazepine, phenobarbital, and phenytoin may lower ethosuximide levels.

Lacosamide (Vimpat)

- Used for focal seizures and generalized tonic-clonic seizures
- Common side effects:
  - Dizziness, sleepiness, double or blurred vision, nausea, headache.
- Rare side effects:
  - Allergic reactions.
- Drug–drug interactions:
  - None reported.

Lamotrigine (Lamictal)

- Used for focal seizures, tonic-clonic seizures, typical and atypical absence, and atonic and myoclonic seizures associated with the Lennox-Gastaut syndrome.
- Common side effects:
  - Dizziness or unsteadiness, headache, double or blurred vision, and nausea. Unlike other AEDs, lamotrigine is more likely to cause insomnia than sleepiness.
- Rare side effects:
  - 5 percent to 10 percent of people who take lamotrigine will develop a skin rash or other sign of allergic reaction. The chance of rash may be higher in children, when the drug is combined with valproate, with a high initial dose, or when the dose is increased too rapidly. As with other drugs, more serious allergic reactions affecting skin, liver, or other organs can occur.

- Drug–drug interactions:
  - Oxcarbazepine, phenytoin, carbamazepine, phenobarbital, and primidone can lower lamotrigine levels. Valproic acid will increase lamotrigine levels. Lamotrigine will decrease valproic acid levels by approximately 25 percent. Oral contraceptives and pregnancy will lower lamotrigine levels.

Levetiracetam (Keppra) and Brivaracetam (Briviact)

- Used for focal and generalized tonic-clonic seizures and myoclonus.
- Brivaracetam is a newer drug that works in a similar way to levetiracetam, but it may have fewer side effects for some persons.
- Common side effects:
  - Irritability, depression, fatigue, dizziness, sleepiness, nausea.
- Rare side effects:
  - Rare allergic reactions. The dose should be adjusted for older people or people with kidney disease.
- Drug–drug interactions:
  - None reported.

Oxcarbazepine (Trileptal) and Eslicarbazepine (Aptiom)

- Used for focal seizures and generalized tonic-clonic seizures. May worsen absence (petit mal) or myoclonic seizures.
- Eslicarbazepine is a newer drug that is an active metabolite (derivative) of oxcarbazepine
- Common side effects:
  - Sedation, dizziness, difficulty with balance and coordination, double vision or abnormal vision, nausea.
- Rare side effects:
  - Oxcarbazepine and eslicarbazepine can reduce the body's ability to regulate water and salt balance, causing a lower-

ing in the blood sodium level; this is called *hyponatremia*. Symptoms of hyponatremia may include nausea, tiredness, headache, sedation, or confusion. People with an allergy to carbamazepine have a 25 percent to 30 percent chance of being allergic to oxcarbazepine.

■ Drug–drug interactions:
  ● Carbamazepine, phenobarbital, phenytoin, and verapamil can lower the effectiveness of these drugs. Oxcarbazepine at higher doses can lower the effectiveness of lamotrigine, and oral contraceptives.

Perampanel (Fycompa)

■ Used as an add-on treatment for focal seizures
■ Common side effects:
  ● Sleepiness, dizziness, irritability, headache.
■ Rare side effects:
  ● Serious allergic reactions, hostility.
■ Drug interactions:
  ● Perampanel levels can be lowered by phenytoin, carbamazepine, phenobarbital, and other drugs.

Phenobarbital (Luminal) and Primidone (Mysoline)

■ Used for focal seizures and generalized tonic-clonic seizures.
■ Most primidone is changed to phenobarbital by the liver.
■ Common side effects:
  ● Sedation, dizziness, difficulty with concentration, irritability, and depression. Children may become hyperactive.
■ Rare side effects:
  ● Allergic reaction, *hepatotoxicity* (liver problems), and blood disorders.

- Potential long-term effects:
  - Osteopenia or osteoporosis, Dupuytren's contractures (thickening of the tendons in the palms), and frozen shoulder.
- Drug–drug interactions:
  - Valproic acid can increase phenobarbital levels. Phenytoin may increase or decrease phenobarbital levels. Phenobarbital can decrease the effectiveness of antipsychotics, carbamazepine, cyclosporine, lamotrigine, narcotics, oral contraceptives, phenytoin, steroids, theophylline, topiramate, valproic acid, and warfarin.

Phenytoin (Dilantin, Phenytek)

- Used for focal seizures and generalized tonic-clonic seizures.
- Common side effects:
  - Double or blurred vision, headache, dizziness, unsteadiness, and drowsiness. Bleeding or swelling of the gums may occur, which may be lessened by good oral hygiene, including brushing and regular visits with the dentist. Acne and hair growth on the body and face may occur.
- Rare side effects:
  - Rash affects 5 percent to 10 percent of people. Rarely, life-threatening skin reactions or failure of organs, including the liver, can occur.
- Potential long-term effects:
  - Osteoporosis (thin bones), *peripheral neuropathy*, and *cerebellar atrophy*.
- Drug–drug interactions:
  - There are many. Phenytoin affects many drugs that are metabolized by the liver. Phenytoin can lower the effectiveness of warfarin, antipsychotics, cancer chemotherapy drugs, antiviral drugs including those used for HIV, narcot-

ics, oral contraceptives, steroids, and other drugs. Antacids, carbamazepine, ciprofloxacin, and phenobarbital can lower phenytoin effectiveness.

- Phenytoin doses can be difficult to adjust and blood levels too low or too high can occur even with small dose changes.

Gabapentin (Neurontin) and Pregabalin (Lyrica)

- Used for focal seizures and generalized tonic-clonic seizures.
- Pregabalin and gabapentin have similar actions in the brain, but pregabalin is better absorbed and can be taken less often.
- Common side effects:
  - Drowsiness, dizziness, unsteadiness, dry mouth, weight gain, and swelling of the feet, legs, or hands.
- Rare side effects:
  - Muscle pain, soreness, or weakness.
- Drug–drug interactions:
  - None known.

Topiramate (Topamax, Qudexy, Trokendi)

- Used for partial seizures, generalized tonic-clonic seizures, atonic, tonic, and tonic-clonic seizures in Lennox-Gastaut syndrome; can be used for myoclonic and absence seizures.
- Common side effects:
  - Difficulty concentrating, drowsiness, slowed speech, depression, decreased appetite and weight loss, tingling of the hands or feet, tremor, nausea, and vomiting.
- Rare side effects:
  - Kidney stones, so adequate fluid intake must be maintained. *Glaucoma* (high pressure in the eye), with symptoms of blurred vision or eye pain, is possible but goes away if the

drug is stopped promptly. Decreased sweating, which can lead rarely to heat stroke in children, has been reported, as has *metabolic acidosis*. Psychosis occurs rarely.

- Drug–drug interactions:
  - Phenytoin, carbamazepine, and phenobarbital can lower topiramate levels. Topiramate can increase phenytoin levels by 25 percent. Topiramate at higher doses can lower the effectiveness of oral contraceptives.

Valproate (Depakote, Depakene)

- Used for all seizure types: focal, tonic-clonic, typical and atypical absence, atonic, and myoclonic seizures.
- Common side effects:
  - Weight gain, nausea, stomachache, drowsiness, difficulty concentrating, dizziness, temporary hair thinning, hand tremor.
- Rare side effects:
  - *Hepatotoxicity* (liver disease), *pancreatitis* (inflammation of the pancreas), *thrombocytopenia* (decreased amount of platelets in the blood). Birth defects in infants born to mothers taking valproate. Allergy is rare.
- Potential long-term effects:
  - Cysts in the ovaries, which may lead to irregular periods and problems with fertility. Sexual dysfunction. Osteoporosis.
- Drug–drug interactions:
  - Fluoxetine (Prozac) can increase valproate levels. Carbamazepine, lamotrigine, phenobarbital, and phenytoin can lower valproate levels. Valproic acid can increase the levels of other drugs, especially lamotrigine.

Zonisamide (Zonegran)

- Used for partial seizures; generalized tonic-clonic seizures, tonic, and myoclonic seizures. May be used for absence seizures.
- Common side effects:
  - Dizziness, difficulty with balance, fatigue, loss of appetite, nausea, headache, and tremor.
- Rare side effects:
  - Kidney stones, so adequate fluid intake must be maintained. Decreased sweating, which can lead rarely to heat stroke in children, has been reported. Allergic reactions affecting skin or other organs.
- Drug–drug interactions:
  - Carbamazepine, phenobarbital, and phenytoin can lower zonisamide levels. Grapefruit juice can lower zonisamide levels.

Medications Used Less Often

Other medications may be chosen by your doctor. These drugs are the best choice for some people, but they are not as frequently used as those described earlier. Only the most prominent side effects are listed: you should discuss side effects and possible drug interactions of these medications with your doctor.

Acetazolamide (Diamox)

- This is a mild *diuretic* (increases urination) that has some anti-seizure effect. It is often prescribed to women who typically have seizures just before their menstrual periods. This medication can be used for 1 week, prior to menses, or on an everyday basis. Its effectiveness may wear off if used on a daily basis.

Benzodiazepines

- Benzodiazepines are a large group of chemically similar *psychotropic drugs* (medications that affect behavior) that include diazepam (Valium), rectal diazepam (Diastat), lorazepam (Ativan), clonazepam (Klonopin), clorazepate (Tranxene), alprazolam (Xanax), clobazam (Onfi), and several other brands. They are most often prescribed as mild tranquilizers, but they have some important uses for seizures.
- The most important use of benzodiazepines is for *emergency treatment*. Because these drugs can be given *intravenously* (through a vein) and therefore work within a few minutes, they are commonly used in emergency rooms and hospitals to stop seizures quickly. Some are also available for home use, by mouth, rectal suppository, or nasal spray, to stop severe or recurring seizures.
- These medications are also used daily to prevent seizures for some people, but they have three disadvantages: they tend to make people sleepy, the anti-seizure effect may wear off in a few months, and, if they are stopped suddenly, severe seizures may result. Those benzodiazepines most commonly used for epilepsy are discussed here. Other side effects may include depression, trouble thinking clearly, and slowed reaction times.

Diazepam (Valium, Diastat)

- Diazepam is given intravenously to stop seizures quickly, but the effect wears off in a few minutes, so additional doses or another medication must be added soon. Oral Valium is rarely used for seizures because of sleepiness. Diastat is a diazepam gel in a prefilled tube; it is given in the rectum to stop repetitive seizures. It causes sleepiness, but is very safe and designed only for occasional use. Diastat is an excellent choice for people who tend to have "clusters" of seizures, that is, people who are likely to have more than one seizure in a day. It can be used at home and may prevent the need to go to an emergency room.

Lorazepam (Ativan)

■ This is the first choice of many doctors for use in emergency situations to stop seizures. When given intravenously, it usually stops seizures within a few minutes. Unlike diazepam, the effect lasts several hours. Lorazepam can be used by mouth at home for this purpose, but by mouth it takes at least 30 minutes to have an effect.

Midazolam (Versed, Nayzilam)

■ Midazolam is a very rapid onset drug once given through IV or through the nose or mouth. Over the past years, people have used this IV drug to treat patients having severe seizures or status epilepticus. The drug is approved for use as a nasal spray to stop seizures at home.

Clonazepam (Klonopin)

■ Clonazepam is sometimes useful, especially for absence seizures or myoclonic seizures. It is often used at bedtime for nighttime seizures.

Clorazepate (Tranxene)

■ When taken by mouth, this medication lasts longer than some of the other benzodiazepines. Clorazepate is sometimes used for complex partial seizures and other seizure types.

Clobazam (Onfi)

- This medication is now approved in the United States for seizures associated with the Lennox-Gastaut syndrome, but it may have usefulness for other seizures types. It may have less tendency to lose its effect with time than other benzodiazepines and appears to be less sedating.

Bromides

- Bromides are bitter, salty-tasting liquids containing bromide. Bromide is interesting from a historical standpoint because it was the first medication that worked well to control seizures. It was, therefore, the first real AED. Bromides was discovered by an English physician in 1857 and was the most commonly used drug for seizures until phenobarbital was discovered in 1912. Bromides are almost never used now because they usually cause drowsiness and acne. However, for a few people, they are very effective. Bromides must be made up especially by a pharmacist; they are not commercially available.

Felbamate (Felbamate)

- This is an effective drug that is useful for most seizure types, with the exception of absence seizures. Felbamate is also nonsedating. However, it is only used when most other drugs have failed because there is a one in 4000–8000 chance of severe or fatal blood or liver abnormality. People taking this drug must have regular blood testing.

Rufinamide (Banzel)

- Used for seizure types associated with the Lennox-Gastaut syndrome and sometimes for focal seizures. Rufinamide is particularly useful for atonic seizures ("drop attacks").

Tiagabine (Gabitril)

- Used for focal and generalized tonic-clonic seizures. Sleepiness can be dose-limiting. Rarely, it can cause *nonconvulsive status epilepticus* (a condition of continual staring spells, which can be dangerous).

Vigabatrin (Sabril)

- This is an effective drug for focal seizures and can be taken once daily. In some people who take it for 3 months to several years, a narrowing of the peripheral visual field may occur (trouble seeing off to the sides), which is permanent. Vigabatrin does not cause blindness. For this reason, persons taking vigabatrin should have eye testing regularly.

Experimental Medications

All medications were experimental at first. Experimental does not mean necessarily dangerous or ineffective, just that the drug has not yet been approved for sale by regulatory agencies because more information is needed. In the United States, the Food and Drug Administration (FDA) requires careful testing of all medications before approval is given for sale. This usually requires several years and involves trials with animals, normal human volunteers, and then finally persons with the disease for which the drug is intended.

If standard medications have been unsatisfactory for you, you may want to consider an experimental drug. No one is ever given an experimental drug without their permission, and the possible risks and benefits must be explained in advance. Clinical trials of a new drug are usually free, and persons taking the drug are closely supervised by an experienced physician. These trials are often available through universities or specialized epilepsy clinics. At present, several promising AEDs are in clinical trials. Your doctor may know of clinical trials in your local area. Another source of information is clinicaltrials.gov, a registry of all experimental drugs in testing programs in the United States, or The Epilepsy Foundation.

FREQUENTLY ASKED QUESTIONS

Q   How does my doctor choose a medication to treat my seizures?

Before embarking on potentially long-term antiepileptic medication therapy, a diagnosis of epilepsy must be made. This diagnosis is based on several factors, such as history, a physical and neurologic examination, and diagnostic testing. From this information, your doctor will try to determine what type of epilepsy you have. A medication will then be selected based on seizure type, the presence of other illnesses and medications, the cost of the drug, how often the drug must be dosed, and the potential side effects. Once a medication is selected, the dose will be adjusted at various intervals. Your doctor will try to use one medication, and they may need to increase the dose until your seizures are controlled or until you develop annoying side effects. It may be necessary to try several medications before finding one that causes few side effects and controls your seizures. Occasionally, multiple medications will need to be used together.

Q **Do all antiepileptic medications cause side effects?**

All medications, not just seizure medications, have the potential of causing mild or severe side effects. Many people start a medication and experience no side effects at all, or only mild side effects that are easily resolved by adjusting a dose. As with any medication, more serious side effects can occur and must be addressed immediately.

Q **Will I need to take seizure medication forever?**

The decision to withdraw medication is never an easy one. Your doctor must take into account the likelihood of seizure recurrence off the medication, the risks of injury with seizure recurrence, and the risk of potential long-term drug effects. Some types of epilepsy require lifelong treatment; *juvenile myoclonic epilepsy* is a genetic form of epilepsy that rarely goes away. Other children, however, may experience a benign form of epilepsy that they outgrow.

Q **Can I take the generic form of seizure medication?**

Generic formulations work well for most persons and are usually less expensive than the original brand name drug. However, a particular brand may work better or have fewer side effects in some persons. Persons who have complete seizure control with a particular brand, or a drug from a particular generic manufacturer, should try to keep taking it if financially feasible. This may require a special request from your doctor to your insurance company and a discussion with your pharmacist.

Q **What if I can't afford the medication?**

Financial concerns should be discussed with your doctor, prior to starting a new medication. Your doctor may be able to assist you with obtaining the medication you need. Most pharmaceutical companies participate in patient-assistance programs, which are programs that supply the patient with medication, free or at lower cost, if they meet financial eligibility requirements. Starting samples or coupons are sometimes available. Sometimes, a change in the pill size is all that is needed to make a medication affordable. Frequently, there is little difference between the costs of various pill sizes. For example, instead of using a 100-mg pill twice each day, change the pill size to 200 mg and take half a pill twice a day. Simple things, such as obtaining a 90-day supply rather than three 30-day supplies, can save money. Although most older drugs are less expensive than newer ones and may control seizures just as well, this must be balanced against a possible risk of more side effects or drug interactions.

Q Are timed-release drugs better?

Several common AEDs are now available in so-called "timed release" or "extended release" forms, which can be taken less often than the "immediate release" forms. These include phenytoin, levetiracetam, oxcarbazepine, topiramate, valproate, and others.

There is no clear evidence that the timed-release forms work any better than immediate-release forms of the same drug to control seizures, and they are usually more expensive. However, timed-release drugs may be more convenient because most can be taken just once a day (some twice a day). This may help you to remember to take your medication and may give you more flexibility in dose timing. For a few people, the timed-release drugs lessen side effects because they do not enter the bloodstream as quickly.

Some drugs, such as eslicarbazepine, perampanel, vigabatrin, and zonisamide naturally last a long time in the body after each dose, so that once a day dosing is possible without a timed-release form.

CHAPTER 5

Diet, Nutrition, and Alternative Therapies

■ The ketogenic diet is the only scientifically proven alternative and dietary treatment of seizures. Most patients treated with the ketogenic diet are children, but adults can benefit as well.

■ The ketogenic diet is effective, reducing seizure frequency, in about 50 percent of the people treated.

■ Achieving a healthy body weight and adopting a healthier, more balanced diet can be beneficial for those with epilepsy not willing to use ketogenic diet therapy.

■ Herbs, vitamin and mineral supplements, and Chinese medicine are widely used with standard drugs. However, no scientific study has shown beneficial effects of these therapies.

■ Melatonin can be of help in the management of sleep disorders and epilepsy in some patients.

■ Complementary and alternative therapies and self-care can be useful adjuncts to traditional medical approaches, but they should not be considered a primary treatment for epilepsy.

■ All alternative methods for seizure treatment should be discussed with your doctor before you start.

The Ketogenic Diet: Nutrition Therapy for Epilepsy

Modifying diet to treat and manage disease has been apparent since biblical times. Although the modern medical world has evolved remarkably since then, clinicians continue to use diet and nutrition to manage chronic disease, including epilepsy.

The ketogenic diet exemplifies the use of diet and nutrition to treat and manage disease. The classic *ketogenic diet* (KD) was originally based on the premise that fasting controls seizures in some individuals. The positive effect of dietary modification for epilepsy was discovered in the early 1900s when epilepsy patients were fasted prior to surgery. These fasted patients experienced a drastic decline in their seizures. For this reason, the earliest dietary treatment of epilepsy was prolonged fasting (up to 40 days in some cases). Given the medical dangers and difficulties associated with prolonged fasting, physicians at the Mayo Clinic proposed that a diet mimicking starvation could provide the same seizure control benefits, yet be achieved without complete fasting. A diet limiting dietary protein and carbohydrates forces the body to shift its metabolism from using glucose (sugar) as an energy source to using fat. When the body uses fat to meet energy demands, ketone bodies are produced, creating a state of *ketosis*. During periods of fasting, the body also uses fat as an energy source and, thus, shifts the body into a state of ketosis. The KD shares the same metabolic characteristics of fasting metabolism without actually depriving the body of energy. The KD was named after these ketone bodies used as energy when metabolism shifts from glucose to fat utilization.

Although beneficial, the KD fell out of use in the 1940s after the introduction of antiepileptic drugs. Its popularity was revived in the 1990s by the Johns Hopkins team after the widely publicized success of Charlie Abrahams, who was cured of severe intractable epilepsy while on the diet. This lead to the creation of the Charlie Foundation, clinical trials, and international acceptance that the KD can be highly effective in selected populations. As the diet's popularity grew, so did its restrictive reputation, which fostered the development of alternative, less-restrictive (Modified

Atkins, Low Glycemic Diets) for epilepsy, and the expansion of dietary therapies for epilepsy to include adults. The KD is an alternative to medications or procedures and among "alternative epilepsy therapies," it has the greatest data that demonstrate effectiveness.

The KD's success in controlling epilepsy is well documented, with roughly 50 percent of children achieving >50 percent seizure control with sustained diet therapy. The efficacy of the diet was best summarized in a 1998 study, which found that out of 1084 pediatric patients, 56 percent of them had a >50 percent reduction in seizures, 32 percent had a >90 percent reduction in seizures, and roughly 16 percent became seizure free. This rate of success makes the KD an effective and attractive option when medications and other therapies fail.

There are several variations of the KD and, although no head-to-head clinical trials have compared the efficacy of each variation, they are all considered to have similar success rates. This chapter briefly explores the various KDs and the basics of each one.

The Classic Ketogenic Diet

The KD is a high-fat, restricted carbohydrate, adequate protein diet that encourages the body to use fat as energy instead of glucose. Calories are calculated to provide enough energy to support growth, but to prevent excessive weight gain. The calorie makeup of the diet is based on the selected ratio. Higher ratio diets have more fat, less protein, and less carbohydrate. Ratios range from 1:1 to 4:1. A 4:1 classic diet is roughly 2 percent carbohydrate, 8 percent protein, and 90 percent fat. A 3:1 ratio is roughly 80 percent fat, a 2:1 ratio 70 percent fat, and a 1:1 ratio 60 percent fat. The diet ratio refers to the proportion of fat in the diet to the proportion of carbohydrates and protein. The ratio is selected and the diet is precisely calculated by the RD. Every diet is individualized and based on protein requirements, energy requirements, and the person's dietary habits and preferences. Higher ratios are generally used in younger children, and lower ratios are used in older or larger children who have higher calorie and protein needs.

How the Diet Works

Although we know a great deal about the metabolic changes that occur in the body while on the KD, exactly how the KD works to control seizures is unknown. During fasting, *ketone bodies* (chemicals like acetoacetate, B-hydroxybutyrate, and acetone) are formed in the blood. These chemicals become the brain's source of energy, rather than its usual source, which is *glucose* (a kind of sugar that the body derives from the digestion of carbohydrates).

Scientists think that it's possible that the ketone bodies themselves, particularly acetone, may have anticonvulsant properties. In addition, the KD may alter neurotransmitters, the chemicals that transmit electrical energy within the brain. The diet also may change energy metabolism in the brain or simply provide less energy to the brain so that it won't support seizures. Because the KD is carbohydrate restricted, it provides the brain with a very stable and somewhat low level of glucose, which may also be an important factor in seizure control. It is most likely that the diet, like most drugs, has multiple mechanisms of action that cannot be isolated. This is why all aspects of the diet should be considered of importance when implementing and creating the diet prescription. During the last decade, there has been a substantial increase in the basic science surrounding the KD, and someday we may actually pinpoint how it works.

How Well Does the Ketogenic Diet Work?

The diet is not an easy program to stick with. The largest prospective study showed that about 50 percent of the children who start the diet actually remain on it at 1 year, largely because it has been effective in their controlling seizures. Of those who stayed on the diet for 1 year, 7 percent were

seizure free, 20 percent had more than a 90 percent reduction in their seizures, and 23 percent had a 50 percent to 90 percent decrease in seizures.

Candidates for KD Therapy

There is no strict criterion defining who is and who is not a candidate for the
KD. The diet should be considered for all individuals who have failed more
than two antiepileptic drugs and who are deemed safe candidates for the
KD. Although the diet is used in both children and adults, most scientific
publications providing guidance on the KD are focused on children. The diet
can be extremely effective and practical in very young children and should
be considered sooner rather than later in this population. This is especially
true for children consuming formula, children who have feeding tubes or
children who consume mostly pureed foods. Like with any treatment, there
are groups that have been identified for which the KD is contraindicated and
then groups that the KD can be particularly effective in. An expert consensus defined these groups below (see Table 5.1 on the next page).

Although the cause for seizures is not discovered in most people with
epilepsy, you should be sure that an appropriate metabolic work-up is done
before using the diet. It's important that the doctor and the dietitian who
will be designing your child's diet know of any metabolic problems that
would make the diet dangerous. Most seizure types respond to the diet.
However, some studies suggest that partial or focal seizures might not be
as well controlled. (If your child's seizures are not well controlled, and they
are coming from one part of the brain [focal seizures], it is important to
know if your child is a good candidate for surgery. If surgery is appropriate,
this has a better chance at achieving seizure control than the diet.

Starting the Ketogenic Diet

This is not a do-it-yourself cure for epilepsy! Without proper oversight,
the diet could be very dangerous. The KD should be administered by a

TABLE 5.1   Contraindications to the Use of the KD

Absolute Contraindications	Relative Contraindications	Conditions or Syndromes Which Have Been Associated with Higher Rates of Success with KD
Carnitine deficiency (primary	Inability to maintain adequate nutrition	Glucose transporter protein 1 (GLUT-1) deficiency
Carnitine palmitoyltransferase (CPT) I or II deficiency	Surgical focus identified by neuroimaging and video EEG monitoring	Pyruvate dehydrogenase deficiency (PDHD)
Carnitine translocase deficiency	Parent or caregiver noncompliance	Myoclonic-astatic epilepsy (Doose syndrome)
Beta-oxidation defects		Tuberous sclerosis complex
Medium-chain acyl dehydrogenase deficiency (MCAD)		Rett syndrome
Long-chain acyl dehydrogenase deficiency (LCAD)		Severe myoclonic epilepsy of infancy (Dravet syndrome)
Short-chain acyl dehydrogenase deficiency (SCAD)		Infantile spasms
Long-chain 3-hydroxyacyl-CoA deficiency		Children receiving only formula (infants or enterally fed patients)
Medium-chain 3-hydroxyacyl-CoA deficiency		
Pyruvate carboxylase deficiency		
Porphyria		

(Adapted from Recommendations of the International Ketogenic Diet Study Group, E. H. Kossoff et al.)

team trained and experienced in its use. This team must include, at a minimum, an epilepsy physician and a dietitian with knowledge of the intricacies of administering the diet. The physician should be experienced in working with the diet, monitoring its side effects, and manipulating the diet in collaboration with a dietitian. The keto team must be in place before beginning the program. A list of epilepsy centers that have KD programs or registered dietitians (RDs) and physicians experienced in administering the diet, can be found on The Charlie Foundation's website (http://charliefoundation.org/resources-tools/resources-2/find-hospitals). If you are going to an epilepsy center that does not have a KD program in place, but your physician is experienced and open to monitoring the diet, the Charlie Foundation also has a list of experienced Ketogenic Specialists that can assist your center and epileptologist.

The KD can be started in various ways and the method in which it is initiated varies from center to center. It may be initiated in the hospital or at home, but most major medical centers prefer to initiate the diet in the hospital. Before initiation, the neurologist should assess and examine the patient to make sure the diet is an appropriate therapy. The family should be seen by the RD for counseling, training, and nutrition assessment. In most cases, the diet is gradually introduced over 3 days to allow the body and patient to acclimate. Other centers may begin the diet on an outpatient basis, however, hospitalization allows for careful observation of the child to see how they respond to the metabolic change, a very controlled application of the diet, and a thorough education of the family. Once initiated on the diet, ketone levels should be checked daily via urine ketone testing strips. The urine ketone strips determine if the individual is in a state of ketosis. There is no "magic" ketone number that provides seizure control; however, testing ketone levels allows the RD and the team to determine whether the diet is properly calculated and being correctly followed by the patient. Follow up is required with the physician and RD at 1 month, and then 3 month intervals. Blood work is required at 1 month after starting the diet and every 3 to 6 months thereafter to assess for and correct any abnormalities by modifying the diet or introducing supplements. Frequent follow up with the RD and the KD team is required during diet maintenance, which improves effectiveness and safety.

Family education is very important. The keto education program should include extensive information about the diet, how to calculate and prepare meals, how to monitor the child, how to respond when the child is ill, and how to observe the child for side effects. In preparation for placing your child on the diet, the RD reviews their dietary history, allergies, food preferences, and nutritional status. The RD then calculates and prescribes the appropriate number of calories (usually in the range of 75 percent to 85 percent of the recommended daily allowance), the best meal plan (i.e., 3 meals and 1 snack depending on eating habits), and the appropriate ratio ·(depending on age, nutrient requirements, and eating habits). Once these calculations are complete, the dietitian then creates several meal plans and menus to provide this formulation. With creativity, and the help of good computer programs that can readily calculate meals, appetizing meal plans can be created.

As an example, let's consider that a 15-kg child might require 68 calories (kcal), per kilogram (kg) of body weight, per day. This would amount to a diet of 1,000 calories per day. If this child were placed on a 1,000-calorie diet at a 4:1 ratio, they would require 1,000 ÷ 40, or 25 dietary units. Remember that a dietary unit on a 4:1 ratio has 40 calories in it. The child would need a meal plan that included 25 × 4 = 100 grams of fat. Each day, 900 calories would come from fats, because each gram of fat has 9 calories. The other 100 calories would be from proteins and carbohydrates. The child should eat about 1 gram of protein per kilogram of body weight each day to stay healthy and provide for reasonable growth, so 15 grams of this diet should be consumed as protein. The other 10 grams are then allotted to carbohydrates. That's not much starch or sugar!

Monitoring and Maintaining the Diet

Once the diet has been initiated, you need to maintain contact with the team via phone and email. A good idea is to keep a seizure calendar, a food log, and a ketone log to monitor the impact of the diet on seizure frequency. Children return to their clinic for follow-up on a routine basis, usually at 1, 3, 6, and 12 months. Very young babies, or children who are medically very fragile, are often seen more frequently. During these visits, the team verifies that your child is healthy, reviews the seizure situation, discusses issues related to the diet, and provides appropriate support and changes to the diet as needed. The team also reviews blood work, dietary habits, and any side effects, and then implements the necessary remedies. At these visits, the team also determines whether medications can be discontinued, since it's known that the majority of children on the diet can be weaned successfully from some, and perhaps all, of their anticonvulsant medications. If the diet is successful, it will be continued for a period of 2–3 years, and then weaned slowly. The diet, especially at lower ratios of 1:1 or 2:1, can be continued for longer than the recommended 2 to 3 years with close medical and nutrition monitoring. There is no telling whether seizure control will be maintained once the child is weaned, which is why the diet is weaned slowly. However, experience has shown that most children will continue to maintain the seizure control they achieved on the KD once weaned from the diet.

Side Effects and Challenges

Like most medical therapies, the diet is not without side effects. Families are taught about the various medical issues that can arise while on the diet. During the initiation phase of the diet, common side effects include hypoglycemia (low blood sugar) and acidosis (blood becoming more acidic). The maintenance phase of the diet presents different challenges and side effects. These include constipation, kidney stones, elevated lipid levels, and slowed growth. Most of these side effects can be managed with dietary and lifestyle modification.

Initiation Side Effects: Hypoglycemia and Acidosis

Since the KD is carbohydrate restricted, blood sugar is expected to drop to lower than normal levels (50–70mg/dL, while normal levels are 70–90mg/dL). However, blood sugar can drop very low (<50mg/dL) during the first few days of the diet due to the rapid and drastic reduction in carbohydrates. Generally, patients are not symptomatic and hypoglycemia resolves once the body acclimates to the new metabolism. If hypoglycemia persists past the initiation phase, the RD can re-calculate the diet to contain either more calories or more carbohydrates to manage the hypoglycemia.

Acidosis is more common in children taking certain antiepileptic drugs (AEDs) and can persist throughout the maintenance stages of the diet, but it is most common during initiation and times of illness. Acidosis can only be diagnosed through a blood test. The state of ketosis can create an acidic environment in the blood, and bicarbonate, carbon dioxide, and pH levels are expected to drop. However, if a patient is symptomatic and levels are dropping too quickly, they can be treated with extra fluids and a bicarbonate solution. If a patient is taking an AED that commonly causes acidosis in conjunction with the diet, the RD and doctors will usually prescribe a buffering agent to prevent acidosis. Citrates, baking soda, phosphate, and potassium supplements are common buffering agents.

Usually, acidosis and hypoglycemia are limited to the initiation phase and often self-resolve without intervention as the body adapts to the new diet and metabolic change. If the diet is initiated in a hospital setting, the ketogenic team is able to monitor and treat both hypoglycemia and acidosis.

Maintenance Phase: Constipation, Lipid Levels, Kidney Stones, and Growth

Given the limited carbohydrate options, constipation is the most common side effect of the diet. To prevent constipation, consuming enough high-fiber foods, activity as tolerated, and encouraging liquid intake is key. If constipation persists, meals can be re-calculated by the RD to include more fiber, more fluids, and some oils that help promote regular bowel movements. If modifying the diet doesn't do the trick, several over-the-counter products such as stool softeners, suppositories, and enemas that are "keto-friendly" can be used to help alleviate problems.

The risk of kidney stones is increased while on the diet, but it is very uncommon (1 in 20 children) unless there is a documented family history or if the child is on a carbonic anhydrase inhibitor, such as zonisamide (Zonegran), topiramate (Topamax), or acetazolamide (Diamox), which increase the risk. Encouraging fluids and correcting acidosis by using a buffering agent can usually prevent kidney stones altogether. If a family history of kidney stones exists, tell your KD team and steps will be taken to reduce the risk of developing stones.

Increasing cholesterol and lipid levels are a highly discussed concern among those starting the diet. Unfortunately, increased cholesterol and lipid levels are a reality in some patients on the diet. Although in a recent study at Johns Hopkins, only ~30 percent of children had cholesterol and triglyceride levels that exceeded recommendations for healthy children. In addition, these elevated levels are usually temporary and, in many cases, levels return to normal once a patient is taken off of the diet, despite the length of time they were maintained on the KD. Persistent and extremely high levels of cholesterol and triglycerides often have a genetic tendency (familial hyperlipidemia) aggravated by the diet. In these cases, the diet can be modified to include heart-healthy fats and other components to help reduce triglycerides and cholesterol levels. If these methods don't work, the fat content of the diet can be reduced to help lower levels. It is very rare that a child has to discontinue the diet due to elevated lipids and cholesterol.

Growth and weight gain are monitored closely by the ketogenic team. The dietitian will monitor your child's growth trajectory on a growth chart to make sure they continue to follow the same growth curve they were before starting the diet. Normal growth is expected as long as calorie goals are being achieved, but in some cases, linear (height) growth may slow on the KD. Studies and experience show that children often "catch up" and achieve normal height and weight once the diet is discontinued. If growth does falter, calories and protein can be increased to encourage weight gain and growth while still trying to maintain the same level of seizure control.

The diet's restrictions on carbohydrate intake can cause nutritional imbalances in the diet. The KD is not nutritionally complete; therefore, your dietitian will design a supplement regimen to meet all your child's nutrition needs. Most children can meet all of their micronutrient needs with a varied diet and a low carbohydrate multivitamin and calcium-vitamin D supplement.

Challenges

The diet is a commitment and a life-altering undertaking. Although food can be made to resemble old favorites and there are solutions to holidays and birthdays, the diet is a significant lifestyle change. The patient and family must be fully committed to successfully implementing and maintaining the diet for it to be a successful and manageable treatment. All meals and snacks are carefully calculated and must be weighed on a gram scale in exact portion sizes. The portions are smaller than typical meals because of their caloric density (fat has more calories per gram than carbohydrate or protein). Preparing and planning meals is usually the biggest burden and falls on the caregiver (or the person prepping meals). Most recipes use "homemade" products and whole foods, almost completely avoiding convenience and store bought products. This makes prep work and meal assembly time consuming. Families often prepare multiple meals at a time to help reduce the burden. Many ketogenic meals can be prepared ahead of time and either frozen or safely stored. Your dietitian can provide guidelines on how to safely prepare and store meals ahead of time.

Social events are often challenging for those on the diet. Food is a key component to almost every social outing or event, and planning for these events while on the diet is vital to the diet's success. Ketogenic food is rarely available at weddings, birthday parties, school trips, and so forth so it is important for patients on the diet to plan ahead and make sure to bring their ketogenic meals with them. Maintaining the diet while on vacation can also be challenging, however, many hotels, theme parks, and resorts are more than willing to help patients maintain their diet by providing the appropriate foods. In addition, some patients just decide to bring food with them to avoid sourcing it while on vacation. Be sure to speak with the resort's kitchen prior to leaving, so they can accommodate the diet to the best of their ability. Your RD can provide you with documentation supporting your need for the diet for both airline travel and hotel accommodation.

Variations of the Ketogenic Diet

The classic KD has always been open to modification. This was true even during the first decade of its use, when Peterman, also at the Mayo Clinic, made the first changes to the original plan. Because no one is sure exactly why the KD works, it is reasonable to assume that thoughtful clinicians will continue to make changes, tweaking one element or another to make it more successful, more palatable, or easier to use.

The MCT Ketogenic Diet

One of the first major changes to the original KD was the substitution of MCTs (medium chain triglycerides) for the traditional long- and short-chained fats (such as butter, oil, and cream). MCT fats are absorbed more efficiently than long- and short-chain fats and are carried directly into the liver for metabolism. This metabolic difference makes MCTs highly ketogenic, producing more ketones per gram than long-chain fats. Thus, less fat is needed if MCT is used instead of long-chain fats to produce the same level of ketosis. The classic 4:1 KD provides 90 percent of its calories from fat, but due to its ketogenic potential, the MCT diet can produce a similar ketosis with only 70 percent to 75percent of energy from fat, allowing more carbohydrate and protein. The MCT is usually given in a liquid oil form and is calculated into the diet like any other fat. Like other diets, the diet prescription is individualized and the amount of MCT oil is calculated by the RD. Studies show similar efficacy in seizure control when using the MCT diet compared to the classic KD, but the MCTs are not always well tolerated and often cause bloating, diarrhea, and cramping.

The Modified Atkins Diet

The most significant and widely used modification to the classic KD is the Modified Atkins Diet/Modified Ketogenic Diet (MAD). The diet was pioneered at Johns Hopkins Hospital to create a more palatable and sustainable version of the KD. The MAD can be initiated without fasting or a hospital admission.

On the MAD, carbohydrates (carbs) are strictly limited to 10 g for children and 20 g for adults, while fat and proteins are not limited. This is a very low carbohydrate diet and the MAD meals resemble KD meals (as a reference point, a one-ounce slice of bread has 15 grams of carbohydrate). Therefore, bread, grains, cereals, sweets, baked goods, and other carbohydrate-rich items are excluded on the MAD. Most carbohydrates come from dairy, vegetables, fruits, and nuts. The nutrient breakdown of the MAD resembles a 1:1 or 2:1 KD, and is roughly 60 percent to 80 percent fat. The MAD is similar to the KD in that it is low in carbohydrate and high in fat, however, food is not precisely weighed and measured on a gram scale, which allows for more flexibility. Although no head-to-head studies compared the MAD and classic KD, data suggests that the MAD and KD yield similar results. In the eight published studies on the MAD, 45 percent of patients had a 50 percent to 90 percent seizure reduction and 28 percent had a >90 percent seizure reduction. Unlike the classic KD, which is primarily administered to children, the MAD is used often in adult and pediatric patients.

The Low Glycemic Index Treatment

The last popular modification is based on the premise that blood sugar may play a role in the KD's success. The Low Glycemic Index Treatment (LGIT) was developed at the Massachusetts General Hospital as a liberalized alternative to the KD. The LGIT is lower in fat and higher in carbohydrates than both the MAD and the classic KD, and it resembles roughly a 1:1 ratio (60 percent fat). The LGIT regulates both the quantity and *type* of carbohydrates. Typically 40–60 grams per day of carbohydrate are recommended. Only low glycemic carbohydrates (glycemic index of <50 relative to glucose) are consumed. The LGIT is based on a food's *glycemic index*, which refers to a food's effect on blood sugar as compared to a reference food. Many variables, such as fiber levels, fat content, protein content, and acidity affect a food's glycemic index. The lower the glycemic index, the less effect the food has on raising blood sugar. Further, low glycemic foods cause more gradual elevations in blood sugar as compared to high glycemic foods. Foods with higher fat, protein, acidity, and fiber content usually have low glycemic indexes.

No head-to-head comparisons for the LGIT versus the KD or MAD exist. However, recent studies demonstrate that the LGIT yields results similar to those of KD and MAD. More than half of the patients on LGIT achieve >50 percent seizure reduction.

Modified Diets Summary

The modified diets, although more flexible, require all of the same medical and nutritional monitoring and oversight as the classic KD. All are generally initiated in the outpatient setting with close follow up and supervision by the keto team, which is attractive to patients as it can be started right away. Implementation and monitoring of the modified diets can differ slightly across the healthcare setting. Generally, an outpatient assessment with the KD team covers carbohydrate counting, label reading, recipe making, meal planning, and troubleshooting. The assessment should include instructions for implementing the diet, as well as how to properly calculate the diet, recipes, exchange systems, sample meal plans, and instructions for follow up and monitoring. Recommendations on nutrient intakes for the whole day will be calculated and the patient will be provided with protein, fat, and carbohydrate intake recommendations. The RD will provide counseling to families on how to achieve these goals at each meal. Follow up is encouraged frequently to help individuals adjust the diets to achieve optimal seizure control and maintain nutrition status.

The same follow up and blood work is recommended as the classic KD. Like the classic KD, the modified diets are not a nutritionally complete diet, and the same vitamin and mineral supplementation are used as with the KD. Side effects on the modified diets are similar, but less common, given the flexibility of the modified diets. Patients on the modified diets will be monitored (and treated if needed) for all of the side effects that can occur on the classic KD.

The Future of the Ketogenic Diets

The medical community has become increasingly interested in implementing the KD for seizure control, and in finding better ways to do it. In the last decade, many centers in the United States and around the world have developed ways to make the keto diet available to their patients, but many patients still have no access to it. Wider availability and easier methods will be important, as will the studies that demonstrate which patients are most likely to be helped. It will be important to know when the diet should be used earlier, rather than later, in treatment. Scientists must continue to explore how the diet works. It's important that the elements of the diet that make it effective are identified and used.

The KDs are the only scientifically proven nutrition therapies for epilepsy. While the classic KD is considered the original gold standard, the alternative diets are being used successfully around the world. These diets offer effective and more liberal approaches to dietary treatment of epilepsy. Regardless of which diet you choose, dietary therapy requires commitment from the patient, family, and clinicians. If successful, the diets can improve or fully control seizures, while allowing a reduction and, in some cases, elimination of antiepileptic medications. The diet's implementation requires a team of experienced clinicians, and as with any treatment, your physician should be consulted.

Alternative Therapies:
General Nutrition, Vitamins, and Minerals

General Nutrition

Identifying, preventing, and treating nutritional deficiencies are crucial for optimum health. Although the KDs are the only scientifically proven diets to treat epilepsy, epilepsy patients often ask if other dietary changes, other than the strict KDs, can be beneficial. To date, no evidence suggests that simple alterations in diet, without producing ketosis, are beneficial for controlling seizures. However, proper nutrition and a healthy body weight are essential for health. Proper nutrition can improve other disease states; therefore, epilepsy patients may benefit from a healthy body weight and optimal nutrition.

Many views exist on how to achieve and maintain good nutrition. What diet is the best diet? How do we achieve optimal nutrition? The answer is balance. Balance is best achieved by eating a variety of foods to maximize nutrient intake. There is no consensus among nutritional experts on the "best" diet. Some hold sugar as the main culprit in promoting disease, while others hold fat, meat, and animal-based diets responsible. Some argue calories are key, while others argue specific types of calories are more harmful or beneficial. There is evidence to support most arguments. Regardless, we are facing an obesity epidemic that has given way to a rise in heart disease and other comorbidities. Despite this excess, deficiencies still exist.

Achieving and maintaining a healthy weight improves health outcomes, but a healthy weight does not always assure optimal nutrition. Good nutrition requires micro and macronutrient balance, and consumption of all nutrients in moderation.

Achieving balance can be difficult with all of the conflicting nutrition information available. The American Academy of Nutrition and Dietetics and MyPlate.gov offer the public information on maintaining and achieving good nutrition. The selected dietary messages for consumers based on the 2010 Dietary Guidelines are as follows:

- Balance calories
- Enjoy your food, but eat less
- Avoid oversized portions
- Foods to Increase:
- Make half your plate fruits and vegetables
- Make at least half your grains whole
- Switch to fat-free or low-fat milk
- Foods to Reduce:
- Compare sodium in foods like soup, bread, and frozen meals, and then choose the ones with lower numbers of sodium
- Avoid sugary drinks and drink water instead
  (adapted from Myplate.gov)

In addition, the nutrition recommendations for the general public and those with epilepsy not willing to undertake a therapeutic diet (like the KDs), may benefit from a less restrictive diet lower in carbohydrates and, notably, refined sugars. Most dietitians who counsel patients with epilepsy have noticed that even small changes, such as adopting a natural/whole foods diet that limits simple and refined sugars, have resulted in improvement in seizures. Making these changes by adopting a healthier, lower glycemic lifestyle can be done without medical supervision by anyone willing to improve their diet. A low glycemic diet means choosing carbohydrates with an advantageous (low) glycemic index to improve your body's metabolic response to carbohydrate digestion, which is favorable for weight loss and a variety of other conditions. Foods with a high glycemic index (like refined sugars, breads, and so forth) make your blood sugar increase rapidly because they are easily and quickly digested. Slowly digested carbohydrates, like those in vegetables and whole grains, are changed into glucose much slower, making them low glycemic. The slower digestion and absorption of carbohydrates creates favorable metabolic conditions, such as blood sugar stability and metabolic conditions for combating weight gain. Lowering simple sugar intake and transitioning to a lower glycemic diet is healthy for everyone, not just those with epilepsy. Therefore, this endeavor may be something in which the whole family can participate.

Supplements: Vitamins and Minerals

As previously discussed, consuming a variety of foods is a key component for good nutrition. It is best to try to get the vitamins and minerals the body needs by eating the proper foods. However, when taking certain epilepsy medications, it might be necessary to supplement the diet with specific nutrients. It is important to note that to date, no scientific studies have identified strong evidence for the use of vitamins, minerals, or other compounds in the treatment of epilepsy.

Vitamins

Publications dating back to the 1970s raised concerns of *osteomalacia* or bone weakness caused by the use of anticonvulsant medications. Vitamin D is an antioxidant and key regulator of bone metabolism. AEDs that increase (carbamazepine, phenobarbital, phenytoin, and primidone) or otherwise alter (valproic acid) liver metabolism can increase vitamin D metabolism, which can lead to *osteopenia* (mild reduction in bone mineral density) or *osteoporosis* (modest to severe reduction in bone mineral density associated with increased risk of fracture) in some taking these drugs.

Therefore, combined calcium and vitamin D supplementation might be warranted for those taking these drugs for several years.

Folate supplementation is particularly important for women of child-bearing potential, as maternal folate levels may be depleted by medication. *Folate* is important to protect against birth defects, including neural tube abnormalities. In principle, we recommend that all women of childbearing potential take folic acid irrespective of pregnancy plans or sexual activity. It is often too late to start folic acid by the time they realize they are pregnant.

Certain children have *pyridoxine-responsive seizures* that are improved by treatment with vitamin B_6. Deficiency of B_6 is the primary characteristic, however, these conditions are very rare and are usually diagnosed in the first year of life by genetic testing. Pyridoxine deficiencies require lifelong supplementation to prevent seizures. Vitamin B_6 is an essential vitamin, meaning it cannot be synthesized by the body; it must be obtained from the diet. Several enzymes require B_6 to convert compounds. Deficiency of B_6 could reduce the conversion of these compounds, increasing levels of seizure-provoking compounds. Therefore, *deficiency* of B_6 could result in an increase in seizures. Without a well-defined deficiency state, there is no solid data that B_6 supplementation improves seizure control. In addition, B_6 is often used to help counteract the behavioral side effects of the AED levetiracetam, but controlled studies lack the evidence to support its benefit. Very high-dose daily B_6 supplements can damage sensory nerves causing neuropathies, as well as decrease the efficacy of phenobarbital and phenytoin, so supplementation should always be discussed with your physician.

Minerals

Minerals play a critical role in the nervous system. People with epilepsy rarely need mineral supplementation for seizure control unless there is a known deficiency. AEDs may contribute to mineral deficiencies. The research shows mixed results. One study found that average copper, magnesium, and zinc levels in hair samples were lower in epilepsy patients than controls. However, serum analysis showed no differences in the average magnesium and zinc levels among patients treated with AEDs and those who were not. These are preliminary studies that need to be confirmed before any conclusions or recommendations can be made.

Very low levels of sodium, calcium, and magnesium can alter the electrical activity of brain cells and cause seizures. Deficiency of these minerals is rare without severe malnutrition, except for low sodium (hyponatremia), which can be caused by medications (e.g., diuretics, carbamazepine, oxcarbazepine), excess water intake, kidney disease, or hormonal imbalances.

Magnesium, along with calcium, is known to affect neuronal function. Mild magnesium deficiency can occur in some people with epilepsy and can contribute to increase seizure susceptibility. Pilot, un-blinded studies suggest that magnesium supplements of ~450mg/day can improve seizure control, however, it remains uncertain if magnesium supplements can reduce seizures in everyone with epilepsy or just those with slightly low blood magnesium levels. In situations where magnesium deficiency is possible (e.g., severe GI illness, malnutrition, cancer) and magnesium intake can be low or magnesium losses can be high (such as chronic diarrhea) supplements are recommended.

Other Compounds

Carnitine is a compound synthesized from amino acids, and it is responsible for transporting fatty acids into the cell when fat is metabolized into energy. We obtain most of our carnitine needs from meat and dairy, and the rest is made by the body. In rodent models, carnitine has been shown to have neuro-protective properties, but this has not been replicated in humans. Valproic acid can inhibit carnitine production in the body, lowering carnitine levels. The reduction in available carnitine can make valproic more toxic to the liver. However, the degree of carnitine deficiency resulting from taking valproic acid is generally mild, and there is no evidence that carnitine definitely benefits the average person on valproic acid.

However, carnitine supplementation is relatively benign and many neurologists prescribe carnitine supplements to those on long-term valproic acid therapy. Since liver toxicity is most common in children under age 2 years, and especially in those under age 6 months, most doctors recommend carnitine supplementation in this group.

Melatonin is a hormone normally produced by the pineal gland, which is located in the middle of the brain, and it is secreted to the base of the brain where it likely promotes sleep. Removing the pineal gland in animals may produce seizures. A small number of children with light-sensitive epilepsy have low melatonin levels. Melatonin is marketed as a dietary supplement because it is found in some plants. It is not Food and Drug Administration (FDA)-approved or regulated.

Melatonin has some reported anticonvulsant effects, but it has been shown to both increase and decrease seizure frequency. Most reports suggest that it may be more effective in children. Melatonin may improve sleep quality and, because sleep has such an important effect on seizures, the improvement in sleep quality alone may reduce seizures. Doses in the range of 2 to 5 mg are commonly used, but no scientific evidence supports this use. Concerns exist regarding its adverse effects. These include drowsiness, sleep disruption, nightmares, low sperm count, and abdominal pain. There are also concerns regarding effects on puberty because animals given melatonin have delayed sexual maturation. Melatonin may also cause vasoconstriction, a particular concern for patients with coronary artery disease.

Omega 3 Fatty Acids

Fats have an undeserved bad reputation after decades of blame as the sole cause of heart disease and obesity. Fats do contribute the most calories per gram, however, they also provide essential compounds for bodily functions. The *type* of fat being consumed determines whether fats help or hurt. Unsaturated fats are healthy, while saturated and trans fats are unhealthy.

Two essential and popular unsaturated "healthy fats" are omega 3 and omega 6 fatty acids. The balance of these two fatty acids in the diet is usually more important than the actual consumption. Omega 3s have anti-inflammatory properties, while omega 6s have pro-inflammatory properties. Balancing foods with both of these fatty acids is associated with lower rates of heart disease. Animal studies have shown that omega-3s reduce seizure threshold and improve seizure activity. Unfortunately, the seizure protection from omega 3 supplementation in animals was not reproduced in human trials. In contrast, a 2014 small randomized control trial suggests that omega 3 fatty acids in the form of fish oil may help decrease the frequency of seizures. In the study, taking 3 fish oil capsules (1080mg of omega 3s) was found to significantly reduce seizures. This study is in contrast to previous studies involving high doses of omega-3s that showed no clear benefits in epilepsy. The group taking this dosage of omega 3s decreased their number of seizures by 33 percent compared to the placebo group. This suggests that taking low doses of fish oil may be a safe, beneficial adjunct therapy in those with treatment-resistant epilepsy. Although this is just a single study, it opens the door for longer, more controlled studies to better understand the role of omega 3 fatty acids in seizure protection.

Nutrition supplementation remains an attractive approach that requires more controlled studies to determine its place in epilepsy treatment. Aside from the ketogenic and related diets, no evidence supports dietary supplementation to improve seizure control. In addition, some supplements may be dangerous or interact with medications; therefore, discuss dietary supplements with your physician. If you are seeking a dietary therapy other than the KDs, we recommend following a healthy balanced diet, rich in all nutrients and food sources while making sure to maintain a healthy weight.

Complementary and Alternative Therapies

The role of complementary and alternative medicine (CAM) in today's medical world is becoming increasingly more popular. The therapies included continue to evolve. More people are seeking CAM in addition, or instead of, traditional medical approaches, such as medications, surgery, and dietary therapy. Traditional medical approaches are considered evidence-based practice, as they are supported by science's gold standard: Class I research. However, traditional medical approaches, although successful, may come with unwanted side effects or not completely eliminate seizures. Therefore, CAM can be an attractive option for those who have not been completely satisfied with traditional medical treatments.

Relaxation and Alternative Stress Relievers

People with epilepsy report numerous triggers for their seizures, some of which appear to be highly individualized. Some common seizure triggers include poor sleep hygiene, fevers or illness, flashing lights (photosensitivity), and certain foods. The association between stress and seizures is not clearly documented, yet patients have often reported an increase in seizures when stressed. Stress can manifest in many different ways, including altering sleep patterns, decreasing or increasing appetite, and increasing the risk of infection. Therefore, a person with epilepsy who is stressed may experience a lower *seizure threshold* than another person with epilepsy who is practicing some basic stress-management strategies. Some stress management strategies include exercise, massage, yoga and tranquil exercise practices, craniosacral therapy, and biofeedback.

Biofeedback

Epilepsy can often cause people to feel a loss of control and, therefore, increased anxiety and depression. *Biofeedback* or *neurofeedback* involves the use of some instrument (like an electroencephalogram [EEG] that measures brain rhythms) to provide feedback. This is a technique that involves learning to control bodily functions that are normally not under voluntary control, such as your heart rate. These techniques rarely make a person seizure-free, but they can help reduce stress, which can be a seizure trigger. However, biofeedback can be time-consuming as well as expensive and, therefore, its use should be evaluated on an individual basis. *Neuro-EEG biofeedback*, which works by obtaining an EEG to identify abnormal brain rhythms, has been successfully used in epilepsy patients. These rhythms are then targeted with biofeedback and conditioning to make them more normal and, thereby, reduce seizure activity. The sessions last about one hour 1–3 times a week for 3–12 months. No studies on biofeedback have been control trials, so it should not be considered a primary treatment for epilepsy. However, in 2009 a meta-analysis of multiple studies looking at the effectiveness of neuro-biofeedback showed that 74 percent of patients with medication-resistant epilepsy reported fewer weekly seizures in response to EEG biofeedback. Finding practitioners who are experienced and certified can be challenging, but the Biofeedback Certification Institute of America certifies and oversees practitioner standards. Visiting their website can be helpful in finding a clinician who is experienced in providing this therapy.

Exercise

The benefits of aerobic exercise and weight-bearing techniques are well-established for the health of the general public. However, the benefits of exercise in those with epilepsy are not as well-established and, as a result, are not routinely recommended by practitioners as an adjunct therapy. Many fear that exercise and physical activity can provoke a seizure or cause physical injury – there are several studies where exercise-induced seizures have occurred. Hyperventilation is a known seizure trigger and a common concern among practitioners when recommending exercise. Several small studies examined the effects of exercise in people with epilepsy. Some found that people who regularly exercised had fewer seizures and another study found that when they enrolled epilepsy patients in a 15-week exercise program, they had a significant reduction in seizures compared to their baseline. However, whether the improvement in seizures from exercise is directly related to the exercise itself or the additional physiological benefits gained from exercise is unknown. Better recommendations for exercise need to be established for people with epilepsy. However, exercise can improve mental and physical health, and if your practitioner has cleared your child for exercise, a moderate program can be beneficial. Exercise programs should be individualized based on the risk of seizures and injury. Mild-to-moderate exercise has been shown to rarely induce seizures and this may be the best place to begin an exercise program. For patients with frequent seizures who lose consciousness or motor control, the safest exercise is the one that uses the safest apparatus (a stationary bike compared to a treadmill would be optimal for someone with impaired balance or at risk of losing consciousness). Helmets and exercising in padded or carpeted areas can also be safer for someone with impaired balance. During exercise, it is important for those with epilepsy to make sure they are well rested (not sleep deprived), well hydrated, and properly cooled. They should pay attention to their body and not ignore warning signs such as auras, light-headedness, and extreme fatigue.

Tranquil exercise such as Tai-Chi and yoga are also great relaxation techniques. Yoga has not been formally studied in treating epilepsy, but it has been touted for its stress reduction. Some effects of yoga on the EEG and autonomic nervous system have been reported, but no controlled data exists. Yoga is generally a safe and healthy therapy, but given the lack of hard data, should not be considered a primary treatment for epilepsy, but rather an adjunct therapy that helps reduce stress and improve overall well-being. Usually, with a supervised program, seizures during yoga classes are rare. Controlled breathing should be learned to avoid hyperventilation, which can cause seizures in some people.

If proper precautions are taken, mild-to-moderate exercise (i.e., walking, using a stationary bike, yoga/movement programs) can be a great adjunct therapy for improving overall health, well-being, and mood.

Craniosacral Therapy

Craniosacral therapy usually involves gentle physical manipulation of the spine and skull. It is based on the premise that disruptions and interferences in the normal flow of cerebrospinal fluid commonly cause medical symptoms. Tapping the skull with the fingertips is believed to free these interferences and restore normal flow of fluid. The taps are administered as solid, sharp, but nonpainful blows to the head. The goal is to optimize the flow of cerebrospinal fluid, open nerve passages that may be restricted, and align bones into their healthy positions. However, studies done in the 1970s did not show any proof that cranial bones move or that craniosacral therapy is effective. In addition, there is no real scientific support for the major elements that support the biological plausibility of the therapy and its mechanisms. Craniosacral therapy is widely practiced, despite limited scientific support for its efficacy. However, it does not appear to yield any dangerous complications. There is no evidence that it helps patients with epilepsy and thus, it can't be recommended.

Self-Care

Self-care strategies that can help with stress management include support groups, counseling, good sleep-hygiene, and recreational activities. When evaluating an appropriate stress-management program, it is important to look at your needs as they relate to the stress in your life. If you are feeling isolated by your seizures and this is causing you to feel depressed, support groups or counseling might be an appropriate stress-management strategy. A person who is feeling isolated might also enjoy joining a bowling league or an art class to meet other people and integrate into the community. Having a psychological evaluation and treatment can help people get to the root of anxiety and depression, which may improve their *quality of life*, as well as seizure control for an individual with epilepsy.

People with seizures report a decreased quality of life when compared with their peers. Actively employing stress-management strategies may help improve quality of life and seizure control. Remember, the key to managing stress is individualizing a program and following through with that self-care plan.

Herbs

Many herbs have been used to treat epilepsy. However, guidelines for these recommendations, studies to support their use, and which herbs are most commonly used to treat seizures are extremely difficult to find. The herbs detailed in the following paragraphs have been described as effective, or possibly effective, for the treatment of seizures. Despite the lack of evidence supporting herbal therapies, nearly 20 percent of all patients who take prescription drugs also take herbal supplements. While some herbals are considered safe, others are considered dangerous for those with epilepsy and can actually cause seizures. In addition, some herbals can interact with AEDs, rendering them less effective, which can also cause seizures

The most popular selling herbs in the United States are ginkgo, St. John's Wort, ginseng, garlic, echinacea, saw palmetto, kava, pycnogenol, cranberry, valerian root, evening primrose, bilberry, and milk thistle. Herbs used specifically for epilepsy are listed in Table 5.2.

TABLE 5.2 Herbs for Epilepsy

Valerian root	Chrysanthemum	European peony
Black cohosh	Burning bush	Ginger
Hyssop	Yew	Forskolin
Geranium	Scullcap	Calotropis
Passion flower	Kava	Lily-of-the-valley
Mugwort	Kelp	European mistletoe
Betony	Carline thistle	Tree of heaven
Flaxseed oil	Lady's slipper	

Valerian Root

Valerian (*Valeriana officinalis*) is an herb native to Europe and Asia, which has been known as a sedative for thousands of years. It was probably named after the Roman emperor Valerian, who reigned from 253 to 260 AD. It is an extremely popular herb in Western Europe, particularly in Germany and Russia. Research has shown it to improve the quality of sleep, and it is used for nervousness and insomnia. Although valerian is the most common herb prescribed for epilepsy, no significant animal or human proof of its usefulness exists for this disorder. Importantly, sudden discontinuation of valerian after chronic use can cause withdrawal symptoms such as confusion, similar to withdrawal from benzodiazepines or alcohol.

Kava

Kava (*Piper methysticum*) is widely used as a calming and sedative herb. Other names for kava include *ava, awa, kava-kava, kawa, kew sakau, tonga,* and *yagona.*

Kava seems to have a positive effect on anxiety. Kava also appears to help with pain, muscle relaxation, and seizures, although these effects have not been scientifically proven in humans. Claims are made for the treatment of many conditions using kava, including asthma, depression, lack of sleep, muscle spasms, and pain. Kava should be avoided by pregnant and lactating women, as well as children and patients with kidney disease and blood disorders. This herb should not be used by depressed patients because the danger of suicide may be increased.

Kava can cause side effects such as sleepiness, loss of balance, headaches, dizziness, vision changes, diarrhea, and other problems. During the past several years, liver disease has also been reported.

American Hellebore

American hellebore (*Veratrum viride*) has been used to induce vomiting and for the treatment of headaches, pneumonia, and seizures. American hellebore is also known as *false hellebore, green hellebore, Indian poke*, and *itchweed*. This herb is a native to North America. American hellebore has multiple actions and can generally lower blood pressure, heart rate, and possibly respiratory rate in normal doses. However, this is a highly toxic compound and should be used with extreme caution.

Side effects include numbness of the extremities, paralysis of eye muscles, weakness, and seizures. Other side effects include nausea and vomiting, shortness of breath, increased salivation, and blood pressure problems. The plant is associated with serious potential for birth malformations, and, thus, it should not be used during pregnancy.

Blue Cohosh

Blue cohosh (*Caulophyllum thalictroides*) has been used as an anticonvulsant, and it is also used to increase menstrual flow and induce labor. In the United States, nurse-midwives commonly use it in labor. The active agent, methylcytosine, is similar to, but less potent than, nicotine. Synonyms for blue cohosh are *blue ginseng, caulophyllum, papoose toot, squawroot*, and *yellow ginseng*. The herb can cause diarrhea, stomach cramps, and chest pain.

Mistletoe

Mistletoe (*Viscum album; Phoradendron serotinum*) is also known as *all-heal, birdlime, devil's fuge, European mistletoe, golden bough*, and *viscum*. Mistletoe is widely used, despite its known toxic effects. It is used as a remedy for various ailments, however, it is a highly toxic substance. Mistletoe can cause cardiac, brain, and gastrointestinal problems. Although one study in animals showed some protective effect against seizure-causing agents, no clinical studies have been done on its use as an antiepileptic drug. Mistletoe can cause sedation, seizures, heart problems, low blood pressure, and liver damage, among other side effects.

Scullcap

Scullcap (*Scutellaria lateriflora*), also known as *helmet flower* and *hoodwort*, is a North American herb used as a nerve tonic for the treatment of restlessness, poor sleep, spasms, and alcohol addiction. It has been used to treat epilepsy, but no scientific studies and experiments support its use. Scullcap may be used as the dried herb or liquid extract. Side effects may include giddiness, confusion, and twitching. Preparations of scullcap may be contaminated by other herbs, which may cause liver damage. It should be used with great caution during pregnancy and lactation.

Seizure Provoking Herbs and Compounds

Although herbal medicines are used to treat seizures, several herbal medicines may actually worsen or provoke seizures. Many of these compounds are stimulants and, thus, can increase the likelihood of seizures. The following herbs should be avoided or, if taken, you should tell your doctor about them.

Ephedra

Ephedra is a traditional medicine that has been used for many years in Asia and by Native Americans in the Midwest. The main active ingredient in ephedra is *ephedrine*. Ephedrine is a stimulant, and some reports have surfaced of people experiencing seizures after taking ephedra. Ephedra should be avoided by people who have experienced seizures.

Caffeine

Caffeine is one of the most commonly used stimulants. Coffee and tea have caffeine in them, but several other foods, beverages, and herbs also contain caffeine. Cocoa, which is the main ingredient in chocolate, contains caffeine, as does the cola nut, which is used to make soft drinks. Two other popular drinks containing large amounts of caffeine are maté and guarana. *Maté* is a bushy plant whose leaves are used to prepare a sort of tea that is very popular in Argentina, Paraguay, and Brazil. Guarana is made from the seed of a climbing shrub that grows in the Amazon. *Guarana* is popular in soft drinks beverages in South America. Caffeine acts by stimulating the release of neurotransmitters in the brain, thus increasing brain activity and creating a mentally stimulating effect. Several animal studies have shown that caffeine can prolong seizure activity. Caffeine can also prolong seizures in people who are given electroshock treatments for depression. So, it is probably best for people with seizures to avoid, or at least minimize, their use of caffeine-containing products.

Essential Oils

Essential oils are highly concentrated extracts from a variety of plants used for aromatherapy, massage, and other purposes. Essential oils contain many chemicals, and these chemicals can gain entry into the body and the brain through the skin or the lungs.

Several essential oils have been reported to cause seizures, either in patients who never had a seizure before or to make seizures worse in patients with epilepsy. The essential oils of greatest concern are eucalyptus, fennel, hyssop, pennyroyal, rosemary, sage, savin, turpentine, and wormwood. Wormwood is the active ingredient in the alcoholic beverage absinthe, which contains the convulsant chemical thujone. These essential oils should be avoided by people who have seizures.

Ginkgo

Ginkgo (*Ginkgo biloba*) is a popular herbal medicine used to improve memory. It is uncertain how ginkgo improves memory, but it may increase brain *acetylcholine* levels, an important brain chemical that begins to deteriorate as aging occurs. The FDA has received reports of people experiencing seizures after taking ginkgo. However, it is difficult to determine whether ginkgo actually caused these seizures or whether this was due to chance. It may be safer for people diagnosed with epilepsy to avoid taking gingko until more is known about its effects.

Ginseng

Ginseng is a popular drink in Asia, and it has a reputation for treating many different ailments, including memory loss. Although animal research indicates that ginseng may improve memory, very little research has been done to prove or disprove this in humans.

Ginseng activates the stress hormone system. Stress hormones can worsen seizures, so it may best for people with epilepsy to avoid ginseng.

Evening Primrose and Borage

Evening primrose (*Oenothera biennis*) is used as an herbal remedy for premenstrual syndrome, although it is uncertain if it has any benefits. Borage (*Borago officinalis*) has a reputation for treating depression, inflammation, fevers, and coughs, but these effects have never been tested. Some research suggests that these herbs may reduce seizures, while some suggests they may increase them. It may be safest for people with seizures to avoid either.

Summary: Complementary and Alternative Therapies

An estimated nearly 50 percent of patients with chronic diseases use alternative treatments. In the United States, about 20 percent of people tak-

ing prescription medications also take herbal remedies or high-dose vitamins. There is a natural tendency to trust alternative therapies because
they are "natural" and, therefore "safer" than traditional medical therapies.
However, it's important to realize that just because a treatment is "natural,"
does not mean it is "better" or "safer." The benefits—and risks—of any of
these therapies are unknown, because few scientific studies have looked at
their safety and how well these treatments work.

More important than the potential benefits of natural products, these
forms of treatment may carry certain risks. These risks include the possible
direct toxic effects of the preparations and their ingredients. Another risk
is that, since herbs, vitamins, minerals, and supplements are not regulated
by the FDA, toxic impurities, such as herbicides, may be present. Finally,
herbs can interfere with the way other medicines, including anticonvulsant drugs, work. Your doctor must be aware of any herbs, supplements, or
other alternative treatments that you are taking to prevent dangerous interactions between your antiepileptic (or other prescription) medications and
the alternative treatment. Many doctors believe that alternative therapies
are acceptable as long as the patient also continue taking traditional therapies, and the intended alternative and traditional therapies do not conflict.
The problem is that we know very little about some of these unproven therapies and, thus, the risk might outweigh the benefits.

FREQUENTLY ASKED QUESTIONS

Q   **How soon will I know if the ketogenic diet is going to work?**

It seems to vary a great deal. There are some children for whom it is clear
that the diet will work almost immediately. Seizures seem to evaporate as
they are fasted, and they virtually disappear before the children are discharged from the hospital. This certainly doesn't happen as often as we
would want, and parents shouldn't be disappointed if they see other children initially doing better than their child. Parents are encouraged to work

with the diet for about 3 months before they abandon it. Rarely, children improve even more gradually, and the full effect of the diet isn't seen for as long as 6 months. Generally, encouraging signs along the way enables families and children to persist. These include changes such as shorter seizures or the child having more energy and being more alert. During that time, many adjustments can be made that make all the difference: Calories are increased or decreased, depending on the nutritional needs of the child. The ratio can be changed to try to induce better ketosis or better control may even involve decreasing anticonvulsant medications. A variety of strategies may maximize the effect of the diet, which is why it is important to work closely with experienced dieticians and physicians.

Q **If my child starts the keto diet, can his anticonvulsants be discontinued right away?**

Many families choose the KD because they see it as a more natural way to control seizures. They are frightened about the side effects of medications and, in many instances, they believe that these side effects are badly affecting their child's behavior or learning ability. These parents believe that, if only the medications were stopped, their children would function more normally. However, the KD is certainly not a "natural" way of eating, and side effects certainly are associated with its use. Generally, it is not wise to stop anticonvulsants as soon as the diet is initiated. Some medications, like phenobarbital, probably should be reduced. Others, like topiramate and zonisamide, are associated with an increased risk of kidney stones and, although no evidence suggests that children on these medications and the KD have an even higher risk of stones, these medications are routinely tapered first. Studies have shown that children can be tapered off (or weaned) from some of their medication even during the first month of the diet, but parents are typically encouraged to keep medications steady until the diet has been stabilized. This means that most medications aren't tapered until the child has been on the diet for at least 1 to 3 months. There are many advantages to weaning a child off anticonvulsants that have not been successful, including ending or avoiding unpleasant side effects, and saving money. You should develop a plan with your treatment team that is committed to trying to eliminate medications that are not clearly helpful to your child.

Q **Is my child really getting enough to eat on the keto diet? She seems to be hungry, but she doesn't always finish the meals that I make for her.**

Many issues are involved in this question. Children won't voluntarily starve themselves. If your child is not eating, first make certain that you've worked with your child's dietician to find meal plans that are satisfying and appropriate for your child. If the meal plans are appropriate, but behavioral issues continue, such as fights over mealtime, then you might also need the help of a behavioral therapist. Sometimes, just substituting another family member to supervise mealtime helps by removing the upsetting interactions between parent and child.

If you child seems genuinely hungry all the time, her dietician can sometimes add more bulk to the meal, so that your child will feel fuller. This also involves making sure your child is consuming all the liquids needed as well.

The most important issue in this question, however, is whether your child is getting adequate nutrition. This is best answered by knowing whether your child is healthy and has enough energy to participate in all their various activities. If your child is not getting ill, is growing at a slowed but steady pace, and can do the things expected of her in school and at play, then she is likely getting enough to eat. (It may not look like enough to eat on a big plate, but it may look much better on a special, smaller plate reserved only for the child on the diet.)

Parents must maintain a positive attitude that the nutrition they are providing is really right for the child. Too many children are overfed. Love doesn't depend on the size of a meal.

Q Does stress cause children to have seizures?

We are often asked this question by parents, perhaps for a variety of different reasons. It may be that some parents harbor feelings of guilt or concern that something they did brought on seizures. In other circumstances, it may be that parents are concerned that they are "pushing the child too hard," either in school or with regard to other expectations. Finally, other family strife may also be present.

All these concerns are important to address. It is not possible, to the best of our knowledge, to directly cause seizures in the vast majority of cases. There are very rare seizures that occur in response to specific environmental stimuli (*reflex seizures*) but, by and large, parents cannot cause seizures by their actions.

A natural reaction on behalf of most parents is to become overprotective and somewhat overindulgent once their child has shown a vulnerability to seizures. In this regard, it is helpful to keep in mind that children with epilepsy should be treated similarly to any other child, to the greatest extent possible. Appropriate discipline is actually helpful in providing the child with easily understood guidelines of acceptable behavior. Children like to know their limits and are reassured by understanding the rules. Overindulgence, for fear of creating a stressful situation, becomes counterproductive in the long run. If this overindulgence leads to bad behavior, your child may have problems socializing with others or doing well in school. In the long run, these issues end up producing more stress for the child.

Family problems, like unhappy marriages or other dysfunctional relationships, are important to recognize. Although these are obviously not the direct cause of seizures, they may contribute to misunderstanding and often seem to create the very opposite of a therapeutic environment. Family counseling may be appropriate and beneficial in these cases.

School-related problems can cause substantial stress, both for the child and their family. Fortunately, many resources can be brought to bear on the situation. A useful tip is to schedule time with the child's educators to express concern and to learn more about the school's assessment. If significant concerns are present, a formal evaluation can be called for, including *neuropsychological testing*. Sometimes, all that is required are some adaptations. In other circumstances, more resources are needed, even a change in the school setting. *Individualized education plans* (IEPs) summarize the results of the evaluation and make specific recommendations. These evaluations are commonly repeated every 3 years, but they can be updated more frequently if the need arises. Educators benefit from detailed medical information that is specific to the child. An up-to-date medical summary is very helpful information to have at the IEP. An alignment between the abilities of the child and their scholastic expectations can lead to reduction in stress and improvement in the child's self-esteem.

Q   **What vitamins or other supplements should I take if I am taking antiepileptic drugs?**

Talk to your doctor. In general, a multivitamin is appropriate. Folate is particularly important for women of childbearing age. Vitamin D and calcium may also be indicated, particularly in those at risk for bone problems.

As a special note of caution, herbal supplements may have potent effects, particularly on drug metabolism. It is important to inform your doctor and pharmacist of concurrent supplements, so they can check for possible drug-on-drug interactions.

CHAPTER 6

Surgical Treatment of Epilepsy

■ Brain surgery is safe and effective in selected patients with intractable epilepsy.

■ Surgery should be considered by anyone whose seizures are not completely controlled by antiepileptic medication.

■ Epilepsy is, in some people, a serious and potentially life-threatening illness.

■ When undergoing tests before surgery, the ideal result is to identify a single, abnormal part of the brain that produces the seizures and can be safely removed.

■ After all the tests are completed before surgery, the neurologist will review the results with you, and then have you meet with a neurosurgeon.

■ Seizure outcome after brain surgery depends on the specific epilepsy syndrome, the type of pathology causing the epilepsy, the surgical procedure used, and other factors.

■ For some patients who are not optimal brain surgery candidates, neuromodulatory devices can be implanted, but they are unlikely to render a patient seizure-free or cure a patient.

Epilepsy surgery is not new or experimental. In fact, the first few operations were performed by pioneering surgeons beginning in the 1860s. Once neurosurgery became safer, epilepsy surgery really developed after the 1930s. Epilepsy surgery is now performed at hundreds of centers around the world, and many thousands of patients have been operated on with good outcome. In this chapter, we describe the indications, procedures, testing, and outcome related to epilepsy surgery.

Reasons for Epilepsy Surgery

The goals of antiepileptic drug (AED) therapy are both to produce seizure-freedom and also no side-effects. If that is not possible, then AEDs are used to minimize the severity and reduce the frequency of seizures as much as possible, which would enable people with epilepsy to lead as normal a life as possible. The goal of surgical therapy is no different because it aims at the same target.

When should someone consider having surgery as a treatment for epilepsy? Surgery should be considered by anyone whose seizures are not completely controlled by medication—that is, when seizures continue to occur despite properly taking appropriate AEDs. In this circumstance, surgery often offers a relatively safe and effective means of either completely stopping seizures, or at least reducing their severity or lessening their frequency. In practice, surgery is a reasonable option only if stopping or reducing seizures would improve a patient's quality of life or reduce their risk of injury or death from recurring seizures.

Surgery may seem a drastic step for symptoms that rarely occur in some patients, especially when many individuals are able to have happy and fulfilling lives for themselves despite having epilepsy. However, uncontrolled epilepsy can cause many problems, some mild and others quite serious. These problems can appear at any time, often long after epilepsy has begun. These complications may be medical or psychosocial, and are discussed later in this book. Surgery is considered precisely because it is effective in treating some forms of epilepsy, and the risks of surgery are often lower than the long-term risks of uncontrolled seizures.

People come to an epilepsy center for a variety of reasons. Often, they are unhappy either with the seizure control provided by their current treatment or with the unacceptable side effects of their AEDs. Some patients come to get a more precise diagnosis. Whatever the reason, when first arriving at an epilepsy center, you should not be surprised if your physician discusses brain surgery with you. This is because many epilepsy specialists want to inform patients about all their possible treatment options when they begin to care for them. A doctor may describe treatments that are appropriate now, some that may be needed in the future, and others that may ultimately never be recommended.

Many patients coming to an epilepsy specialist for the first time have already thought about surgery. Some mistakenly think that brain surgery will change their personality or paralyze them. The truth is that the risks of brain surgery are very small. As a result, patients are afraid to discuss surgery or become upset if the doctor brings it up. Nevertheless, most people appreciate an honest discussion about surgery.

Who Is a Candidate for Surgery?

 What kinds of seizures and types of epilepsy lead people to consider having surgery?

Seizures that lead people to consider surgery are usually those that cause alterations of awareness because these have the potential to produce injury and disrupt the quality of life. Most commonly, people who have surgery have either *focal seizures with altered awareness* (formerly known as "complex partial seizures"), which may or may not progress to tonic-clonic (formerly called "convulsions" or "grand mal") seizures (see Chapters 1 and 2). These seizures, by virtue of interrupting awareness, have adverse psychosocial and medical repercussions. Loss of awareness prevents the legal operation of a motor vehicle, forces people to rely on others for transport, limits independence, reduces employment opportunities, reduces educational choices, and imposes psychological burdens. Simple acts, such as riding a public bus, are burdened in ways that people who have not experienced seizures cannot imagine. In addition, if seizures cause someone to suddenly, and with little warning, fall to the ground (for example, tonic-clonic seizures or *drop attacks*), then serious injury might occur. Lastly, some seizures, although they might not cause falling or loss of awareness, might be so unpleasant or upsetting that surgery could still be an option. For example, a seizure that periodically gives rise to intense nausea and vomiting, or one that leads to socially unacceptable behavior, might warrant consideration of surgical therapy. In general, the individual who suffers from the seizures is the only one who can state with certainty whether the residual symptoms are inadequately controlled and might warrant surgical treatment.

Q   How often should seizures occur to consider surgery?

There is no scientifically determined seizure frequency required to consider surgery. While most people who have surgery have seizures at least once per month, others have had fewer seizures and decided that surgery was worthwhile. After all, having just 1 or 2 seizures per year prevents someone from driving and can have serious medical and psychosocial consequences. Some patients may have only a few seizures per year, but these episodes are severe and serious every time they occur. In our experience, some patients with as few as 2 or 3 seizures per year have had surgery and viewed it as worthwhile. Careful preoperative counseling should always be done, so that patients will have realistic expectations.

The time of day at which seizures occur might also influence the decision to have surgery. Seizures that occur at predictable times pose fewer problems than randomly occurring seizures. For example, a person who has seizures consistently only while asleep (*nocturnal seizures*) may (in some states) drive an automobile and live a relatively unrestricted life. However, it should be noted that these seizures might still be psychologically disturbing to the patient and their family and still pose a risk of injury or *sudden unexpected death in epilepsy* (SUDEP). Unfortunately, most patients have seizures that occur in an unpredictable way.

Lastly, the type of epilepsy influences the decision to consider surgery. A few types of epilepsy are known to disappear with age, so surgery would not be appropriate. Other types of epilepsy get worse over time (for example, *progressive myoclonic epilepsy*), so surgery will not produce a long-term benefit. Other types of epilepsy (for example, *medial temporal lobe epilepsy*) are usually resistant to medical therapy and do not go away. The latter types often respond favorably to surgical treatment, so surgery might therefore be offered in those conditions.

Risks of Epilepsy

In this section, we will review the risks posed by epilepsy. Not every complication occurs in all people. The severity of the problems varies from person to person, and some fortunate individuals may live full lives without difficulty. Scientists do not completely understand why and how many of these complications happen, but the simple fact remains that epilepsy is, for some people, a serious and potentially life-threatening illness. The adverse consequences of epilepsy can occur in people with mild seizures as well as severe seizures, and it is impossible to predict when they might occur.

By and large, complications occur in people who have uncontrolled seizures. People whose epilepsy is completely under control—that is, people who are not having any seizures have little to fear from their condition. However, ongoing seizures (*recurrent seizures*) often pose risk, which depends on the type of seizure and the rate at which they occur. The major determinants are: severity of seizures, how often they occur, whether consciousness is altered, whether seizures cause falling, whether they produce psychologically or physically unpleasant symptoms, and whether they cause socially unacceptable or embarrassing behavior (e.g., disrobing, incontinence).

The medical risks can be placed into one of several broad categories: bodily injury, brain injury, and death.

Seizures can cause direct bodily injury such as lacerations (cuts), bruises, fractures (broken bones), joint dislocations, burns, and internal injury. For example, if a seizure causes a person to fall, they might break a bone or suffer a laceration of the skin. If the seizure happens while driving a motor vehicle or vessel, a more serious injury might occur, not only affecting the driver, but possibly affecting other occupants of the vehicle, as well as pedestrians and/or persons in other vehicles.

Brain injury arises for two reasons. First, seizures may cause brain damage due to the excessive release of certain neurochemicals like glutamate within the brain. In addition, some seizures, especially tonic-clonic seizures lead to lower levels of oxygen in the blood, which can also cause brain injury. Seizures may place stresses on other parts of the body and it is not uncommon to find heart damage in people with epilepsy who have uncontrolled tonic-clonic seizures. Lastly, people with uncontrolled seizures are at greater risk for dying than people whose seizures are controlled. The causes of death vary, but it is known that about half of these deaths are from SUDEP, and the other half are from ordinary causes, including pneumonia, heart disease, and cancer. SUDEP is believed to be caused by either *respiratory arrest* (stopping breathing) or heart rhythm abnormalities that are either provoked by seizures or occur in the aftermath of a seizure. Evidence suggests that the risk of death in people who have successful surgery (with complete seizure control after surgery) becomes lower, reverting to that of the general population.

The psychosocial consequences of uncontrolled epilepsy are many. People are more apt to experience depression, anxiety, and other psychological problems when seizures occur on a frequent basis. This may be due to several factors, including changes in the way the *neurons* (brain cells) communicate with one another, changes in brain chemistry, and behavioral reasons (e.g., losing a job because of a seizure would make anyone unhappy). Socially, people with uncontrolled seizures experience a variety of difficulties because of their seizures. The degree of educational attainment is often lower, and occupational opportunities are more limited. When children have seizures, parents naturally tend to be overprotective, which can limit psychological development and restrict independence. Inability to drive limits independence as well in the modern world, with resulting restrictions on social activities and employment. People with uncontrolled seizures are less likely to marry, and they earn less money than people whose seizures are controlled. Evidence suggests that surgery can reverse some of these detrimental effects if patients become seizure-free. After successful surgery, patients are most likely to socialize and change marital status, earn more money, drive a vehicle, and engage in a wider range of social activities than people who continue to experience uncontrolled seizures.

Pre-surgical Evaluation

Once it is decided that surgery should be considered, patients will undergo outpatient and inpatient testing (see the next sections). This could be quite time-consuming and may spread out over several months. Time must be scheduled away from home or work to complete the testing. Family or friends may also need to take time off to accompany patients to the testing and to provide care at home after testing is complete. Many epilepsy centers expect patients to set aside at least 1 week, and to be ready to take part or all of a second week for monitoring by video and electroencephalogram (EEG) with scalp electrodes; this is known as scalp *video-EEG* (VEEG) monitoring. If VEEG monitoring with scalp electrodes cannot precisely identify the brain focus from which seizures arise, then intracranial VEEG monitoring is done using subdural electrodes surgically placed on the surface of the brain or depth electrodes inserted into certain brain areas (stereo-EEG). If intracranial VEEG monitoring is required, up to 6 weeks off work may be required. Patients must carefully follow the instructions given about how and when to take AEDs before and after V-EEG monitoring.

The purpose of this evaluation is to identify a single, abnormal part of the brain that is the epileptic focus and can be safely removed. For example, physicians might find scar tissue (a structural *lesion*) that is electrically abnormal by EEG testing in a brain area that can be safely removed. Finding a single abnormal region offers the best chance of success if the patient is considering removal of part of their brain to treat seizures (Table 6.1).

TABLE 6.1   Preoperative Evaluation for Epilepsy Surgery

When done?	Always performed	Sometimes performed
Clinical information	History and examination	
Interictal EEG	Routine EEG	Electrocorticography, MEG
Neuroimaging	MRI head	FDG-PET, MRS, SISCOM, PET receptor studies
Ictal EEG	Video-EEG (scalp)	Video-EEG (intracranial)
Cognitive evaluation	Neuropsychology	Intracarotid amobarbital study

History and Physical Examination

Despite all the amazing advances in medical technology, nothing surpasses the importance of the office examination. The history and physical examination are the most important tools that exist, especially the history, which provides critical information. The office evaluation helps establish what kind of seizures are present, assesses the potential causes of the seizure disorder, and help the physician establish a diagnosis and plan of treatment. After taking a history and examination, an experienced physician can usually decide whether surgery is a reasonable idea. The history and physical examination often contain important clues regarding the area of the brain that might be causing seizures. Sometimes, a physician can even form a preliminary opinion as to the potential benefits and risks of surgery.

A doctor may begin taking a patient's history by asking about their birth and development. Any difficulties that occurred with the mother's pregnancy and the patient's delivery may indicate an early insult to the brain or a congenital malformation of brain development that may result in epilepsy. Prematurity, infections while in the womb, brain hemorrhages, strokes, and disordered brain development may all cause epilepsy. These problems may be identified when infants and children do not meet expected milestones, such as walking and talking at appropriate ages, or after seizures appear. Any neurologic symptom, such as memory difficulty, weakness, walking difficulty, visual disturbances, and the like may provide clues to abnormal function in a particular part of the brain. This might indicate which part of the brain is producing seizures.

A detailed history about the seizures you have also provides important clues. The seizure's initial sensations or movements *(auras)* may indicate where in the brain seizures start, but some symptoms are not specific. For example, a seizure beginning with tingling in one hand usually occurs in the opposite parietal lobe. Visual symptoms, such as flashing lights or colors, suggest that seizures originate in the occipital lobe (visual area). In contrast, déjà vu and fear often occur in temporal lobe epilepsy, but can also happen in seizures starting elsewhere, such as in the frontal lobe. The description of the movements that occur during a seizure may also help identify where seizures start. Seizures that cause lip smacking and swallowing often arise in a temporal lobe, while stiffening of one side might indicate the seizure has begun on the opposite side of the brain. One side of the brain controls the other side of the body.

A physician performs a physical examination to search for signs that may help determine the diagnosis. The general examination may sometimes be as important as the neurologic examination. Analysis of vital signs like heart rate and blood pressure, skin examination, and inspection of the head, eyes, chest, and abdomen may reveal evidence of a disorder that can affect multiple organ systems, including the brain. For instance, birthmarks on the skin may be characteristic of a genetic disorder like *tuberous sclerosis* or *neurofibromatosis,* disorders commonly associated with brain abnormalities and seizures. An elevated blood pressure is a risk factor for a stroke, and strokes can cause later epilepsy.

The neurologic examination detects abnormal function of the nervous system. For example, weakness or spasticity of a limb or abnormal tendon reflexes may indicate brain injury. Temporal lobe seizures are usually associated with memory impairment. Any abnormal finding may help the neurologist pinpoint the source of your seizures. However, the examination is usually normal or nonspecific, even when seizures occur frequently, and further testing is required.

Neurologic Testing

Electroencephalogram

The brain produces electrical activity that may be analyzed using an EEG instrument. A routine EEG is typically collected for 30 to 60 minutes by the application of metal electrodes glued onto the scalp with a conducting paste. The electrodes are attached to wires that connect to the input box of the EEG machine. The EEG instrument displays the electrical activity as a series of waveforms on a computer screen. Specially trained neurologists (*electroencephalographers*) read the recorded waveforms and interpret the findings. For patients considering surgery, the EEG is often reviewed and the information analyzed in conjunction with all other tests (see Chapter 2 for details).

Video-EEG Monitoring

To gather more evidence for seizure localization before surgery, most physicians prefer to record and observe seizures. This is typically done in the setting of a specialized *epilepsy monitoring unit* (EMU) in a hospital. EEG and video are recorded continuously for many days to correlate the physical manifestations of the seizure with the brain's electrical activity. Trained nurses or EEG technologists can also perform testing during the seizure. Because seizures may occur relatively infrequently in some people, AED doses are often reduced or stopped to allow seizures to occur. This reduction in dose may lead to seizures being stronger than usual, so close observation is required. An intravenous port is usually placed when AEDs are stopped to allow for the rapid delivery of medication if seizures must be stopped quickly. If people fall to the ground with their seizures, restraints (such as padding, bed rails, or vests) may be used to prevent injury. To conduct VEEG, patients are usually admitted to the hospital for several days or up to a few weeks, depending on how often their seizures occur and how many need to be recorded.

Physicians usually need to study several seizures to fully determine the precise location of seizures origin in the brain. The EEG and video are carefully analyzed to determine which side and lobe of the brain is likely to be responsible for seizures.

Magnetic Resonance Imaging

Nearly all patients being evaluated for epilepsy surgery require *magnetic resonance imaging* (MRI). The MRI supplies detailed anatomic information about the structure of the brain. It is highly sensitive for localizing strokes, tumors, birth defects *(malformations of cortical development)*, scar tissue from traumatic injury, and other abnormalities associated with seizures. In temporal lobe epilepsy, which is the most common type of epilepsy treated with surgery, shrinkage of the inner (medial) part of the temporal lobe *(hippocampus)* can be seen. More sophisticated MRI techniques like *volumetric MRI* (which measures the size of specific regions of the brain) are employed at some epilepsy centers to supplement the basic MRI information. MRI is a safe technique, although it may be uncomfortable for people who suffer from claustrophobia because the MRI machine is a long, hollow cylinder in which the patient lies while his brain is being scanned.

Functional MRI

Functional MRI (fMRI) is useful in some people who are having epilepsy surgery. fMRI measures changes in blood oxygen during the performance of certain tasks, such as reading, speaking, and moving, to identify which areas of the brain are responsible for those functions. By localizing these important functions, fMRI may help guide the surgeon to avoid removing parts of the brain that are necessary for critical functions.

SPECT and PET

Positron emission tomography (PET) and *single photon emission computed tomography* (SPECT) imaging tell us about the function of the brain. Both techniques use radioactive tracers that are injected into a vein. The radiation dose is very low and safe. PET measures brain metabolism when patients are not having seizures, studying how much *glucose* (a form of sugar) is used. Areas of the brain that trigger seizures typically require less energy, so less glucose is seen in that area on the scan. PET scans take approximately 75 minutes. The most common study used in the evaluation of intractable partial epilepsy is the ^{18}F-*deoxyglucose* (FDG)-PET. The disadvantages of PET include the difficulty obtaining *ictal* (during seizures) scans, the cost of the procedure, the short-lived radioactive exposure, and the limited number of scanners available. However, interictal PET is very sensitive in patients with temporal lobe epilepsy and can aid in the decision-making process. The use of a radioactive compound precludes the performance of this study in pregnant women.

SPECT scans measure blood flow and, like PET, may be done between seizures, but they are most accurate when performed during or immediately after seizures. During seizures, blood flow is selectively increased in the area that triggers seizures. The injection of radioactive tracer must take place very early in the seizure in order to reliably localize the brain region responsible. Ictal SPECT studies are more sensitive and specific than are *interictal* (between-seizures) examinations for indicating the site of seizure onset. In selected patients, ictal SPECT is very valuable for the surgical decision-making process. SPECT scans take about an hour. The disadvantage of ictal SPECT is due to the difficulty of injecting during a seizure, meaning that hospitalization, multiple daily seizures, and special personnel are required. If an ictal SPECT scan can be obtained, then many epilepsy centers obtain an interictal SPECT scan, subtract the two images on a computer, and carefully overlay the resulting images onto the patient's own brain MR images to show the area of increased blood flow in the brain lobe(s) involved. This is called, *subtraction ictal-interictal SPECT co-registered to MRI* (SISCOM).

Magnetoencephalography

The same electrical currents that generate EEG output also produce very small magnetic fields. These magnetic fields are measured in a special device called the *magnetoencephalograph* (MEG), which is placed with the patient in a specially designed room that is shielded from external electrical sources. The MEG is used with increasing frequency because it sometimes provides unique information about seizures. It can be easily correlated with the anatomic information provided by the MRI. MEG can also be used to map vital regions of the brain responsible for movement, sensation, vision, and language. All the mapped brain functions are displayed on the MRI and given to the surgeon to help them plan a safe surgical procedure. MEG's are less commonly utilized currently as the units are expensive and difficult to maintain.

Neuropsychological Testing and the Intracarotid Amobarbital Test (Wada Test)

Neuropsychological testing consists of a complex battery of cognitive assessments. These include standardized IQ tests, memory tests (both verbal and nonverbal memory), language tests, learning tasks, mental flexibility tasks, attention tests, and an assessment of emotional and personality traits. This testing can last from 4 to 6 hours. The neuropsychologist will analyze this information to characterize cognitive and emotional function, and, in some cases, to make inferences about a region of the brain that may not be working well. Sometimes this region is also the place where seizures are originating.

Often, the last test done before surgery (especially temporal lobe surgery) is the *intracarotid amobarbital test* (ICAT; Wada test). This test helps identify which side of the brain is responsible for language (speech, comprehension), and assesses the memory capabilities of the temporal lobes. It takes about 2 hours and is done on an outpatient basis in a radiology angiography lab with the patient awake. A catheter is inserted into the femoral artery after local anesthetic is injected in the skin of the groin overlying the artery. The catheter is directed upward into the internal carotid artery in the neck. A short-acting sedative drug, *amobarbital,* is injected to temporarily anesthetize one side of the brain. Then, language and memory can be assessed from the still-functioning, non-anesthetized side of the brain. For example, if the left carotid artery is injected, and you cannot speak, then language is located on the left side of the brain. This is the case in most right-handed, and some left-handed, people. During the period of amobarbital anesthesia (typically lasting several minutes) objects, pictures, or words may be presented to the patient. After the sedative wears off (usually about 6 minutes after injection), a patient is asked to recall what was shown. In this way, doctors are able to assess the patient's memory for each side of the brain. Knowledge of this information helps assess the risks of surgery and may confirm that a suspect temporal lobe functions abnormally. The Wada test is not necessarily required, and different epilepsy centers have different criteria for determining when it is used. The Wada test carries a very small risk of stroke in epilepsy centers that regularly perform it. It is most helpful when planning a left temporal lobectomy in a right-handed individual or if the side controlling language is uncertain and must be known. In some centers, this final language and memory assessment is performed using fMRI instead.

Intracranial Video-EEG

After all the aforementioned studies are performed, the exact origin of seizures may still be uncertain in some patients. In carefully selected individuals, placing EEG electrodes directly on the surface of the brain or within the brain may help pinpoint where seizures start. These electrodes are inserted by a neurosurgeon, with the patient under general anesthesia in

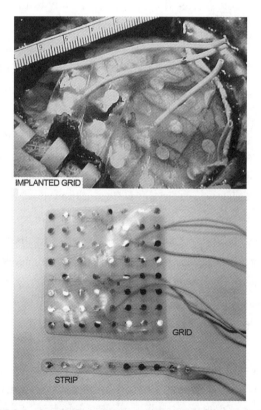

FIGURE 6.1 Surgically implanted subdural electrode grid (top). Picture of new subdural electrode grid and strip (bottom).

the operating room. *Subdural electrodes* are flat plastic strips containing EEG electrodes that are placed on the surface of the brain. Two types of subdural electrodes are used: grids and strips. *Grids* are rectangular plates, varying in size, but usually no bigger than 8 × 8 cm. *Strips* are narrower, about 1 cm wide, and from 4 to 12 cm long (Figure 6.1). *Depth electrodes* are inserted using computer-MRI stereotaxic guidance into sites that are situated deep within the brain to record *stereo-EEG* (SEEG). Subdural and depth electrodes may be placed on one or both sides of the brain, depending upon need. The wires are connected to an EEG instrument after the head is carefully wrapped with a sterile dressing. VEEG monitoring can then be performed in the same way as scalp electrodes. This is a neurosurgical procedure, so it carries the same risks as any brain surgery, including bleeding, infection, stroke, and death. Chances of a permanent serious complication are small, but this possibility means this procedure should be done only when absolutely necessary. Intracranial VEEG recording is needed in a minority of patients, but it is essential in some to determine where to operate. Paradoxically, it is sometimes safer to use intracranial electrodes than to proceed directly to surgery. This is because better definition of the area to be removed might reduce the chances of producing a permanent neurologic complication and improve chances of success.

When electrodes are placed on the brain, they may be stimulated with a small electrical current to *map* brain function. For example, if a small current is applied to an electrode on top of your brain's language area, you will suddenly stop speaking until the current was turned off. If a current were applied to an electrode lying over the motor region of your hand, your hand muscles might contract or twitch. By mapping these areas, the surgeon can then avoid removing them during surgical removal of the epileptic focus.

Intracranial VEEG monitoring can take as little as several days or as long as a few weeks. Depending on individual circumstances, surgery might be performed immediately upon concluding the monitoring, or electrodes might be removed and surgery scheduled several weeks later.

Surgical Procedures

Three types of operations are offered to treat epilepsy. Most commonly, the part of the brain responsible for producing seizures is removed. This is called *resective surgery,* and it includes *focal cortical resection, anterior temporal lobectomy,* and *hemispherectomy.* These surgeries can make patients seizure-free. If seizures come from a single place that cannot be safely removed, then a procedure called *subpial transection* is done, in which small parallel cuts are placed in the brain epileptic focus; this may reduce, but not completely stop, seizures. Last, when multiple areas of the brain cause seizures, a disconnection procedure called *corpus callosotomy* (or anterior corpus callosotomy) might be performed. This is a *palliative* procedure, used to reduce the number of seizures and their severity, although it does not completely eliminate seizures.

Surgical Discussion

After these *preoperative tests* are completed, the neurologist will review all test results with you, and then have you meet with a neurosurgeon. This is the time to be sure to clearly understand the chance of benefit, as well as the risks of a complication or undesired outcome, with surgery. Patients should compare the risks and benefits of surgery against the risk of problems (injury, death, side effects) and likelihood of acceptable seizure control if they continue with nonsurgical treatments. Patients should also review with the surgeon all the medications taken, discuss any problems they have had with anesthesia or previous operations, and tell the surgeon about any other serious medical problems they may have. For example, patients often ask how long it will take to recover and how much personal assistance they will need from others once they get home.

Doctors usually prefer that you bring along the person who will care for you at home after surgery. This allows your caregiver to hear and help you remember the discussion. This person should also ask questions.

After discussing the risks, goals, rationale, and alternatives associated with the surgery, you or your legally authorized representative will be required to sign a form stating that you have been informed about and understand these issues and consent to undergo the surgery. After signing an *informed consent* form, patients must make certain that they follow the preoperative instructions exactly. Some of these instructions may include where and when to report on the day of surgery, when to get certain blood tests, what medications to avoid before surgery (for example, aspirin and ibuprofen), what to do if another illness arises, what to bring to the hospital, or what to leave at home. Usually patients are asked not to eat anything after midnight the day before surgery, although medications can usually be taken with a sip of water on the day of surgery.

Surgical Procedures

Focal Cortical Resection

When a localized (*focal*) area of the brain is found to cause seizures, it may be possible to remove this area and eliminate the seizures, however, this area of brain must be dispensable. In other words, the tissue to be removed should not be one of the critical brain areas (*cortex*) that are required for movement, sensation, language, or vision. Removal of these important areas can lead to permanent impairments. Fortunately, other brain functions such as personality, intelligence, and the senses of taste and hearing are spread over large areas of cortex. As a result, small focal cortical resections are not likely to cause major deficits in those brain functions.

Focal cortical resections often involve brain surface areas that are found, through testing, to contain physically abnormal tissue. Abnormalities can include scar tissue, benign or malignant tumors, blood vessel malformations, congenital brain malformations, and other abnormalities. MRI and other imaging techniques may not find a visible *anatomic abnormality*. In these situations, EEG recordings, PET scans, and fMRI are used to show the area of brain *functional abnormality*. The surgery, often ideally, is planned to remove the entire anatomic lesion, the functionally abnormal cortex, or both. However, the presence of nearby critical brain areas, blood vessels, and numerous other factors may limit the size of the resection that can be safely performed.

Anteromedial Temporal Resection or Anterior Temporal Lobectomy

For patients with epilepsy in whom seizures appear to arise in the deep part (*medial area*) of the temporal lobe, partial removal of the temporal lobe is performed. This is called anteromedial temporal resection (AMTR). In this case, a removal of the front (*anterior*) portion of the temporal lobe is often the first step of the surgery. This part is similar to a focal cortical resection. This may be done in a standard fashion under general anesthesia, or while awake. In this surgery, the surgeon may remove the lobe to a certain distance back from the tip. A direct recording of the electrical activity of the brain cortex (an *electrocorticogram* (ECoG) may also be performed. Some surgeons prefer to perform this step when the patient has been awakened from light general anesthesia, so that many different areas of the exposed brain cortex can be stimulated with low electrical currents. This is done to find areas that might be important for language. In that case, the surgeon will remove the cortex from the tip back as far as they can, without removing language areas. Either way, the next step is for the surgeon to remove the inner (*medial*) area of the lobe that contains deeper brain structures known as the *hippocampus* and part of the *amygdala*. Some surgeons remove these medial tissues as a whole unit, and others remove them piece-by-piece.

Short-term memory is the main brain function supported by the temporal lobe. Indeed, many patients with temporal lobe epilepsy have problems with their verbal or visual-spatial short-term memory before surgery. At a few epilepsy centers, surgeons may prefer to primarily remove the medial structures. This variation of medial temporal lobe surgery is called an *amygdalohippocampectomy,* and is often a more difficult surgery to perform. It may be done on the belief that it might minimize the chance of memory impairment, which can occur with temporal lobe resections. However, many studies suggest that several things predict a low risk of substantial worsening of memory with temporal lobe resections. These include visible abnormal tissue in the hippocampus on MRI, onset of epilepsy as a young child, and surgery on the side of the brain opposite to the one in which language function is mainly located. Specifically, in most right-handed people, language is localized to the left hemisphere of the brain, so that right temporal lobe surgeries seldom significantly worsen language and verbal memory abilities. As a result, AMTR is more commonly performed than amygdalohippocampectomy.

After temporal lobe surgery, some patients will lose a small portion of their upper visual field on the side opposite from surgery. This is usually unnoticeable by the patient. Visual testing may reveal that the patient is not able to see objects well in the upper quadrant of their peripheral vision (pie in the sky) on the side opposite the surgery. This usually does not pose a problem for people who want to drive after surgery.

For about 20 years, doctors around the world looked at a more non-invasive way to remove the medial temporal lobe. Many different centers researched a technique called *stereotaxic radiosurgery (gamma knife surgery)*. In late 2016, it was announced that a research study that compared this technique to conventional AMTR showed that gamma knife surgery was inferior. So, this technique is no longer offered as a replacement for standard temporal lobectomy.

Laser Interstitial Thermal Therapy

Another promising, less invasive technique has been under research over the last several years and now is approved by the Food and Drug Administration (FDA). This is known as *laser interstitial thermal treatment*

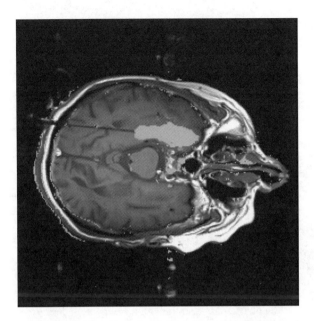

FIGURE 6.2   Laser interstitial thermal therapy.
MRI image showing depth fiberoptic cable in left medial temporal lobe
and the calculated area removed by the laser heating.

(LITT). It involves first placing a fiberoptic cable through a hole in the rear
of the skull deep into the medial temporal lobe using computer navigation.
Then, laser light is passed through the fiberoptic cable, and the hippocampus and amygdala or any other lesion is heated (under MRI observation)
to a point that they are removed (Figure 6.2).

For the procedure, the patient is placed either under conscious sedation or general anesthesia. An incision is made, followed by a twist drill
hole using a small bit. Navigation to plan the laser insertion is performed
using either a special frame or MRI guidance and a plastic bone anchor
secures the device in place (Figure 6.3). The catheter is then introduced
through the bone anchor and passed to the appropriate length to reach
the target under XR guidance. Finally, the laser fiber is placed within the
cooling catheter in the operating room. Laser fibers containing one of two
types of diffusing tips are used.

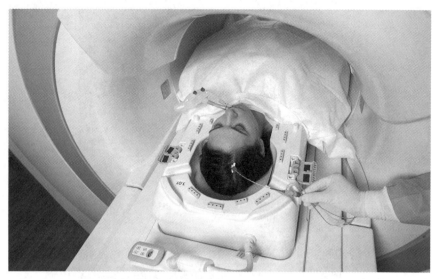

FIGURE 6.3 Patient in the MRI unit with laser catheter placed and anchor to skull. The fibers are placed through the anchoring device.

Then the patient is taken to the MRI for imaging. Once localization of the probe is confirmed, the ablation is performed and observed in real time for the length of time deemed appropriate by the surgeon (1 to 3 minutes). LITT is performed using the laser system with temperature measurements done every 10 seconds. Temperature usually reach 90 degrees C at the lesion center and are programmed to treat the tissue. The software estimates the amount of tissue that is destroyed. If additional treatment is indicated, the fiber is manually retracted several times as needed in the MRI suite and a test dose is repeated to assess the location of the tip using MR thermometry. When the desired volume is fully treated, the implanted device is removed and the incision site is closed with staples.

The long-term effectiveness at seizure control using LITT is not yet determined, but early research shows that it has fewer detrimental effects on verbal memory and language function. As a result, LITT is now increasingly being considered as an alternative to AMTR in patients with very good dominant (usually left) temporal lobe language and memory function in preoperative tests. LITT has also been used to treat small epileptic lesions. The main advantage of LITT is that patients can be discharged home the next day, or even on the same day, making the procedure much more tolerable than open surgery (Figure 6.4).

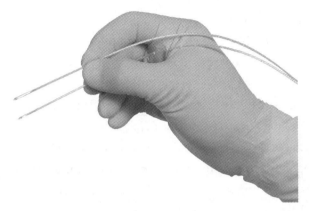

FIGURE 6.4   Example of the laser fibers.

Corpus Callosotomy

The *corpus callosum* is a very large bundle of white matter that connects the right and left hemispheres of the brain. *White matter* is made up of very long, thin, tube-like extensions of brain cells (*axons*) surrounded by an insulating material (*myelin*). When brain cells (*neurons*) make electrical signals, axons move the signals over long distances where they can then interact with a second group of neurons. This is how the brain transmits signals, or communicates, across distances. In generalized epilepsies, long axons connecting the left and right sides of the brain allow epileptic electrical discharges to rapidly spread throughout the brain.

Corpus callosotomy was first performed in 1939 to treat epilepsy. It was based on the observation of a patient whose generalized seizures improved as a tumor involving the corpus callosum grew larger. There was little interest in callosotomy until the 1960s, when a neurosurgeon published findings on the clinical and neuropsychological outcome of the surgery. Since then, many corpus callosotomies have been performed, and the technique has been improved to reduce neurologic problems after surgery. The technique now involves an initial incision in the scalp at the top of the head. The surgeon then separates the two hemispheres of the brain. Looking into the fissure between the two hemispheres, the surgeon can see the corpus callosum. In patients who do not have severe neurologic handicaps, the structure is then cut, beginning at the front end, and often extending 75 percent to 90 percent toward the back end. Usually, the entire callosum is not cut in order to minimize neurologic disconnection syndromes, such as inability to read, left arm and leg clumsiness resembling weakness, and inability to name things felt only with the left hand. In some patients with severe pre-existing disabilities, such as severe mental retardation and inability to read, the entire corpus callosum may be cut.

Corpus callosotomy is often used when other treatments have failed to reduce the number of seizures in patients who have severe generalized epilepsies with neurologic impairments due to a variety of conditions. A callosotomy can reduce, but almost never completely eliminate, seizures that cause sudden loss of muscle strength and falls (*atonic seizures*). It may also reduce the number of generalized tonic-clonic seizures (convulsions) and seizures causing sudden body stiffening (*tonic seizures*).

After callosotomy, patients usually recover overnight in an intensive care unit (ICU). Right after surgery, fever can occur, seizure frequency may increase, temporary left-sided weakness may be present, and patients may temporarily talk less. With newer techniques, leg weakness and bladder incontinence are less common compared to the past.

Multiple Subpial Transection

The most effective surgical treatment for partial seizures is a removal (resection) of part of the brain. As mentioned earlier, this cannot be performed if the seizure focus lies within indispensable cortex. For this reason, the technique of *multiple subpial transections* (MST) was developed. Some of the underlying conditions for which MST has been used are *Landau-*

Kleffner syndrome, *Rasmussen syndrome*, scars, and birth malformations of brain cortex.

The technique was first described in a large group of patients in 1989. Since then, many physicians have reported reduction of seizures with little or no neurologic deficits using MST. The procedure involves placing surgical cuts parallel to each other through the cortex, perpendicular to the long axis of an out-folding (*gyrus*) of the brain. MST can be performed as the sole surgical procedure, or it can be accompanied by focal cortical resection. How MST reduces the number of seizures is not fully known, but it is thought to be related to cross-cutting of nerve fibers that run horizontally across the cortex, thereby limiting the spread of electrical seizure discharges.

Patients who undergo MST must understand that this procedure reduces the number of seizures, but it usually does not completely eliminate them. Some patients can have new or worsened neurologic problems after MST, but these are usually only mild and temporary. These temporary problems are usually related to the area of cortex that undergoes MST. MST is being used less often in the last 15 years because its effectiveness has been thought by some doctors to be less than originally hoped and because of the development of *responsive neurostimulation* (RNS). See the following.

Hemispherectomy

A small percentage of persons have seizures that arise from a large area of only one *hemisphere* (one-half) of the brain. This is usually related to a physical condition in one hemisphere of the brain that is present since the time of birth or early childhood. Examples of brain disorders causing medically refractory seizures are birth malformations of cortical development, strokes occurring before or just after birth, tuberous sclerosis, and Rasmussen syndrome. Patients who are candidates for hemispherectomy typically have significant weakness on the opposite side of the body (*hemiparesis*). Generally, the more severe the hemiparesis, the less likely patients will have significant worsening of the weakness after surgery.

In the past, the offending hemisphere was completely removed surgically. However, this sometimes led to long-term complications in which repeated low-level bleeding developed in the remaining brain structures. Therefore, the surgery performed today is known as a modified, or *functional hemispherectomy*. This involves separating the upper lobes of the hemisphere from the deep (central) core of the brain and from the opposite hemisphere. This upper-separated hemisphere is left in place, connected to its blood vessels, but all the white matter bundles passing up and down on that side, and the corpus callosum, are severed.

Vagus Nerve Stimulation

Vagus nerve stimulation (VNS) is not epilepsy surgery at all. It is a type of neuromodulation using a device. VNS is designed to treat seizures by sending mild pulses of electrical energy to the brain through the vagus nerve. Experimental work showed that long-term stimulation of the vagus nerve in animals and humans can reduce the frequency of seizures. The *vagus nerve* itself is a part of the autonomic nervous system, which controls bodily functions that are not under conscious control, such as heartbeat, breathing, and sweating. Exactly how the VNS helps with seizures is probably through the spread of the electrical stimulus up the left vagus nerve to the brainstem. From there, nerve cells spread the stimulating signals widely through the upper brain (cerebral hemispheres) where they modulate the brain to reduce seizures in some persons.

The VNS device was approved in the United States in 1997, and has been used worldwide in adults and children.

The major indications for VNS are:

1. Patients with intractable seizures who are not candidates for brain surgery.
2. Patients who have failed brain surgery for epilepsy. All potential patients should undergo testing to be absolutely sure that they are good adequate candidates for VNS (see Chapter 2).

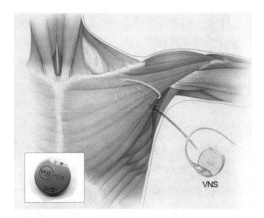

FIGURE 6.5   Example of the VNS device and location of insertion
under the skin on the chest.

The device consist of two parts: a generator (similar to a pacemaker) and a lead with 3 wires. During surgery, two incisions are made—one for the implantation of the generator device under the skin in the upper-left chest, and the second to tunnel the lead under the skin up to the mid-neck area to the left of the voice box—and then the wires are wrapped around the vagus nerve. The process generally is completed in 1 or 2 hours and the brain is not involved during the surgery (Figure 6.5).

Stimulation is produced by a small generator that is flat and round, like a silver dollar, 4cm wide and 10 to 13 millimeters thick, depending on the model used. Newer models may be somewhat smaller or have heart-rate sensing features.

The generator sends impulses from the vagus nerve in the neck to the brain and delivers therapy in two ways. A doctor can program a 24-hour a day, seven-day a week "dose" of intermittent stimulation. One dosage frequently used is 30 seconds of stimulation, followed by a five-minute period of no stimulation. The stimulation is automatically delivered. The second use of the device is when a patient or family member senses a seizure coming on (an aura), they can swipe a magnet over the area in the chest where the generator is implanted, activating extra stimulation to suppress the seizure. In some patients, this may stop a seizure.

The battery for the stimulator lasts approximately 5 to 10 years. Although the surgery is relatively safe, a small number of patients may have vagus nerve injury that can result in voice changes and hoarseness. In addition, some patients may cough or have difficulty talking while the stimulator is on.

The VNS has been shown to reduce seizures by at least half in about 30 percent to 40 percent of patients. Significant seizure reductions are seen in about 20 percent to 25 percent of patients, while very few become seizure free (<5%). This is about the same effectiveness as seen with AEDs. Patients who have tried a number of AEDs and experienced medication side effects, (and those who are not optimal candidates for brain surgery) sometimes are interested in trying a device like the VNS or the RNS (see the following).

Responsive Neural Stimulation

In the United States, responsive neural stimulation (RNS) received FDA approval in 2014. RNS uses a device that delivers a short burst of repeated electrical shocks to the brain area or areas that trigger seizures, in an attempt to shut down the seizure as it is starting. The RNS device uses 2 leads, each of which has 4 electrodes. These can be either 4-electrode subdural strips or 4-electrode depth electrodes that are placed directly on the brain surface or inserted stereotaxically into deep structures like the hippocampus. These 8 electrodes are attached to the device that is in the skull. The device is recessed into the skull, so there is no visible lump under the skin. The device contains 4 things: an EEG amplifier and recorder, a battery, a computer that reads the EEG and is programmed by the neurologist to recognize the patient's own electrical seizure patterns, and a stimulator that "shocks" the epileptic focus when an electrical seizure is recognized. In many cases, the RNS device may recognize and "treat" the beginning of electrical seizure patterns many times during the day, even though the patient may not be having an outward clinical seizure. Effectiveness is moderate: about 40 percent of patients have their seizures reduced by about half, but almost no one becomes seizure-free. This is about the same as with VNS and with new AED trials. Side effects are essentially only related to the risks of the surgical implantation of the device and the electrodes. Patient typically feel no side effects once the RNS is in place (Figure 6.6).

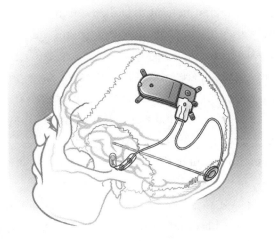

FIGURE 6.6 The RNS device consist of a computer and battery which is implanted on the bone. Electrodes are attached to the device and are implanted in the brain surface or brain tissue. The device is able to detect seizures and applies small currents to the area to stop them.

Stereotactic Radiosurgery

Stereotactic radiosurgery is not really surgery in the traditional sense. The procedure involves administering beams of radiation from outside the skull, at various angles, which are all aimed at the same small target deep in the brain. The objective is to use radiation to destroy epileptic tissue instead of doing an operation to remove it. As previously discussed, this technique is no longer offered as a replacement for standard temporal lobectomy. Nevertheless, gamma knife surgery is used to treat certain tumors and blood vessel malformations that cause epilepsy (see the following).

Postsurgical Recovery

Most operations for epilepsy take 4 to 6 hours. Before entering the operating room, the patient goes to a preanesthesia area to meet the anesthesiologist and see the neurosurgeon. From there, the patient is taken to the operating room, where they are moved onto the operating table. After anesthesia is started, the operation begins. Many surgeons have a nurse call the family midway during the operation to update them on the progress of surgery.

Immediately after leaving the operating room, the patient is taken to the postanesthesia recovery area for a few hours. After recovering from anesthesia, some patients are taken to an ICU for close observation until the next day or longer. After that, patients are transferred to an intermediate care unit or a regular hospital ward with other neurologic and neurosurgical patients, until they are ready to go home.

The length of time spent in the hospital depends a lot on the type of surgery, side effects, age, presence of other medical problems, and any complications from surgery. Pain is the most common symptom that occurs after surgery, but it usually becomes relatively mild within 3 days. Nausea and vomiting may occur within the first 24 hours, and occasionally for a longer time. Sometimes, a seizure occurs after surgery. This can be upsetting, but studies suggest that a postoperative seizure does not necessarily indicate that epilepsy will continue. This may be especially true if it occurs right after surgery. After a typical operation, many patients can be discharged 3 days after surgery.

When epilepsy patients are discharged from the hospital, they usually feel quite tired and complain of head pain. The neurosurgeon instructs patients about activity restrictions, when they should be seen, and what kinds of symptoms and signs need to be reported right away. Some things that should be reported are fever, worsened headache, vomiting, seizures, scalp swelling, and leakage of fluid or blood from the incision.

After returning home, the rate at which patients return to normal activities again depends on type of surgery and individual age, level of general health and fitness, and pain tolerance. After focal cortical resections or anteromedial temporal resections, most patients can walk well within the first week after surgery; require some assistance with feeding, bathing, or dressing for 2 to 3 weeks; can resume part-time work with no lifting after about 4 weeks; and can return to full-time light duty work at 6 weeks after surgery. Many surgeons advise avoiding lifting or exertion for 6 weeks.

Seizure Outcome after Epilepsy Surgery

Surgery can result in complete seizure control or cure, reduction in number of seizures, decreased seizure intensity or duration, or no benefit. Rarely, some patients may experience worsened seizure control after surgery. Seizure outcome depends on the specific epilepsy syndrome, the type of pathology causing the epilepsy, the surgical procedure used, and other factors. (In this section, when an approximate percentage for seizure freedom is given, it applies to those groups of patients treated with that surgery who, for the most part, continue to take at least one medication for seizure control.)

In general, the most effective procedure is a focal resection of small benign tumors. Most reports in the scientific literature estimate a 90-percent chance of seizure freedom 1 year after this particular type of surgery. The procedure with the next highest seizure-free rate is anteromedial temporal resection (AMTR) or anterior temporal lobectomy. When this surgery is done in patients who have an early risk factor (febrile seizure as an infant or toddler) or when a detailed brain MRI scan shows scarring in the hippocampus of the medial temporal lobe, the seizure-free rate 1 year later is approximately 65 percent to 80 percent. Two randomized-controlled research studies comparing AMTR to continued AED-only treatment were done. In 2001, a Canadian study showed a seizure-free rate of 64 percent in patients who had uncontrolled temporal lobe epilepsy for many years. In 2014, an American study called ERSET showed a 2-year seizure-free rate of 85 percent with surgery compared to a 0 percent rate with continued AEDs-only among patients who had seizures uncontrolled with AEDs for up to 2 years. A review of the scientific literature found that only one-quarter of adults and one-third of children have discontinued medication and remain seizure-free 5 years after AMTR. Most patients who are seizure-free choose to remain on at least one drug for many years. This may be because about half of patients who are seizure-free on drugs after surgery will have a seizure recurrence if they stop all medication. When AMTR is performed in patients with no early childhood risk factor, adult age of onset, or completely normal temporal lobes on MRI scan, then the seizure-free rate is roughly 50 percent. Some recent studies have found evidence that the seizure-free rate measured 1 year after surgery declines slightly when again measured at 5- and 10-year time intervals after AMTR. The seizure-free rates cited here refer to current seizure status—that is, the proportion of patients who have been seizure-free for at least 1 or 2 years when last examined. The proportion of patients who never have another seizure after surgery may be as low as 40 percent to 50 percent once 10 years have passed since surgery Some patients may still experience auras, although complex partial seizures have stopped.

After focal cortical resections in frontal, parietal, or occipital lobes in which no physical abnormality is seen on MRI, about 50 percent or less of patients stop having seizures. For resections in these areas when lesions such as birth malformations of the cortex, blood vessel malformations, old strokes, or other scar tissue are present, the seizure-free rate depends on how completely the abnormal tissue can be safely removed and how large or widespread the pathologic tissue area. For brains that have more than one damaged area (for example, with traumatic brain injury or infections), the seizure-free outcome may be much less than 50 percent. Physicians must give patients the best estimate of the likelihood of seizure-freedom, which must be individualized.

With corpus callosotomy, some 70 percent to 80 percent of patients experience a decrease in seizure numbers by at least half their previous rate. Certain types of seizures may be reduced at higher rates, including tonic, atonic (drop attacks), and tonic-clonic seizures. Focal seizures with altered awareness, myoclonic, and atypical absence seizures are often not helped by corpus callosotomy.

As mentioned earlier, MST is considered a treatment to reduce, but not to eliminate seizures. A research study in 2001 that gathered data from many different American epilepsy centers reported that two-thirds of patients had a worthwhile reduction in complex partial seizures. Seizures may return in perhaps 20 percent of cases. Complete seizure freedom is rare. Seizure-free results can be better for Landau-Kleffner syndrome, and many of these children show improved language development. The results for Rasmussen syndrome, however, are poorer because of the progressive nature of the disorder. Seizure-free rates may be as high as 90 percent for hemispherectomy in children with epileptic areas confined to the hemisphere being treated with surgery.

Operative Complications

With any surgery, there is a risk of bleeding or infection. The chances of these are minimized in various ways, and usually there is about a 1 percent to 2 percent risk of each of these complications. Infections are nearly always successfully treated with antibiotics, and most bleeding does not cause significant problems. On occasion, however, bleeding can be life-threatening. When the skull and the coverings of the brain (*meninges*) are opened to allow for the operation, a small chance exists that the cerebrospinal fluid surrounding the brain can leak out and collect under the scalp. This can be treated in a few ways, but sometimes it requires repeat surgery to stop the leak. A small and uncertain percentage of patients experience persistent headaches that occasionally are hard to treat. This can occur in persons with a long history of migraine, or it can occur for the first time. The treatment is the same as it is for other migraine patients.

During surgery, nearby critical brain areas could be damaged either directly if a clot develops in a blood vessel (*ischemic stroke*) or if bleeding occurs (*hemorrhage* or *hematoma*). The chance of these occurrences depends on the type of operation and other factors. If the resection involves the anteromedial temporal lobe, then special complications may occur. These include difficulties with naming and with memory. In most right-handed persons, there may be language problems and problems remembering verbal material after a left-sided AMTR. After a right-sided AMTR, there may be difficulty remembering visuospatial or other nonverbal material, but this is usually only detected with sophisticated neuropsychological testing and is rarely apparent to patients. In left-handed or ambidextrous persons, language can be located in either hemisphere, and right-sided surgery could cause naming or verbal memory difficulty.

Psychiatric disturbances may follow AMTR. Depression is probably the most common psychiatric problem after surgery. It may occur more often in people with a history of depression before surgery, but can also be seen in people with no history of depression. It typically occurs 2 to 6 weeks after surgery, and improves within a few months. In a small number of patients, *anxiety* (nervousness or panic attacks) or *psychosis* (unusual thinking) can occur after surgery. This occurs more commonly in people with a history of these problems before surgery. Although these symptoms usually respond to medication, at times they can be difficult to treat. For all of these psychiatric concerns, medications may be prescribed, and the patient's AEDs may be adjusted.

After surgery that renders patients seizure-free, close relationships and marriages may experience strain. This happens because patients feel better, and they are more energetic and independent. This changes relationships, especially ones in which the patient has been very dependent on the spouse. Often this is temporary, but occasionally it can produce long-lasting problems in the relationship. Conversely, many relationships improve. The improvement in energy level fosters better interactions with the spouse, stronger sexual drive, and less depression over the long run.

Immediately after corpus callosotomy, some patients experience fever or temporary leg weakness. Depending on the amount of corpus callosum that is sectioned and the degree of developmental disability of the patient, there may be some permanent signs of a disconnection syndrome after surgery. This can be seen in various ways, but it can include difficulty following commands to perform tasks using one arm (usually the left), not using that arm as much as the other, unintentionally doing different things with one hand or leg, and difficulty reading.

After MST, neurologic problems occur in about 20 percent of patients. The vast majority of the time, these are temporary and, if permanent, they are mild.

After hemispherectomy, marked weakness and complete loss of vision on the side opposite surgery will result if the patient has good use of the hand, fingers, or foot, or has good vision. However, often, there is moderately good recovery of strength in the leg. This usually means that the patient can walk fairly well after hemispherectomy, although they may not perform fine movements with the toes and foot.

Future Directions

Deep Brain Stimulation

Deep brain stimulation (DBS) was tried in the early 1970s to control epilepsy, and it has been used for almost 20 years to treat Parkinson's disease and essential tremor. It is now being studied for epilepsy again. It involves placing electrodes into the various areas of the brain and delivering intermittent electrical stimulation, whether seizures occur or not. Stimulation may help prevent seizures, perhaps both in partial and in generalized epilepsies. The Stimulation of the Anterior Nucleus of the Thalamus for Epilepsy (SANTE) study in the United States was ruled not to show enough effectiveness to grant FDA approval, but DBS is now approved in the USA and Europe. The target is deep brain structures, such as thalamus.

Conclusion

Epilepsy surgery is a good treatment choice for many people. It is a reasonably safe and effective therapy when medications do not completely control seizures. Surgery is underutilized because of lack of knowledge on the part of patients. It is important to recognize that the consequences of uncontrolled epilepsy can be dire, and that seizures might not be inevitable. Surgery affords properly selected patients a good chance of achieving seizure control, thereby helping them gain independence and improve their quality of life. People should discuss this option with their physicians or with an epilepsy specialist when seizures are not controlled by medication.

FREQUENTLY ASKED QUESTIONS

Q   What types of epilepsy respond best to surgery?

Several types of epilepsy respond well to surgical treatment. Medial temporal lobe epilepsy, in which seizures begin in the deep part of the temporal lobe, called the hippocampus or amygdala, is often successfully treated by surgery. Surgery is also usually successful when seizures come from an obvious lesion that is seen in the MRI, provided the EEG also shows an epileptic abnormality in the same area. Lastly, drop attacks, known as atonic or tonic seizures, also respond nicely to surgery.

Q   What types of presurgical testing are performed to determine if I am a candidate for surgery?

The medical history is the most important part of the evaluation process. The physician obtains information regarding the seizure symptoms, type of seizure, seizure frequency, background neurological history, and details of medical treatment. The testing that is performed serves to confirm the diagnosis made by the physician. The tests aim to find a structural lesion in the brain, show that the lesion is epileptic, and must be consistent with the background historical information. MRI and EEG are the tests that usually provide the most information. However, other tests can help establish whether surgery is possible, including PET scans, SPECT scans, MEG, the Wada test, and neuropsychological testing.

Q **Will I be able to quit taking my antiepileptic medications after I have surgery?**

Physicians typically advise that patients continue to take their medications for a period of time after surgery. Opinions differ regarding the length of therapy after surgery. Some recommend as little as 1 year, while others advise remaining on medication indefinitely. Most advise continuing medication for 2–5 years. Medication doses, or the number of AEDs, are often reduced sooner, upon physician discretion. We have found that most patients who are seizure-free and taking only 1 AED with no side effects are happy to remain on the medication long-term, because they are satisfied with their outcome and do not wish to risk a relapse of seizures.

Q **Can surgery eliminate all my seizures?**

Surgery eliminates all seizures in some people, but many continue to experience some seizures after surgery. Your doctor can estimate the chances of complete seizure relief for you. This depends on the type of epilepsy, the type of operation, and other factors. Even when seizures are not completely stopped, most patients experience a major reduction in the number of seizures that they experience.

Q **What are some of the side effects I might have after surgery?**

The side effects depend on the type of operation that is being considered and your present neurological state. The most common operation, anterior temporal lobectomy, has the potential to adversely affect memory, mainly when done on the side of the brain that controls language. However, the chances of a serious, disabling memory decline after surgery is relatively small, and some of the preoperative tests can predict who is at greatest risk. Also, a small, usually insignificant visual field loss can occur that does not usually cause symptoms or disability. Operations in other lobes of the brain have the potential to affect language abilities, or cause weakness, impairment of sensation, or partial loss of vision. Since operations in these areas are individualized, no general statements can be made, and patients should discuss specific risks with their physicians. In general, however, efforts are made to minimize the chance of causing a permanent neurological deficit since the goal of surgery is to make life better, not worse.

CHAPTER 7

Epilepsy and Marijuana

- Early use of therapeutic marijuana (*cannabis*) dates back to the 1800s, when it was used by some to treat migraines and seizures.
- Animal studies in the mid-twentieth century suggested anti-seizure effects of CBD and THC, two of the many cannabinoids, or chemically related compounds, that cannabis produces.
- In the 2010s, early reports of cannabis's efficacy came from case reports, surveys, and case-series, as more people began to use cannabis in Colorado, California, and other states where it was legalized for medicinal purpose.
- In 2017, the first blinded, randomized, placebo-controlled trial of a purified CBD extract called Epidiolex™ was published and demonstrated efficacy for treating children with Dravet syndrome and Lennox-Gastaut syndrome.
- More studies are needed to understand how cannabis can help treat seizures, what safety measures must be taken, and what long-term risks there may be.

The cannabis plant has been cultivated by humans since the dawn of agriculture, around 12,000 BCE, when its fibrous stalks were grown for use in rope and cloth. Prehistoric peoples also used the plant as medicine, and archaeological records suggest that cannabis was used to treat human disease over four thousand years ago. Seizures and epilepsy were among the conditions that healers treated with extracts of the cannabis plant throughout the Middle East, North Africa, India, and China. Therapeutic cannabis was introduced to European medicine by William O'Shaughnessy, an Irish physician who traveled to India to study its medical traditions. He wrote about the use of extracts of the plant to treat many different ailments including seizures, headaches, cramps, and cholera. One of his earliest reports was on the successful use of "hemp tincture" to treat a young girl with frequent seizures. His reports were widely read by Victorian-era physicians and many began using cannabis extracts to treat neurological conditions, such as migraines and seizures. However, as chemists began to isolate and purify single molecules that had therapeutic uses, such as morphine and salicylic acid (aspirin), physicians began to view the tinctures and extracts of plants as primitive and unscientific. Therapeutic cannabis became unfashionable. This also coincided with laws prohibiting the use of recreational cannabis in the 1920s. Mainstream medicine abandoned cannabis and research into its potential use as disease treatment for many decades, and scientific studies instead focused on the abuse potential of recreational marijuana (Figure 7.1).

The cannabis plant is native to central Asia and India, and it has traditionally been divided into two subspecies—C. indica and C. sativa—although centuries of selective breeding have blurred the distinctions. The plants produce a family of chemically related compounds, called cannabinoids. Over 100 unique cannabinoids have been identified and many can act on the brain. Perhaps the best-known cannabinoid is Δ-9 tetrahydrocannabinol (THC), the compound that is most responsible for the "high" of recreational cannabis. Cannabidiol (CBD) is the most abundant non-psychoactive cannabinoid found in the plant. Both compounds were

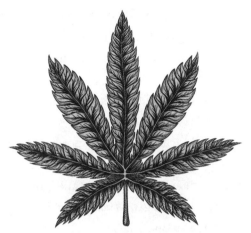

FIGURE 7.1   Please provide a caption.

isolated and synthesized in the middle of the twentieth century. Other cannabinoids, such as cannabinol, cannabidivarin, Δ 9-tetrahydrocannabivarin, and Δ 9-tetrahydrocannabinolic acid, were isolated later. As early as 1949, researchers have proposed studying the uses of isolated cannabinoids for treating seizures based on the observations of the prior century. Animal studies in the 1960s and 1970s suggested antiseizure effects of both THC and CBD, although scientists realized that the "high" associated with THC limited its use as human medicine.

In the late 1980s and early 1990s, there was a renewed interest in cannabinoids for brain diseases when scientists identified the brain receptor for THC and molecules that are made in the body that bind to these receptors. This signaling system, called the *endocannabinoid* (endogenous cannabinoid) system is now known to be important for regulating how brain cells communicate with each other and immune function in and out of the brain. Experiments performed in the lab and with samples of human tissue demonstrated that this system is involved in seizures and epilepsy. However, laboratory experiments targeting the endocannabinoid system using THC or synthetic activators of the receptor showed mixed results. In some, receptor activation had anti-seizure effects, no effects in others, and worsening of seizures in some. Some of the other cannabinoids, such as CBD and cannabidivarin, act on other targets than the endocannabinoid receptors, yet demonstrated more consistent antiseizure effects in laboratory experiments.

While there was growing evidence for antiseizure effects of cannabinoids in the laboratory, proof that it worked in humans was difficult to come by for many years. Much of the early reports of the efficacy of cannabis or compounds derived from cannabis were case reports, surveys, and case-series. As states, such as Colorado and California, legalized cannabis for medical use, more patients began to use cannabis for epilepsy treatment and discuss their experiences on social media. In the early 2010s, word that a strain of cannabis extract high in CBD and low in THC was particularly beneficial for severe childhood seizures spread through parent groups and gained widespread awareness in the mainstream. This lead to an outcry by families of children with severe epilepsy for access and pharmaceutical industry interest in developing CBD as a medication for epilepsy treatment. In 2017, the first blinded, randomized, placebo-controlled trial—the highest standard for scientific evidence in medicine—of a purified (less than 98 percent) CBD extract called Epidiolex™ (GW Pharmaceuticals) was published and demonstrated a benefit of this compound over placebo for reducing seizures in Dravet syndrome, a severe form of childhood-onset genetic epilepsy. Many more trials of both extracted and synthetic CBD are currently in progress.

There is an increasing amount of data to suggest that some cannabinoids may improve seizures in some people with epilepsy, but there remains much that is unknown. To add to the confusion, as of this writing, 40 states and the District of Columbia have legalized some form of medical cannabis use; 8 states have also legalized recreational use. Epilepsy is among the approved medical conditions in all states to qualify patients to get medical cannabis. In addition, there are many companies that are selling CBD-rich cannabis extracts, marketed as nutritional supplements, over the Internet. However, to date, there is no FDA-approved cannabinoid for the treatment of epilepsy and the US Drug Enforcement Administration (DEA) still considers any product derived from the cannabis plant a Schedule I compound, meaning there is a high-abuse potential and no acceptable medical use because of the paucity of well-controlled data. Because of lack of standardization of cannabis strain, delivery methods, preparation, and local quality control, there is no uniformity as to the agents patients get from medical cannabis dispensaries. There are even greater concerns about products obtained from the Internet. In an analysis performed by the FDA in 2016, many samples labeled as CBD extracts obtained online actually contained little or no detectable CBD.

Pharmacology

When used medicinally, cannabis is typically ingested as a liquid extract or as a prepared capsule, or vaporized into the lungs, although many patients have also made their own preparation as butters or baked into edibles. Cannabinoids taken through the mouth are poorly absorbed. On average, about 6 percent of the dose taken by mouth gets into the bloodstream. This is often erratic and home-made preparations have even more issues with dose-to-dose variability. Cannabinoids are extensively metabolized by the liver and in clinical studies, have been given twice daily.

The effective and best-tolerated doses of cannabinoids are currently not well known. In the clinical trials of purified CBD doses ranged from 5–25 mg/kg/day with doses of 10 and 20 mg/kg/day used in the randomized trials as they appeared most effective in preliminary studies. Little is known about dosing for cannabis extracts available through state dispensaries because of lack of standardization of preparations, accurate and reliable measurement of individual cannabinoids in preparations, and variation in cannabinoid levels seen in even genetically identical plant clones because of subtle variations in growing conditions.

Cannabinoids are broken down and eliminated from the body by the liver through a specialized set of enzymes called the *cytochrome P450 sys-*

tem, the main method by which the body rids itself of toxins, hormones, and medications. This system is dynamic and adaptable. The activity of these enzymes is influenced by concentrations of the chemicals to which they bind. Many medications, including antiseizure medications, are also broken down by this system and the presence of one drug in the bloodstream may affect the speed at which another is broken down. This can lead to potentially harmful drug–drug interactions when drug levels are inadvertently too high or too low, leading to side effects or loss of effectiveness. Cannabinoids like THC and CBD are *inhibitors* of some of these cytochrome P450 enzymes, leading to a buildup of other drugs in the blood. This has been seen in patients with a metabolite of clobazam (Onfi™), where adding CBD to a regimen including clobazam leads to high levels of a clobazam metabolite that also has potent effects on the brain, leading to greater than expected sleepiness.

Safety

Much of what has been known about the safety of cannabinoids comes from studying recreational cannabis. It is well known that acute use of recreational cannabis can cause euphoria, paranoia, psychosis, impaired judgment, and slowed motor skills, effects that are mostly due to THC. Long-term cannabis use has been associated with increased rates of psychosis, decreased motivation and attention, and decreased verbal IQ, but it is difficult to tease these effects out from the factors that cause people to use cannabis in the first place. There have also been cases of stroke and heart disease associated with cannabis use. CBD, when studied in isolation, appears relatively safe in the acute setting. In controlled studies with healthy volunteers receiving single doses, there have been no psychiatric effects, no changes in heart rate, blood pressure or breathing, or significant effects on motor performance. When used medicinally, cannabis appears relatively safe as well. Pooled data from cannabinoids (primarily a mixture of THC and CBD) used for various neurological conditions, including multiple sclerosis, pain, spasticity, and movement disorders (a total of ~1600 exposures in adults for < 6 mo) showed that only about 7 percent stopped the drug due to side effects. Common side effects included nausea, behavioral changes, mood changes, suicidality, hallucinations, dizziness, and weakness. Preparations containing higher THC were more likely to cause psychiatric side effects. In studies of CBD for severe childhood epilepsies, minor side effects were common, occurring in 2/3–3/4 of patients. Most of these were related to sleepiness, gastrointestinal, or appetite problems. However, some patients experienced worsening seizures, including prolonged seizures and liver function abnormalities. Some of these side effects may be related to drug–drug interactions and some may be due to the CBD itself. In all of the studies of CBD for treating disease, there have been no deaths related directly to treatment.

Efficacy for Seizures

To date, there have been limited studies to examine cannabinoids for the treatment of seizures. Most have focused on CBD or cannabis extracts high in CBD. Early controlled studies in the 1980s were inconclusive because they were very small. Retrospective, uncontrolled studies of children receiving various cannabis extracts in Colorado and Israel suggested that 33 percent to 50 percent had a greater than 50 percent reduction in seizures. Similar results were seen in a prospective trial of purified CBD (Epidiolex®) that was performed at multiple centers as part of an expanded access, compassionate use program in the United States. More recently, several randomized, placebo-controlled trials, the highest quality of scientific study for medications, were performed and showed that purified CBD was more effective than placebo for the treatment of seizures in patients with Dravet syndrome and Lennox-Gastaut syndrome. In one study of children with Dravet syndrome, 53 percent of patients on CBD had a 50 percent or higher reduction in seizure frequency compared to only 22 percent of patients who received placebo. In two studies of CBD for seizures in Lennox-Gastaut syndrome, 36–44 percent of patients receiving 10 or 20 mg/kg CBD had a 50 percent or higher reduction in seizures, whereas only 14–24 percent of patients receiving placebo had such a response. Based on these studies, Epidiolex® was approved by the FDA in 2018 as an add-on treatment for seizures in these two conditions. It is not clear if the benefits of CBD are limited to specific causes of epilepsy. Studies are in progress to determine if this cannabinoid is effective in other forms of epilepsy, including focal epilepsy in adults. All of the studies performed so far have looked at patients with epilepsy that was not adequately controlled by medications and the patients took CBD in addition to their other medications. It is not currently known if CBD (or any other cannabinoid) can protect against seizures when taken on its own.

Conclusions

After thousands of years of anecdotes about the benefits of cannabis for the treatment of epilepsy, there is now growing high-quality, scientific evidence that specific cannabinoids can reduce seizures. However, the compounds are not a panacea—effects are moderate and side effects can occur. Further research is needed to understand who benefits the most, as well as the most effective dosages and long-term side effects, especially in the developing brain.

CHAPTER 8

Seizure and Epilepsy in Infants and Children

- Because of the immature condition of the baby's brain, neonatal seizures often appear different from seizures in older individuals.

- *Febrile seizures* are seizures that occur in association *only* with fever, in children between the ages of 18 months and 3 years, and without evidence of a serious infection (such as meningitis) or other central nervous system cause.

- *Benign rolandic epilepsy* (BRE) is the most common type of childhood epilepsy in children between ages 2 and 12 years. Affected children experience seizures soon after falling asleep, during daytime naps, or upon awakening.

- Children are especially vulnerable to the side effects of certain medications and, conversely, seem resistant to others.

- Children with epilepsy are prone to learning problems in school.

Neonatal Seizures

Seizures are more common in newborn infants (*neonates*) than in older children or adults (Figure 8.1). Seizures occur in 1 to 5 babies per 1,000. The incidence is highest in the very low-birth-weight infants (those who weigh less than 1,500 grams or about 3 pounds).

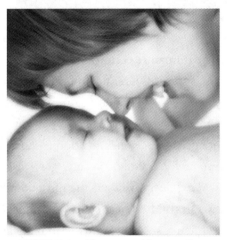

FIGURE 8.1   Please provide a caption.

Newborns are more likely to have seizures for several reasons, including an immature nervous system, birth defects affecting the brain, biochemical or *metabolic problems*, and many diseases that affect newborn infants. Although most brain development occurs before birth, further developmental changes happen during early childhood, leaving the newborn especially susceptible to seizures. These changes include insulation of nerve fibers (*myelination*), formation of new connections (*synapses* between neurons), and the normal loss of some neurons (*apoptosis*), as well as changes in the balance between the chemicals called *neurotransmitters* that help to control the brain's activity.

Risk factors for neonatal seizures include:

- Premature age, especially infants born before 30 weeks of gestation
- Male gender

- *Intraventricular hemorrhage* (bleeding inside the ventricles of the brain)
- *Necrotizing enterocolitis,* a condition that causes parts of the infant's bowel to die, leading to infection (*sepsis*)
- *Patent ductus arteriosus,* a congenital heart defect that can affect brain circulation
- Lack of oxygen at birth and birth defects (mostly in full-term infants)

Types of Neonatal Seizures

Because of the immature condition of the baby's brain, neonatal seizures often appear different from seizures in older individuals. Neonatal seizures may be difficult to recognize, even by trained doctors and nurses. Without continuous *video-electroencephalogram* (video-EEG) monitoring, neonatal seizures may be misinterpreted as normal newborn behavior or missed altogether, especially if they lack outward signs. Unlike older individuals, newborns do not have typical, generalized tonic-clonic (grand mal) seizures.

Seizures in newborns can be classified into several types:

- **Clonic seizures,** characterized by either *focal,* with repetitive jerking of a single region of the body (face, arm, trunk, or leg) or *multifocal,* involving several body regions.
- **Tonic seizures,** characterized by sustained stiffening of a limb or the whole body, lasting a few seconds
- **Myoclonic seizures,** characterized by rapid jerks occurring singly or repeatedly
- **Subtle seizures,** characterized by lip smacking or chewing; roving eye movements; eyes turned up, down, or to the side for a prolonged period (known as *eye deviation*); or eye opening and staring. Infants may also manifest "bicycling" movements of the legs, "swimming" movements of the arms, or abrupt changes in pupil size or heart rate. Difficulty breathing (*apnea*) as the only

sign of a seizure is uncommon and usually is caused by something else, such as a still-developing breath-regulation system, infection, or respiratory, cardiac, or metabolic disturbances. In near-term infants, apnea may be accompanied by other seizure phenomena such as eye deviation, eye opening, or repetitive mouth movements.

■ *Subclinical seizures*, which are detected only by EEG, because they have no outward signs.

Diagnosis

Neonatal seizures are usually diagnosed when a caregiver identifies an unusual pattern of behavior, such as those just described. The most commonly used diagnostic procedure is the EEG, which records brain electrical activity and can determine whether the pattern is normal or abnormal. In the newborn, the EEG is typically recorded for at least an hour. However, this interval may be insufficient, and more prolonged video-EEG recording for hours or days may be required to make a positive diagnosis. Subtle seizures and certain seizure types may not have abnormalities detectable in the scalp-recorded EEG. In this situation, the trained eye of a neurologist may be necessary to recognize if seizures are occurring. In contrast, sick newborns, many of whom are paralyzed and on breathing machines, may have seizures that can only be detected by EEG.

Additional tests to determine the cause of the seizures include blood tests to check for abnormalities in sugar and *electrolyte* (sodium, calcium, magnesium) levels, which can be corrected relatively easily. Additional tests for metabolic disorders may be necessary in some newborns. Examples include blood tests for lactic and pyruvic acid levels, or blood or urine testing for amino acids and urine organic acids. A *lumbar puncture* (spinal tap) can check spinal fluid sugar and protein levels. A family history of seizures, especially during the newborn period or infancy, should be identified because genetic factors can be responsible for seizures in the newborn.

Imaging tests, such as ultrasound, *computed tomography* (CT), or *magnetic resonance imaging* (MRI) scans of the brain can show malformations or other structural abnormalities, such as hemorrhage (bleeding in the brain), enlarged ventricles, birth defects, or stroke. Ultrasound of the head can be performed at the bedside, but CT and MRI scans require that the infant be transported by a medical team to the radiology department. MRI scans, which take a much longer time than CT scans, are usually done when the infant is medically stable.

Genetic Testing in Neonatal Seizures

Genetic and metabolic testing is required if the newborn has a very abnormal EEG background that is discontinuous in term infants (burst suppression pattern). Although very rare, there are conditions termed EIEE (early infantile epileptic encephalopathy or Ohtahara syndrome) and EME (early myoclonic epilepsy) that may start in the neonatal period or very early infancy that are caused by metabolic disorders like NKH (nonketotic hyperglycinemia) or structural brain lesions, but they also have a genetic mutation. Another important genetic cause of seizures in the neonatal period are pyridoxine dependency seizures, caused by mutation in a gene called ALDH7A1. This condition needs treatment with high dose of vitamin B6. Another genetic condition caused by mutation in KCNQ2 gene, a potassium channel gene, causes seizures around the third day of life. Often there is a family history of seizures in neonatal period. This condition is called Benign Familial Neonatal Seizures as most children stop having seizures in a few months although developmental delay is common.

Treatment

The treatment of neonatal seizures depends in part on establishing the cause. Biochemical disturbances are common in newborns with seizures, and some are easily corrected. Phenobarbital and fosphenytoin (Cerebyx) are primary agents administered intravenously for recurrent seizures. To stop seizures quickly, physicians may also administer lorazepam (Ativan) or diazepam (Valium) intravenously, orally, or rectally. Less commonly used antiepileptic drugs (AEDs) include valproic acid (Depakene), lamotrigine (Lamictal), levetiracetam (Keppra), topiramate (Topamax), and zonisamide (Zonegran).

Although no AED has been extensively tested in newborns, and none has been approved by the U.S. Food and Drug Administration (FDA) for use in infants, physicians use these medications because of their known safety and effectiveness in older children and adults.

Newborns with extremely frequent or prolonged seizures are referred to as having *status epilepticus*, a life-threatening condition that requires aggressive treatment with antiepileptic medications, usually in an intensive-care setting.

Outcome

Medical treatment with phenobarbital and phenytoin stops seizures in approximately 70 percent of children. Status epilepticus that does not respond to medications is particularly serious in newborns and carries a high risk of death.

Fortunately, most infants with easily correctable metabolic disturbances or brain hemorrhage have a good outcome and do need antiepileptic medication. Prompt recognition and treatment of more serious metabolic disorders, like certain chemical imbalances or vitamin deficiencies (for example, vitamin B6), can also result in normal outcome. Infants who have a few isolated seizures after experiencing a lack of oxygen (*hypoxic-ischemic injury*) or mild infection may have an excellent outcome, without the need for antiepileptic medication. Quite often, infants are discharged from the nursery without seizure medications, or their AEDs are discontinued by 1 or 2 months of age, if there have been no further seizures.

Two-thirds of infants who have frequent neonatal seizures or status epilepticus are at risk for serious problems, including cerebral palsy or developmental delay. In a large group of newborns followed from birth to 7 years, 61 percent developed epilepsy, most within the first 2 years of life. The outcome is poor in children with severe brain malformations and certain metabolic disorders.

Febrile Seizures

Febrile seizures are seizures that occur in association *only* with fever, in children between the ages of 18 months and 3 years, and without evidence of a serious infection (such as meningitis) or other central nervous system cause. This definition is important because febrile seizures are not related to infections of the brain or nervous system and are *not* true epilepsy, because affected children are not at risk for seizures unless they have a fever.

Febrile seizures run in families. They are approximately two to three times more common among the family members of affected children, and having an affected parent increases the risk of occurrence. (A higher incidence of epilepsy has been reported in close relatives, such as parents or siblings.) Ninety percent of children with febrile seizures will have them within the first 3 years of life, 4 percent before 6 months, and 6 percent after 3 years of age. Approximately half of these seizures appear during the second year of life, with a peak between 18 and 24 months.

A febrile seizure typically occurs early in the course of an infectious illness, usually on the rising phase of the temperature curve. Rectal temperatures often exceed 102°F (39.2°C), and one-fourth of seizures occur at temperatures above 104°F (40.2°C). However, febrile seizures aren't more likely to appear the higher the child's temperature. What's more is that they're usually uncommon in the later stages of a fever-producing illness.

Febrile seizures are typically associated with common childhood illnesses, usually viral upper respiratory, middle ear, and gastrointestinal infections. Bacterial infections, including pneumonia and meningitis, are less common causes.

Types of Febrile Seizures

Simple Febrile Seizures

Simple febrile convulsions are single "events" lasting less than 15 minutes. These seizures don't involve any weakness of a limb, vision changes, or other serious effects. They usually involve shaking, jerking, or kicking movements, and the child may appear to lose consciousness briefly. These simple febrile convulsions occur in normal children who do not have brain-related conditions, defects, or injuries. Between 80 percent and 90 percent of all febrile seizures are simple episodes. The American Academy of Pediatrics recommends a lumbar puncture (spinal tap) as a standard test in a febrile baby presenting with a seizure under the age of 6 months. In older babies and toddlers, a lumbar puncture is usually not necessary unless the child appears lethargic or has received antibiotics that may be masking clinical signs of meningitis. Tests like EEG, CT scan, and extensive blood work are deemed unnecessary in most cases.

Complex Febrile Seizures

The concept of a *complex febrile seizure* originated with studies indicating that some patient- and seizure-related variables are associated with higher rates of developing epilepsy at a later stage. These include seizure that last longer than 15 minutes, seizures with a focal pattern, seizures that recur within 24 hours, seizures occurring in a child who has a brain or nervous system abnormality, and seizures occurring in a child who has a parent or sibling with seizures that are not related to fevers (*afebrile seizures*).

In general, complex febrile seizures have a less favorable outcome than simple febrile convulsions. Seventeen percent of neurologically impaired children with complex febrile seizures develop epilepsy by 30 years old, compared with 2.5 percent of children who lack risk factors. If a child has focal seizures, multiple episodes, and prolonged seizures, they have nearly a 50 percent chance of developing afebrile seizures later.

Recurrence of Febrile Seizures

Approximately 30 percent of patients with a first febrile seizure will experience additional attacks, and 50 percent will have a third seizure. Only 9 percent experience three or more attacks.

Age at the onset is the most important predictor of febrile seizure recurrence. Fifty percent of all infants younger than 1 year of age at the time of their first febrile seizure will have another febrile seizure, compared with 20 percent of children older than 3 years of age. Young age at onset, febrile seizures in a first-degree relative, low-grade fever in the emergency department, and a brief interval between fever onset and seizure onset are all indicators of febrile seizure recurrence. Recurrences generally occur within 1 year, but they are no more likely in children who have had a complex febrile seizure versus a simple febrile seizure.

Treatment

When your child has a fever, it's important to give them anti-fever medications, such as acetaminophen (Tylenol), and tepid sponge baths to control body temperature. Unfortunately, in some children, it's hard to tell when they have a fever until they have a seizure. This is why it's especially important to watch for other signs of infection, such as lack of appetite, diarrhea, or rash, and to consult your doctor immediately if you see anything out of the ordinary.

Although medication can be given to *stop* a febrile seizure, AEDs should not be given to children to *prevent* simple febrile seizures. Recurrent febrile seizures and later afebrile epilepsy are fortunately both rare occurrences, and the risks of a child routinely taking an AED far outweigh the benefit in the case of febrile seizures.

Doctors sometimes consider medication for complex febrile seizures that carry an increased risk for later epilepsy. However, even seemingly life-threatening seizures must be treated cautiously. Since neurologic impairment and death are extremely unlikely, most children do not require long-term medication.

Febrile seizures often stop by the time the child is examined in the emergency room. If the seizure continues, the physician can give intravenous medication to stop the seizure. At home, rectally administered diazepam gel is safe and easy to use. Respiratory depression (shallow breathing) can occur, but this is rare. Some studies have shown an increased chance of damage to an area of the brain called the hippocampus when febrile seizures last a very long time. This is why it's highly recommended to administer the rescue medication after carefully timing the seizure and to call 911 if the seizure does not subside.

Common Childhood Epilepsy Syndrome

In a discussion about childhood epilepsy syndromes, it's important to understand the difference among epileptic seizures, epilepsy, and epilepsy syndromes.

- **Epileptic seizures** are the symptoms resulting from an abnormal electrical discharge in the brain. There are many types of seizures, and children may have more than one seizure type.
- **Epilepsy** is a disorder in which an individual has recurrent unprovoked seizures. According to the recent International League Against Epilepsy (ILAE) definition, two unprovoked seizures are necessary for an epilepsy diagnosis, unless the child has an underlying condition predisposing them to seizures, in which case epilepsy is diagnosed even with one unprovoked seizure.

■ *Epilepsy syndrome* refers to a cluster of specific signs and symptoms occurring in addition to epileptic seizures in the same child. For example, children with Lennox-Gastaut syndrome have multiple seizure types, but they have intellectual impairment and a specific EEG pattern. In some, but not all syndromes, the specific cause, type of seizures, and outcome are well-established. An example is *juvenile myoclonic epilepsy* (JME), which is known to be a genetic disease starting in adolescence or young adulthood, featuring specific seizure types that persist throughout the person's life. Other epilepsy syndromes may not have a clear cause or may have several causes. The Lennox-Gastaut syndrome may occur after lack of oxygen at birth (*asphyxia*), from a head injury or metabolic disorder, or from many other factors, but likely genetic mutations account for a third of the cases.

Common Epilepsy Syndromes

Benign rolandic epilepsy (BRE) is the most common type of childhood epilepsy in children between ages 2 and 12 years. Affected children experience seizures soon after falling asleep, during daytime naps, or upon awakening. Focal motor seizures are most common, while generalized tonic-clonic seizures are rare. Seizures often involve the tongue, lips, and mouth, and they produce drooling and vocalizations. Younger children (under 5 years) are more likely to have a *hemiconvulsion*, affecting one side of the body, or a grand mal seizure. Their neurologic examination is typically normal.

The EEG helps confirm the diagnosis of BRE by demonstrating epileptic electrical activity in the central and temporal regions of the brain. This activity increases during sleep and has a characteristic appearance. Brain scans are typically normal, so that when these EEG patterns are present, imaging studies are often unnecessary.

Children with BRE may experience a single seizure (50 percent will have fewer than 5), or seizures may occur more regularly. Doctors believe

BRE is a genetic disorder. However, although many children (and their siblings) show the characteristic EEG patterns, 90 percent never have seizures. BRE epileptiform discharges are common in children who are undergoing EEGs to evaluate other conditions. Unless they are having seizures, it's OK to ignore these EEG findings.

Medical treatment may not be necessary when seizures are rare and occur during sleep. If treatment is indicated, BRE seizures are easily controlled with medications like gabapentin (Neurontin), carbamazepine (Tegretol or Carbatrol), or oxcarbazepine (Trileptal). In Europe, sulthiame (Ospolot) or valproic acid (Depakote) are also used. The outcome of BRE is excellent, as both seizures and EEG abnormalities disappear between ages 12 and 16 years. AEDs can be withdrawn if no seizures are observed for 2 years. Even if the EEG shows persistent epileptic activity, most neurologists will still attempt to wean the child from medication. A higher chance of academic difficulties, including poor focus and processing speed, has been shown in the children with this condition. As such, they are not entirely "benign."

Childhood absence epilepsy is the second most common form of childhood epilepsy. It usually begins in healthy children between the ages of 4 to 10 years. It is genetically inherited. Absence seizures (often called *petit mal* seizures) consist of brief episodes of staring and arrest of ongoing activity lasting 3 to 10 seconds, but these episodes may occasionally last as long as 20 or 30 seconds. Absence seizures may be accompanied by lip-smacking, blinking, or gestural movements, and they typically occur many times daily. Shorter seizures may go unrecognized or be mistaken for inattentiveness, and school performance may suffer.

Seizures are usually noticed in the daytime and can be evoked by hyperventilation. Grand mal seizures are rare and are more commonly observed in older children. Absence seizures in children between 10 and 17 years represent a different disorder due to their more frequent association with grand mal (80 percent) and myoclonic (15 percent) seizures.

The EEG is almost always abnormal, even in children taking AEDs. Hyperventilation may be employed in the doctor's office or EEG laboratory to trigger an absence seizure and confirm the diagnosis. In such a case, consciousness is impaired during seizures that last longer than 3 seconds, but with even longer seizures, children may remain partly responsive.

Unlike BRE, where treatment may not be required, absence seizures should be treated promptly because these seizures impair attention and learning, and they compromise overall safety on the playground, at school, at home, on the street, or elsewhere. The most commonly used medications include ethosuximide (Zarontin), valproic acid (Depakene or Depakote), and lamotrigine (Lamictal). Newer potential drugs include topiramate (Topamax) and zonisamide (Zonegran). Most absence seizures can be controlled. Hyperventilation testing and repeat EEG studies may be used to verify the effectiveness of treatment.

After a seizure-free interval of 2 years, medication may be safely discontinued. Most children outgrow absence seizures, but a small proportion continues to require medication and may evolve into juvenile myoclonic epilepsy.

A subset of absence epilepsy begins in very young children, less than 4 years of age. The early onset of absence epilepsy may be caused by a genetic defect in a transporter molecule that helps transfer glucose to the brain. Genetic testing for a gene called SLC2A1 and lifelong treatment with ketogenic diet is key as medications usually do not work in this condition. Other genes associated with absence epilepsy include: CACNA1H, GABRA1, GABRB3, GABRG2, and JRK.

Early onset occipital lobe epilepsy or *Panayiotopoulos syndrome* is relatively common and a benign type of childhood epilepsy syndrome, typically occurring between 3 and 10 years of age. The seizures are infrequent, but they may be long, with the child staring off, vomiting, and becoming pale in the face with dilated eyes as some prominent features. EEG shows typical spikes in the occipital region, accentuated by drowsiness and sleep. Late onset occipital epilepsy is usually associated with visual auras and may persist into adulthood.

Juvenile myoclonic epilepsy (JME) starts during adolescence, typically between 12 and 18 years of age. It is a genetic disorder. Myoclonic seizures predominate, consisting of abrupt jerks usually involving the shoulders and upper extremities. They typically occur in the morning after awakening. Myoclonic seizures may make the individual drop or fling objects from their hands. Grand mal seizures occur in over 90 percent of patients and occur soon after waking in the morning. Repetitive myoclonic jerks can lead into a grand mal seizure. Jerking may be predominantly one-sided.

Patients with JME have normal neurologic examinations and normal brain MRI scans, but their EEGs reveals rapid *spike-wave discharges*. In approximately one-third of JME patients, seizures or EEG spike-wave discharges can be triggered by flickering lights. Absence seizures occur in 10 percent to 33 percent of patients with JME.

Mutations in genes like GABRA1 and EFHC1 gene can cause JME.

Effective seizure control is possible in over 90 percent of patients. Valproic acid (Depakote) is the most effective AED, but it is associated with weight gain and hormonal changes in women. Other medications such as topiramate (Topamax), zonisamide (Zonegran), lamotrigine (Lamictal), and levetiracetam (Keppra) are effective treatments and have fewer side effects. The treatment of JME is typically life-long, as attempts to reduce AEDs result in seizure recurrence in most individuals. It is important for patients to take their medications regularly, get enough sleep, and refrain from drinking alcohol.

Psychiatric disorders like depression and cognitive deficits in executive functions, memory, and processing speed are likely to be associated with JME.

Infantile spasms (*West syndrome*) is an age-related epilepsy syndrome occurring in infants younger than 2 years. The peak incidence is between 3 and 7 months. There are many different causes, some of which occur prior to birth (brain malformations, infections while in the womb), at birth, or just after birth (lack of blood supply and oxygen, stroke, brain infections, trauma, brain tumors, metabolic and genetic disorders). *Tuberous sclerosis* is an additional cause. Brain scans are abnormal in about 75 percent of infants with West syndrome. Advanced genetic testing is now able to find a cause in many cases of infantile spasms previously called "idiopathic." Genes like ARX, CDKL5, FOXG1, and GABRB3, among others, may show changes called *mutations* that alter the function of important proteins in the young brain. The spasms consist of an abrupt flexing of the arms, legs, and trunk, often followed by a more prolonged tonic phase lasting for about 2 seconds. Spasms typically occur numerous times over several minutes and "cluster" throughout the day, most often occurring while the child is falling asleep or waking up. Between spasms, infants appear quiet or irritable. Although 90 percent of children with infantile spasms are developmentally delayed prior to seizure onset, nearly all will show a loss of development once the spasms begin. Most of the individuals in these cases will continue to have seizures and significant developmental delays.

The EEG in West syndrome is very characteristic, showing multifocal spikes over both cerebral hemispheres and a disorganized high-voltage background—a pattern called *hypsarrhythmia*. Hypsarrhythmia typically evolves into other EEG patterns as the spasms transform into other seizure types. The majority of infants with West syndrome remain neurologically abnormal and continue to have seizures, but in 10 percent the spasms cease and the EEG returns to normal.

Prompt recognition and treatment of infantile spasms is mandatory. Treatment options include high-dose oral steroids or intramuscular injections of ACTH (adrenocorticotrophic hormone) or vigabatrin. The latter is the first-line treatment in children with tuberous sclerosis. Other antiepileptic medications, such as clonazepam (Klonopin), valproic acid (Depakene or Depakote), topiramate (Topamax), or zonisamide (Zonegran) may be needed. Some infants respond to pyridoxine (vitamin B6) or the ketogenic diet (see Chapter 5). Unfortunately, complete control of seizures is difficult to achieve, and less than 50 percent of infants are completely seizure-free with these treatments.

Some infants with infantile spasms have a particular area of brain damage that causes their spasms, and surgical removal of the epileptic tissue may be the only way to stop the spasms.

Lennox-Gastaut syndrome (LGS) refers to the occurrence of multiple seizure types (most often generalized tonic, atonic, generalized tonic-clonic, myoclonic, or atypical absence seizures) in patients with intellectual impairment and a characteristic EEG consisting of slow spike-wave discharges. Seizures usually begin between ages 1 and 8 years. In contrast to the typical absence seizures seen in childhood absence epilepsy, the atypical absence seizures of LGS occur in neurologically and developmentally impaired children, often do not have an abrupt onset or end, and usually last longer than 15 seconds. LGS is produced by conditions similar to those associated with infantile spasms, but the cause is undetermined in nearly 30 percent of children. About 40 percent of LGS patients start out having infantile spasms. In addition to requiring an MRI and EEG, children with LGS should be evaluated for metabolic or *degenerative illnesses* of the brain. Seizures in LGS are often difficult to fully control with medications. Genetic panels testing for channel mutations like Dravet syndrome (sodium channel mutations), GABA receptor mutations, and many others may be helpful in determining the cause of LGS.

Temporal lobe epilepsy (TLE) in children differs from TLE in adults. Young children rarely describe auras occurring before their seizures start—such as abdominal sensations, nausea, altered taste, smell, déjà vu experiences, or visual or auditory hallucinations—but adult TLE patients often do. Children are more likely to have motor seizures, and infants and very young children are especially prone to spasms and myoclonic seizures—patterns that are rare in later life. Infants with temporal lobe seizures may also have a subtle reduction of activity (referred to as *hypomotor seizures*), pale skin, or changes in breathing.

In children younger than 6 years, malformations of the brain's *cerebral cortex*, such as tumors, are common. Older children and adolescents, on the other hand, usually have causes that are more similar to adults, such as *hippocampal sclerosis*, which is scarring of the temporal lobe. This condition has been linked to prolonged febrile convulsions in infancy. Genetic causes of temporal lobe epilepsy include mutations in LGI1 gene (Autosomal Dominant Partial Epilepsy with Auditory Features), DEPDC5 (Familial Focal Epilepsy with Variable Foci).

The EEG may show focal slowing and sharp waves in the temporal region in approximately 50 percent of the cases, and the MRI is abnormal in nearly 80 percent. Treating with AEDs for focal seizures is effective in approximately half the children. TLE should be treated aggressively, and if seizures are not controlled in a reasonable time period, an evaluation for epilepsy surgery can be the next step. *Temporal lobectomy*, the removal of the diseased temporal lobe, leads to complete seizure freedom in 60 percent to 80 percent of children with TLE. If a temporal lobe tumor is present, early removal is advised because recurring seizures may lead to learning and behavioral problems.

Frontal lobe epilepsy (FLE) starts typically in adolescence and seizures occur in sleep. These seizures can be violent with hypermotor behavior. Some children may be misdiagnosed as sleep walkers. A familial form exists and is caused by mutations in genes like CHRNA2, CHRN4, and CHNRB2.

Landau-Kleffner syndrome is characterized by the loss of previously acquired language and is frequently associated with behavioral and cognitive abnormalities. In the typical patient, a near-complete loss of spoken and understood language takes place slowly over a period of weeks or months between the ages of 18 months and 5 years. Affected children have autistic-like behavior with a profound loss of attention. Seizures occur in a high proportion of patients and show a diverse pattern of both frequency and severity. The neurologic examination rarely shows a specific problem, but the EEG will often reveal a characteristic pattern consisting of nearly continuous epileptic activity during slow-wave (non-REM) sleep. Some children may have a genetic mutation in a gene called GRIN2A.

Conventional antiepileptic therapy is often unsatisfactory in the Landau-Kleffner syndrome, although numerous medications have been tried. Corticosteroid therapy with prednisone and intravenous immuno-globulin has been used successfully to cause a remission in seizures. High-dose diazepam is also reported to be effective in a small number of cases. Unfortunately, remission of seizures does not mean improved behavior or cognitive activity.

Rasmussen syndrome is a serious disorder of childhood that first starts with focal seizures. These are typically followed by progressive continuous focal seizures, cognitive deterioration, paralysis of one side of the body (*hemiparesis*), and shrinkage of one side of the brain (*hemiatrophy*). The seizures and brain damage remain confined to one hemisphere of the brain throughout the duration of the illness, which irreversibly culminates in the destruction of one entire cerebral hemisphere. The cause of Rasmussen syndrome is unknown. Microscopic changes in the brain resemble those seen in *viral encephalitis* (a viral infection of the brain), but no viral agent has ever been identified. Why only one cerebral hemisphere is affected and the other is spared is also an unsolved medical mystery. An autoimmune mechanism has been suspected, but it remains unproven.

The only proven effective therapy for seizures in Rasmussen syndrome is surgical removal of the affected brain hemisphere—half the brain (*hemispherectomy*). Despite the radical nature of this procedure, experience has shown that more limited procedures do not halt progression of the illness and the patient still lives with persistent seizures. Most epilepsy centers perform a *functional hemispherectomy*, which surgically removes the central portion of the hemisphere and disconnects the frontal and occipital poles.

Tuberous sclerosis complex (TSC) is a genetic disorder characterized by light-colored (*hypopigmented*) skin lesions and nodular collections of abnormal cells and tissue in the brain's cerebral cortex. Apart from the brain, abnormally malformed tissue and tumors can occur in multiple organ systems, and there is a tendency for some lesions to become cancerous. Epilepsy affects 90 percent of patients with TSC and typically begins in the first decade of life. There is a significant incidence of infantile spasms, although focal seizures affect a much higher proportion of patients. Seizures are often *refractory* to medication and may be associated with significant developmental regression. Status epilepticus unresponsive to aggressive medical treatment has been observed as early as 2 days of age.

To date, two main genetic forms have been described. TSC1 is caused by fewer than 400 mutations in the TSC1 gene on chromosome 9. TSC2 can be caused by one of the 1100 mutations in the TSC2 gene on chromosome that is located on chromosome 16p.

Infantile spasms in patients with TSC have been shown to be especially responsive to treatment with vigabatrin. The reasons for vigabatrin's good results for infantile spasms in TSC are unknown, because vigabatrin does not offer similar benefit for focal seizures due to other conditions. Conventional AEDs are often ineffective in many TSC patients with epilepsy, and surgery to remove the affected brain tissue offers a significant likelihood of seizure-freedom or improved seizure status. Despite the occurrence of multiple cortical tubers, only one is typically associated with seizure origin. Removal of the offending tuber can produce long-standing relief from seizures. Given the known natural progression of the disorder, prompt referral for surgical consideration should be carried out relatively early. *Everolimus*, an inhibitor of an important pathway called mTOR, is now FDA-approved for use in TSC for treatment of brain tumors and also for reduction of seizures.

Antiepileptic Drugs in Children: Special Considerations

Children are treated with antiepileptic medications similar to those used in adults. These effectively control most seizures in childhood, although children may not always respond to medications in the same way that adults do. For example, children typically require a higher proportional dosage compared to adults because their brain weight is proportionally larger, and children are extremely efficient at removing medications from their bodies.

The liver and the kidneys, which play critical roles in eliminating medications, are at their peak performance in childhood. It may be necessary to divide daily medication into more frequent doses to maintain an even blood level.

The incidence of medication-related side effects is also different for children. Medications that are sedating in adults can have opposite effects in the very young. For example, phenobarbital produces drowsiness in older patients, but it results in hyperactivity in children. Phenobarbital can cause a child to be inattentive at school, and the behavioral side effects of some medications can disrupt normal social interactions like play.

Children are especially vulnerable to the side effects of certain medications and, conversely, seem resistant to others. In children, phenytoin (Dilantin) produces gum overgrowth, excessive body hair growth, and coarsening of facial features. The risk of liver toxicity by valproic acid (Depakote, Depakene) is greater in children, especially those younger than 2 years. Children are also at higher risk of serious rash from lamotrigine (Lamictal). On the other hand, children seldom experience nausea from carbamazepine (Tegretol), and it is rare to encounter lowered sodium levels in children treated with carbamazepine (Tegretol) or oxcarbazepine (Trileptal). Abnormal numbness and tingling of the fingertips is reported by adult patients started on topiramate (Topamax), but this symptom is unknown in children.

Childhood is also a time when healthy bones are forming. Medications can influence the metabolic aspects of bone mineralization and may adversely affect bone health by causing diminished physical activity. Some medications are more likely to produce obesity, while others lead to modest weight loss.

Some *formulations* of medication are better tolerated by children than by adults. Good-tasting liquid preparations are better tolerated in very young children and are easily administered via a gastric tube in the disabled. Sprinkle preparations can be mixed with applesauce, yogurt, or ice cream. Chewable and dissolvable tablets are also favored by children.

Tablets with special coatings to make them less irritating to the stomach (Depakote tablets) or extended-release formulations (Tegretol-XR, Depakote-ER) may not need to be divided or broken into smaller doses. Special preparations that lack sugar are available for children whose carbohydrate intake is restricted by special treatments such as the ketogenic diet (see Chapter 5).

Because of these special concerns about AEDs in children, it's important to talk to your child's physician about the choice of medication, formulation and dosage, and potential side effects. No physician can fully predict all possible medication effects, but patients and their families should promptly communicate any unexpected or bothersome side effects.

Initiating and Stopping a Medication

The occurrence of a single seizure does not mean that a child has epilepsy. Isolated seizures can be provoked by a wide variety of stresses such as low blood sugar (glucose) levels, abnormal sodium levels, or a febrile illness. Other children may be experiencing a benign childhood seizure disorder with a low probability of recurrence. In these situations, treatment with daily medications is rarely indicated.

The decision to start medication in children with recurrent seizures is ultimately based on the overall presentation, rather than on any single test finding. Thus, one child may have an abnormal EEG with epileptic activity, yet treatment is withheld. In contrast, another child with a different seizure type and a normal EEG may be started on medication because the seizure is typical of an epilepsy syndrome with a poor prognosis, or one that originates deep within the brain, so that the scalp EEG does not show abnormal electrical activity. As a rule, whenever seizures recur, the likelihood of an additional recurrence increases significantly. At this point, most physicians will start AED treatment, using the best medication for the particular seizure. The EEG helps determine whether the seizure began in one area of the brain (focal seizures) or in both cerebral hemispheres simultaneously (generalized seizure). Specific AEDs are available for each category. The advantages and liabilities of each medicine must also be considered.

The risk of immediate recurrence after a first seizure is generally low. Thus, medication should not be administered rapidly. Most doctors like to "start low and go slow," beginning with a small dose and slowly increasing the dose until the seizures are controlled. This gradual escalation in dose also allows sufficient time to recognize potential side effects. Some medications, such as topiramate (Topamax), are better tolerated if the starting dose is low and the dose escalation is slow. The "start low, go slow" approach is also more likely to achieve the lowest effective AED dose.

When should medication be discontinued? Many childhood epilepsies and epilepsy syndromes are associated with a favorable prognosis characterized by seizures that do not recur after initial treatment. Children who remain seizure-free for 2 years and have a normal EEG can be safely weaned off AEDs. However, seizure freedom after 2 years does not guarantee a reduced likelihood of seizure occurrence in certain epilepsy syndromes such as JME. Withdrawal of medications will trigger seizure recurrence in this syndrome and lead to a loss of highly prized mobility and the accompanying sense of freedom, especially if seizures restrict operation of a motor vehicle.

Learning and Epilepsy

Children with epilepsy are prone to significant trouble in school. Any underlying brain dysfunction that causes seizures may also contribute to problems with attention, memory, and learning. Studies of children with epilepsy have consistently shown a higher frequency of attention deficit-hyperactivity disorder (ADHD), autism, learning and behavioral problems, and psychiatric disorders. The success or failure in controlling the frequency and severity of seizures will also affect the way in which a child or adolescent learns. The effects of AEDs themselves can also have a significant impact on attention, memory, and other domains of cognitive function.

It is difficult to calculate the overall impact of pre-existing structural brain abnormalities on learning. Although absence of brain damage is associated with a better prognosis for intellectual functioning, some children with brain damage and cerebral palsy perform at an acceptable academic level. Many autistic children with epilepsy, cognitive, and social disabilities may have normal MRI scans. The presence of severe behavioral and cognitive abnormalities prior to seizure onset suggests that learning problems may result from underlying brain dysfunction.

Role of AEDs

Antiepileptic medications can affect alertness, concentration, memory, and learning. Certain medications have a more severe impact on learning. Barbiturates, such as phenobarbital, and the benzodiazepine class of medications, such as clonazepam (Klonopin), diazepam (Valium), lorazepam (Ativan), and clorazepate (Tranxene), impair attention at high doses and reduce school performance at moderately high doses. Barbiturates may cause depression in some patients.

In some children, AEDs can influence a child's capacity to learn. Carbamazepine (Tegretol) and oxcarbazepine (Trileptal) have not been associated with diminished school performance when administered in moderate doses, but among the newer medications, diminished word fluency is associated with topiramate (Topamax) and this effect is encountered with other AEDs as well. Irritability and anger outbursts are described in some children treated with gabapentin (Neurontin) and levetiracetam (Keppra). Behavioral changes are encountered rarely with zonisamide (Zonegran). In contrast, lamotrigine (Lamictal) has not been shown to affect intellectual or social ability in young adults.

Because all children are different, each may respond to medication differently. It's important to closely monitor your child while they are taking AEDs and report to their physician any changes in their behavior or attitude. Problems with attention, memory, and learning can be pre-existing conditions, or they can occur as treatment-related side effects. As a general rule, fewer problems are encountered when medications are started at a low dose and increased slowly. Gradual adjustment also ensures that the medication is given at the lowest effective dose. Using several AEDs at once (combination therapy) may lead to a higher risk of side effects, although recent research suggests that some combinations of newer-generation medications may work better and produce fewer side effects when used together.

Treating Other Problems

Treatment of associated problems can improve a child's learning ability and quality of life. For example, the use of stimulant medications for ADHD does not worsen seizures. Thus, a careful choice of anticonvulsant medications and an open mind toward the treatment of ADHD symptoms may have a positive effect on schooling. Some anticonvulsant medications, such as carbamazepine (Tegretol), lamotrigine (Lamictal), valproic acid (Depakote, Depakene), and occasionally gabapentin (Neurontin), have a beneficial effect on mood. The added use of medications such as fluoxetine (Prozac) or sertraline (Zoloft) may further improve depression and anxiety.

Children who are not seizure-free on medication should be considered for epilepsy surgery. Successful surgery can eliminate seizures and have a favorable effect on later cognitive functioning.

Epilepsy Surgery and Children

The principles of epilepsy surgery in children are not much different from those in adults, as described in Chapter 6. The decision to refer patients for epilepsy surgery rests on the belief that medical treatment has failed. This occurs only if the physician has exercised *due diligence*—he has given the best possible medications at the highest safe concentrations. However, there are few established guidelines to assist the physician's choice of medications, dosing interval, duration of treatment, monitoring of serum concentration, and withdrawal of therapy. Thus, medical treatment of seizures is still largely individualized, and there is no unique point in time when seizures can be positively identified as intractable to medication.

Two broad categories of surgical therapy exist for epilepsy—curative and palliative. *Curative surgery* eradicates seizures and the need for medication, whereas *palliative surgery* lessens seizure severity or frequency or prevents the occurrence of some seizure types. These outcome measures are similar to the goals of surgery in other conditions (e.g., for cancer surgery, complete tumor removal vs. reducing the size of a tumor).

Curative procedures involve removing a portion of the brain responsible for the epilepsy. Examples include removing a portion of a lobe of the brain, or more extensive procedures that remove multiple lobes or one cerebral hemisphere.

Because curative surgery also eliminates the psychosocial disability associated with seizures, surgery is the best hope for achieving a "normal" life, including improved schooling, greater personal independence, enhanced employment opportunities, and attainment of a driver's license. Return to a normal lifestyle rarely occurs in patients who do not achieve seizure freedom.

In some individuals, only one of several seizure types is cured by surgery, but this outcome may still be worthwhile. For example, children usually benefit from the elimination or marked reduction in the frequency of tonic or atonic seizures, due to the reduction in medical risk and injuries (e.g., fractures, lacerations from falls). Similarly, children may benefit from the stopping of focal seizures with impaired awareness, and they will tolerate occasional auras without loss of consciousness. This type of palliative surgery requires a clear definition of the treatment objectives *before* the surgery begins, so that the results can be realistically appreciated.

Whenever surgery for epilepsy is contemplated, its risks and benefits must be weighed carefully. As in adults, the risks are usually acceptably low, with overall complications occurring in between 1 percent and 5 percent of patients. Surgical complications include stroke, hemorrhage, infection, and direct brain injury, possibly resulting in temporary or permanent neurologic deficits. Complications and death vary according to age and type of surgery; the risks of surgery appear to be slightly higher in children compared to adults and for larger procedures, such as hemispherectomy.

Any risk of surgery must also be compared to the risk of continued medical treatment. At present, few studies compare the relative risks of medical versus surgical treatment. The risks associated with ongoing epilepsy and its medical treatments include death, injury, status epilepticus, possible detrimental effects of seizures, and the adverse side effects of medication. People with epilepsy have increased mortality rates compared with the general population. Risk of sudden unexpected death in epilepsy patients (SUDEP) was previously thought to be much lower in children, but more recent research suggests that it may be almost equal to that in adults. Nocturnal seizures, multiple AEDs, generalized tonic-clonic seizures are associated with higher risk of SUDEP.

It is important to remember that despite a generalized EEG pattern like hypsarrhythmia, a focal lesion may be the cause of network disruption in childhood epilepsy, and early surgery may modify the course of not only the epilepsy, but it may also allow for a better cognitive profile in children due to the "plasticity" of the developing brain. This means that any deficits induced by a surgical procedure are less likely to be permanent with the other areas of the young brain taking over that particular function. Hence, if epilepsy surgery is determined to be the best route for seizure freedom and overall health of the child, it shouldn't be unduly delayed.

Corpus callosotomy is a type of palliative epilepsy surgery used in some children with Lennox-Gestaut syndrome. This procedure involves disconnection of the two halves of the brain by cutting a structure called *corpus callosum*, which is a thick band of nerve fibers connecting the two sides. This procedure is particularly effective for atonic or drop seizures.

Vagus nerve stimulation is another option for palliation. FDA has approved the use of VNS in children 4 years and older. The newer versions of the implantable device have additional features like the autostimulation (automatic delivery of a higher strength impulse in response to the sudden increase in the heart rate that precedes most seizures) and flexibility in dosing differently for the day or the night, based on whether the child's seizures are worse during the day or at night.

Another palliative treatment used particularly in children with intractable epilepsy is dietary therapy. The most stringent of these is the ketogenic diet where the child is placed on a carbohydrate-free diet (including sugar-free medications), and the diet is high in fats and proteins. Modified Atkins diet is a more permissive version based on the same idea. The child's urine and blood is then monitored periodically to ensure that they have achieved a state of ketosis. Although difficult to enforce in younger children who may self-feed, the dietary treatments may be a valid option in tube-fed infants or older children who can cooperate with the dietary changes. For detailed information about the diet, please see Chapter 5.

FREQUENTLY ASKED QUESTIONS

Q Are seizures in the newborn harmful to its brain?

It is now becoming clear that frequent, prolonged seizures or status epilepticus that do not respond readily to seizure medications are often indications of an underlying structural brain abnormality or birth defect, a severe lack of blood supply or oxygen to the brain, or a metabolic disorder that is preventing brain cells from obtaining energy in the normal way from food.

Prolonged seizures also cause excessive release of excitatory neurotransmitters, like glutamate and aspartate, which may make it easier for the brain to experience further seizures. In experimental animals, *recurrent* seizures can produce lasting changes that make the animal more prone to more seizures and make it harder for the animal to learn and remember. On the other hand, experimental data from immature rats found that after a *single* prolonged seizure, their brains were relatively resistant to such adverse effects. Repeated neonatal seizures and status epilepticus in experimental animals, however, are clearly detrimental to learning, memory, and activity levels. This outcome is influenced by the overlapping effects of the underlying brain abnormality, injury from various causes, and the effect of the seizures.

Q   How can I tell if my newborn is experiencing a seizure?

Seizures in the newborn may be difficult to detect. Abnormal movements or other manifestations of seizures may be subtle. Repetitive stereotyped movements should arouse concern for seizures, especially if the movements are associated with a change in behavior. Repetitive jerking of the eyes is another possible sign of possible seizures. In rare circumstances, a newborn may transiently stop breathing as the only manifestation of a seizure. If you suspect that your child is having seizures, contact your doctor. It may be helpful to record the manifestations and show the video to your doctor.

Q   What should I do if my child experiences a convulsion during a high fever?

Febrile seizures typically begin without warning at the onset of various childhood illnesses accompanied by fever (e.g., ear or throat infection). Because of their sudden occurrence, it is very difficult to prevent them. Once the febrile seizure begins, the child should be placed on their side until the seizure is over. Most febrile seizures are brief and last only a few minutes. Do not place anything in the child's mouth, as this may cause irritation or break teeth. Placing your finger in the child's mouth could traumatically damage your finger if the child involuntarily bites down during the seizure. If your child is prone to recurrent febrile seizures, rectal diazepam can be administered for seizures that have not stopped on their own by three minutes.

Q **My child's AEDs make her irritable and hard to control. I am worried about her behavior when she starts school next year. What should I do?**

AEDs affect children differently and some produce noticeable changes in behavior and mood. These changes may become apparent immediately after starting the medicine (*idiosyncratic reaction*) or may develop when the dose is increased (toxicity). If your child's behavior changes immediately upon starting a new AED, it is best to bring this to your doctor's attention, who will probably consider stopping the AED and trying something different. If behavioral changes occur only after the AED dose is increased, your doctor may first consider lowering the dosage to eliminate the problem. This may not be possible without causing an increase in seizures. In this case, the AED should be discontinued and a different medicine tried.

Q **My child's physician has tried three different medications, but nothing seems to be working. What are our options now?**

Children who continue to have seizures despite trying three different medications are considered to have intractable epilepsy. Unfortunately, the likelihood of controlling intractable seizures with a fourth or fifth AED is low. Several options exist at this point. The child may be a candidate for a specialized diet, either the ketogenic diet or a Modified Atkins diet. Approximately 20 percent to 30 percent of children with intractable epilepsy will obtain seizure control by dietary manipulation. If dietary therapy is not an option, surgical therapy should be considered. Surgical removal of epileptic brain tissue represents an effective therapy if a well-defined target can be identified. This requires a battery of tests that are typically undertaken at specialized pediatric epilepsy surgery centers. The presence of a well-defined focal abnormality on the child's MRI scan often assists the surgical team in identifying the area of seizure origination. Epilepsy surgery offers the possibility or seizure freedom or improvement in a high proportion of children.

Q   My child has epilepsy. Does she need to have genetic testing?

Most children with well-controlled epilepsy or a recognizable epilepsy syndrome do not need genetic testing. However, if there are associated abnormalities like an abnormal skull shape or size, autism, low tone or global developmental delay, the yield of obtaining a positive result of the genetic testing increases. The genetic testing includes *karyotype*, which counts and looks at the chromosomes. Although this test is not very useful, it can pick up ring chromosomes, which can cause epilepsy. More commonly done tests include microarray *comparative genomic hybridization* (CGH) and epilepsy gene panels. The CGH looks for any missing (deletions) or double (duplications) genes. The results may be reported as normal, pathogenic (which means that the genetic change is the cause of the child's seizures and other symptoms), or variants of unknown significance. The latter need to be analyzed further by obtaining blood samples from both the parents to see if the genetic change seen in the child's sample is merely inherited from one of the parents or is new, or de novo.

The epilepsy gene panels include testing for specific gene mutations known to cause different types of seizures and may be ordered as specific panels (infantile epilepsy panel, JME panel) or comprehensive gene panels looking at hundreds of genes in one sample.

Whole exome sequencing, and now whole genome sequencing, is available as the next generation genetic testing in those cases that do not yield a positive result.

Q   How will finding a genetic cause change my child's treatment?

Although it is true that finding a genetic cause may not result in a "cure" for the child's epilepsy, there are multiple benefits of obtaining genetic work up.

Finding an exact cause for the child's delays or seizures relieves the parents from the burden of guilt or avoids further expensive and invasive diagnostic testing. Parents may be able to monitor for other associated illnesses of that particular syndrome or join support groups and research trials dealing with the particular genetic disease. Also, in some cases, finding a genetic cause has direct implications on the treatment. As an example, finding a mutation in a gene called SLC2 can lead to the diagnosis of glucose transporter deficiency and early institution of dietary treatment. Certain seizure medications, like lamotrigine or phenytoin, may worsen seizure control in sodium channel mutations or mitochondrial disorders. Finally, genetic counseling may be helpful in establishing carrier status for certain genetic conditions for future pregnancies for the parents or siblings.

CHAPTER 9

Concerns for Women with Epilepsy of All Ages

Women of all ages with epilepsy have special concerns. These concerns include the relationship of seizures and antiseizure medicines with pregnancy, menstruation, birth control, sexuality, fertility, polycystic ovary syndrome, perimenopause and menopause, and bone health. This chapter explores these concerns and provides some straight-forward answers to the most frequently asked questions.

Q **Is it common for epilepsy to start at puberty, when menses also start?**

Several types of seizure disorders often begin in the early teenage years when menstrual periods also begin for many young women. Two examples of epilepsy syndromes that start at this age include juvenile myoclonic epilepsy (JME) and juvenile absence epilepsy (JAE).

Q **Are the hormonal changes that happen during puberty the reason why seizures can begin at this time of life?**

Although JME is slightly more common in females than in males, there is no clear scientific evidence that gender-related reproductive hormones such as testosterone, estrogen, or progesterone are associated with the timing of the onset of these seizure types for either young women or men.

Q   Can the menstrual cycle affect seizure occurrence?

Yes, approximately one-third of women with epilepsy can have an increase in seizures at specific times of the month in relationship to their menstrual cycle. The term used for seizures that occur in relationship to the menstrual cycle is *catamenial epilepsy*. "Catamenial epilepsy refers only to the timing of the seizures and not to a specific seizure type or epilepsy syndrome. In fact, catamenial epilepsy can occur with all seizure types, including focal-onset and generalized-onset seizures. The most frequent timing of seizure exacerbation for women with a catamenial pattern is three days prior to menstrual bleeding through the first three days of menstrual flow. The second most common pattern is increased seizures around ovulation, in the middle of the menstrual cycle (approximately 14 days prior to the next menstrual period).

The times of seizure worsening for women with epilepsy of reproductive age is related to normal hormonal changes throughout the month. One of the main female reproductive hormones, *estrogen*, is active in the brain and has various functions in the brain. These functions include regulating reproductive and sexual activity, and maintaining the interconnectedness of brain cells. Estrogen is a hormone that generally excites brain activity and, therefore, is more seizure-promoting than seizure-preventing. On the other hand, the other main reproductive hormone for women, *progesterone*, tends to be calming and sedating. Progesterone, therefore, promotes inhibition of brain activity in general and it is thought that it can inhibit seizure activity as well. The timing of seizure occurrence in relationship to the menstrual cycle is probably related to normal fluctuations in these two hormones throughout the month. For example, progesterone levels decline dramatically just before menstrual onset, resulting in "progesterone withdrawal" effects on the brain. This progesterone withdrawal is thought to make women with epilepsy more likely to have seizures just prior to their period and through the first three days of bleeding. On the other hand, estrogen levels rise and reach a peak just before ovulation at the middle of the menstrual cycle. This "estrogen peak" is thought to influence the occurrence of seizures at mid cycle when ovulation occurs. Interestingly, women who have catamenial seizures may have improved seizure frequency when they are pregnant because of the hormonal changes in pregnancy.

Q   What treatments are available for catamenial seizure worsening?

There is no medicine specifically proven for catamenial seizure exacerbations. Interventions that have been tried for catamenial seizure patterns are discussed in the following.

Natural progesterone: Since the progesterone produced in the body has anti-seizure properties, progesterone has been used to prevent catamenial seizure exacerbations. Progesterone is more often used for obstetrical and gynecological purposes. Natural progesterone can be given in a pill (Prometrium) or a lozenge form to reach the levels needed in the brain to affect seizures. The use of natural progesterone to treat seizures has been studied in a randomized, double-blind, placebo-controlled multicenter clinical trial. The progesterone was added on to the baseline antiseizure medicine(s) for each woman. Progesterone was given as 200 mg lozenges three times per day beginning on day 14 of the menstrual cycle (13 days after the first day of menstrual bleeding) and continued until tapering, which occurred over menstrual days 26–28. The progesterone lozenges were stopped until the next menstrual cycle on day 14. A response to the treatment with a 50 percent reduction in seizures occurred only in the subset of women who had 3-fold or greater seizure frequency during the perimenstrual phase (days –3 to +3 of menses) compared to the other phases of their menstrual cycles. Although natural progesterone is the same hormone naturally produced in the body, there can still be side effects. These are generally mild and include sedation, depressed mood, breast tenderness, and vaginal spotting. Synthetic progesterone, used in most birth control pills and in hormone replacement therapy, does not prevent seizure activity in the same way as natural progesterone since it is not broken down to the same active neuroactive chemical, allopregnanolone, which directly binds to brain receptors to decrease seizures.

Increasing usual antiseizure medicines: Another possible approach to treating catamenial seizure exacerbations is to increase the dose of the antiseizure medicine already being taken at vulnerable times of the month. Usually, one antiseizure medicine is increased slightly for several days premenstrually.

Q **Can birth control methods that contain hormones (such as the birth control pill or hormonal IUD) be used for women who have epilepsy and who are taking antiseizure medicines?**

Hormonal contraception, such as the *birth control pill* (the pill), is the most common form of contraception used by women in the United States, including women with epilepsy. Neither the pill nor hormonal intrauterine devices (IUD) affect seizure control in a consistent manner. It has, however, been reported that oral contraceptive birth control pills have a higher failure rate and are associated with more unplanned pregnancies, when women are taking certain antiseizure medicines. In contrast, hormonal IUDs are not affected by antiseizure medicines. The failure rate of the oral contraceptive pill for women with epilepsy taking the antiseizure medicines listed in the first column in Table 9.1 is reported to be as high as 6 percent per year, compared to a failure rate in women not taking antiseizure medicines of around 1 percent per year. However, even with this increased rate of birth control failure with oral contraceptive pills, the chance of preventing pregnancy (94 percent) is better than with many other commonly used birth control methods, such as condoms, diaphragms, and the "rhythm method."

The antiseizure medicines listed in the first column of Table 9.1 lower the effectiveness of birth control pills because these medicines lower the level of the hormones in the birth control pills. This interaction needs to be considered when choosing both the antiseizure medicine and type of birth control. Women with epilepsy should discuss the best antiseizure medi-

TABLE 9.1 Antiseizure Medicines and Effects on Liver Enzyme Induction
The enzyme-inducers in the left-hand column can decrease the effectiveness of birth control pills and other hormonal contraceptives.

Enzyme-Inducers	Non-Inducers
phenobarbital	ethosuximide
phenytoin	valproate
carbamazepine	gabapentin
primidone	clonazepam
oxcarbazepine	tiagabine
perampanel	levetiracetam
topiramate	zonisamide
felbamate	pregabalin
eslicarbazepine	vigabatrin
clobazam	lacosamide
rufinamide	ezogabine
	clonazepam
	diazepam
	lorazepam
	lamotrigine*

*Lamotrigine has a mild effect on inducing the enzymes responsible for progestin metabolism and may lower the effectiveness of birth control pills and other hormonal contraceptives. Additionally, the metabolism of lamotrigine increases with estrogen-containing contraceptives.

cine and type of birth control with their neurologist/epilepsy specialist and gynecologist.

Women using one of the antiseizure medicines listed in the first column of Table 9.1, who need effective contraception, should consider these options: 1) avoid low-dose formulations of birth control pills and use a barrier method, such as a condom, diaphragm, or sponge, in combination with the pill, 2) use an IUD or Depo-Provera.

Other forms of hormonal contraception, such as the patch, vaginal ring, and the levonorgestrel implant likely also have the same interactions previously described, but they are not well studied. Intramuscular injections with medroxyprogesterone acetate (Depo-Provera) may have continued contraceptive effectiveness given that it is a relatively high dose of medroxyprogesterone acetate, but it has not been fully studied.

Many antiseizure medicines have no interactions with the birth control pill. However, blood levels of the antiseizure medicines lamotrigine and valproic acid are known to decrease with oral contraceptive pills that contain estrogen. The same is likely true for oxcarbazepine. Therefore, women taking these medicines will likely need to adjust their dose when they start using an estrogen-containing hormonal contraceptive, because they may be at risk for seizure occurrence as the antiseizure medicine level becomes lower. Likewise, when they come off an estrogen-containing hormonal contraceptive, they will need to adjust their antiseizure medicine dosage downward to prevent side effects.

The interactions between antiseizure medicines and hormonal contraceptive are listed in the following using the generic names.

Q   Can problems with sexual functioning occur in women with epilepsy?

The majority of women with epilepsy report normal satisfaction with their sexual lives. However, a larger than expected portion of women with epilepsy report very little interest in sex. The exact reasons for this are unclear; there may be anxiety about having a seizure in an intimate situation, for example. Women with epilepsy do report more anxiety about sexual situations than expected. Further, there is some evidence that the physical sexual response, such as vaginal lubrication, is decreased in women with epilepsy, but it is not known whether this is due to the epilepsy itself or particular antiseizure medicines, such as the enzyme-inducers.

Some antiseizure medicines have a known risk of causing problems with sexuality. These are primarily the sedative medications, phenobarbital and primidone. Sexual side effects have been reported with other antiseizure medicines, however, including phenytoin, carbamazepine, valproate, and gabapentin. The cause of sexual side effects for persons with epilepsy may be related to subtle effects of the antiseizure medicines on reproductive hormone levels, including the main hormone associated with sexual interest, testosterone. However, a direct effect of these medications on brain chemicals that regulate sexual activity may also be occurring.

For most women with epilepsy, sexual lives are normal, with the usual difficulties that many people face in a busy, stressful world. If sexuality is a problem, either interest in sex (libido) or ability to achieve orgasm (sexual functioning) should be brought up to the neurologist. The neurologist can consider changing the antiseizure medicine if the problem occurred in association with a specific medicine, as well as referral to a gynecologist or sexual therapist.

Q Do women with epilepsy have more risk of being infertile?

In some surveys, women with epilepsy were found to have lower rates of having children than their own siblings and the general population. This does not necessarily mean that women with epilepsy have *infertility*, which means a biologic inability to become pregnant. The reasons that women with epilepsy are having fewer children may be partly influenced by their own choice not to have children in the setting of having epilepsy and taking medicines. A recent study performed at U.S. academic epilepsy centers found that there were no differences in the ability to become pregnant, the time to achieve pregnancy, or the rate of miscarriage compared to healthy control women. Most of the women in this study, however, were on one or two antiseizure medicines that are not enzyme-inducers. Other studies performed in other countries or in the past do suggest that fertility may be lower in women on multiple antiseizure medications, especially if the regimen includes enzyme-inducing medications (Table 9.1). If a woman with epilepsy is having difficulty getting pregnant after trying for more than 6 months, she should seek guidance from her gynecologist regarding an infertility evaluation.

Q Will seizure activity change during perimenopause and menopause?

Available information suggests that perimenopause, when women begin to have irregular menses and hot flashes, may be a time of risk for more seizures. The hormonal changes of early perimenopause, when the estrogen levels are generally higher than the progesterone levels, may explain why this is a vulnerable time for women with epilepsy. However, the good news is that women with epilepsy may have a decrease in their seizures when they complete menopause and become post-menopausal. Both of these effects are more likely to occur if a woman previously had a catamenial seizure pattern during her reproductive years, and they suggest that these women in particular are sensitive to hormonal fluctuations.

Women with epilepsy, particularly those who have had frequent seizures in their lifetime, may experience an earlier than expected age at menopause. The usual age at which menstruation ceases is 50–51 years. It has been found that women with frequent seizures may experience a slightly earlier age at which their menstruation ceases, around age 46–47 years. The cause of this is unknown, but it may be due to effects of seizures on the parts of the brain that regulate reproductive functioning.

Q Can women with epilepsy use hormone replacement therapy?

The risks of long-term hormone replacement therapy for women in general include a small increased risk of breast cancer, and of cardiovascular disease and stroke. Therefore, the use of the most common type of hormone replacement therapy, *conjugated equine estrogen combined with medroxyprogesterone acetate* (CEE/MPA or Prempro), has been drastically reduced. Some women have severe and disabling hot flashes during perimenopause and postmenopause. These hot flashes can be relieved by estrogen replacement. Some women will be placed on hormone replacement therapy for a short period, so they do not become too sleep deprived, which will allow them function normally every day. Sleep deprivation caused by hot flashes can also increase the risk of seizures for women with epilepsy. This needs to be balanced against a potential risk of hormone replacement therapy increasing seizure frequency in some women. Worsening of seizure frequency with use of CEE/MPA has been demonstrated in one small study of menopausal women with epilepsy. Treatments other than estrogen replacement therapy can be used for treatment of symptoms, such as hot flashes, and can be considered by the primary care physician/gynecologist.

Q   Is bone health the same in women with epilepsy as other women of the same age?

In addition to the risk of fractures from seizure-related trauma, osteopenia and osteoporosis are more prevalent in women on enzyme inducing antiseizure medicines (Table 9.1). The physiological explanation is that liver enzyme induction accelerates vitamin D metabolism to inactive metabolites and, in addition, it lowers estradiol levels. There is a gradation, however, among enzyme-inducing medicines, with some, such as phenobarbital and phenytoin, being more consistently associated with decreased bone-mineral density.

Q   What are special considerations for pregnancy in women with epilepsy?

Epilepsy is the most common neurologic disorder that requires continuous treatment during pregnancy. Although there are risks due to seizures and antiseizure medicines during pregnancy, over 90 percent of babies born to women with epilepsy will be healthy. Seizure control is essential, and most women will need to be maintained on an antiseizure medicine during pregnancy. The emphasis of current medical practitioners and researchers in this field is how to minimize risks of these medicines to a level that is close to that of the general population (women on no medicines and no underlying illness). In the general population, there is still a 1.6–3.2 percent rate of birth defects in newborns. In infants born to women with epilepsy on antiseizure medicines, the overall combined birth defect rate is higher, but it is now known to be quite low on specific antiseizure medicines and particularly high on others (see the following section and Table 9.2).

The birth defects that require surgery and/or can significantly affect the child's life are called major congenital malformations. The ones most commonly associated with antiseizure medicine exposure include congenital heart defects, cleft lip or cleft palate, defects of the kidney and genital structures, skeletal limb defects, and neural tube defects of the lower spine (often spina bifida). *Spina bifida* can cause the infant not to have strength in their legs and possibly not have control of their urine or bowel movements. The abnormal closure of the neural tube to cause neural tube defects occurs between the third and fourth weeks of pregnancy. *It is important to remember that by the time a woman realizes she is pregnant, it is often too late to make medication adjustments as these key structures have already begun forming.*

Other possible increased risks of children born to women with epilepsy, on at least some of the antiseizure medicines, include intrauterine growth retardation, cognitive dysfunction, and microcephaly. Ideally, antiseizures medicines and vitamin supplementations should be reviewed prior to pregnancy to minimize risks to the developing fetus. Supplemental folic acid beginning prior to conception and continuing throughout pregnancy has been shown to reduce the risk of birth defects and negative neurodevelopmental outcomes. Many doctors will ask all their female patients to get into the habit of taking supplemental folic acid once they reach their reproductive years.

Another consideration is if the antiseizure medicines can be reduced to just one antiseizure medicine (monotherapy) that has ample safety data for use during pregnancy (Table 9.2). Sometimes, the dose can even be reduced going into a planned pregnancy to reduce the risk even further. Any treatment regimen should be considered against the backdrop of which medicines are needed to control the individual woman's seizures. If one anti-seizure medicine with a good teratogenic profile cannot control a

TABLE 9.2 Prevalence of Major Malformations for Each Antiseizure Medicine Taken Alone as Monotherapy in the First Trimester, with 95 Percent Confidence Intervals

Drug	N (sample size for each medication)	%	95% CI
Lamotrigine	1994	2.1	(1.7 to 2.8%)
Carbamazepine	1094	3.0	(2.1 to 4.2%)
Levetiracetam	769	2.0	(1.1 to 3.2%)
Topiramate	451	4.4	(2.7 to 6.8%)
Phenytoin	422	2.8	(1.5 to 4.9%)
Valproate	336	8.9	(6.1 to 12.5%)
Oxcarbazepine	230	1.7	(0.5 to 4.4%)
Phenobarbital	202	5.9	(3.1 to 10.2%)
Gabapentin	169	1.2	(0.14 to 4.2%)
Zonisamide	136	1.5	(0.2 to 5.2%)
Clonazepam	87	2.3	(0.3 to 8.1%)
Internal Control*	532	1.5	(0.47 to 2.5%)
External Control**	69277	1.6	(1.5 to 1.7%)

*Internal controls are women not on any antiseizure medicine during pregnancy and were enrolled through the pregnancy registry.

**External controls include women from the Active Malformations Surveillance Program, and Brigham and Women's Hospital in Boston.

Source: North American AED Pregnancy Registry. Winter 2016 newsletter.

woman's seizures adequately, sometimes two medicines are used in combination to avoid a medicine with a known higher risk to the developing fetus. Obtaining a blood level of the antiseizure medicine prior to pregnancy is also useful as a baseline to maintain during pregnancy.

The best path to a healthy pregnancy is a planned pregnancy with an open dialogue among the patient, the doctor prescribing the antiseizure medicines, and the obstetrician. This dialogue should include a review of the latest findings about specific anti-seizure medicines during pregnancy, and the use of supplemental folic acid and/or prenatal vitamins. A planned pregnancy requires effective birth control. As discussed earlier in this chapter, there are potential interactions between some of the antiseizure medicines and birth control, as well as suggestions of how to help counteract this by using different types of birth control.

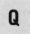 **Q**   ## Which antiseizure medicines may be of higher risk than others?

Researchers have made great progress in determining which anti-seizures medicines are of higher risk to the developing fetus than other medicines. Information from pregnancy registries has helped to define risks of certain seizure medicines when used alone as monotherapy. The risk for birth defects is now known to be quite low on specific antiseizure medicines (e.g., levetiracetam and lamotrigine) (Table 9.2). Conversely, valproic acid/sodium valproate has been shown in multiple different studies, and performed in various geographic regions, to be associated with particularly high rates of birth defects. It should be avoided unless it is the only medicine that controls seizures for a particular woman after trying other medicines. Many of the antiseizure medicines do not have enough data to know if they are of low or high risk during pregnancy. Even fewer combinations of anti-seizure medicines (polytherapy) have been studied. For example, studies recently showed that combining levetiracetam with lamotrigine is not associated with a high risk for birth defects. This may be a preferred option to the use of valproic acid. However, in one study, the rate of major malformations increased to 25 percent for those women on 4 or more antiseizure medicines. Any desired change in antiseizure medicine regimen should be achieved during the preconception planning phase.

Intrauterine Growth Retardation

Intrauterine growth retardation has been associated with some antiseizure medicines, resulting in higher rates of small-for-gestational-age births (topiramate, zonisamide, and phenobarbital) and low-birth weight infants (topiramate). Lower birth weights have been associated with long-term medical risks. Some obstetricians choose to perform serial ultrasounds during pregnancy to assess fetal growth.

Neurodevelopmental Outcome

Studies suggest that some children born to women with epilepsy on seizure medicines during pregnancy are at higher risk of developmental delay and lower verbal abilities. A variety of factors may contribute to this, but different studies have shown a consistently higher risk for valproic acid for lower IQ, lower verbal abilities, and autism and autism spectrum disorder. Conversely, neurodevelopmental studies have shown favorable outcomes following in utero exposure to carbamazepine and lamotrigine. Many other antiseizure medicines have not been fully studied. Use of multiple antiseizure medicines (polytherapy) may increase the risk compared to monotherapy, but this is still unclear and under study. Other contributors can be convulsive seizures during pregnancy. Exposure to the antiseizure medicines during all three trimesters can have effects on the developing fetal brain. Beginning folic acid prior to conception and continuing throughout pregnancy has been shown to be beneficial to child IQ.

Microcephaly

Microcephaly (small head size) has been associated with in utero antiseizure medicine exposure. Studies suggest that the risk for microcephaly is increased for polytherapy, phenobarbital, and primidone (Mysoline).

Risk for Epilepsy

Children of women with epilepsy are at slightly higher risk of developing epilepsy at some point in their lifetime, but the risk is still <10 percent for all children of women with epilepsy, a 2.5-fold increased risk compared to a child without a family history. The risk, however, varies substantially with the many different epilepsy syndromes.

Seizures During Pregnancy

The effect of pregnancy on seizure frequency is variable and unpredictable among patients. The majority of women with epilepsy will not show a change in their seizure control, and seizures are even more likely to stay controlled if a woman was seizure-free in the 9 or 12 months prior to pregnancy. Pregnancy is associated with several physiologic and psychologic changes that can alter seizure frequency, including changes in sex hormone concentrations, changes in drug metabolism, sleep deprivation, and new stresses. Noncompliance with medications can occur during pregnancy due to the strong message that any drugs during pregnancy are harmful to the fetus. However, the risks of anti-seizure medicines are well known, and risks to the fetus are often exaggerated or misrepresented. Proper education about the risks of medicines versus the risks of seizures can be very helpful in assuring women take their antiseizure medicines as prescribed during pregnancy.

During pregnancy, the risk of seizures to the developing fetus is of primary importance. Convulsive (generalized tonic-clonic) seizures can cause low-oxygen levels in the mother and fetus—signs of fetal distress—and have been reported to cause loss of the pregnancy in rare cases. Many types of seizures can cause trauma, which can result in rupture of the membranes protecting the fetus, premature labor, and even fetal death. Extra precautionary measures may need to be taken to minimize risk to the fetus of what could otherwise seem to be a trivial injury.

Management of a woman's antiseizure medicines during pregnancy can be complex. Blood concentrations of almost all the antiseizure medicines decrease during pregnancy due to changes in the body's composition and metabolism. Some studies have examined the effects of the changes in the medicine clearance and demonstrate that monthly monitoring of the antiseizure medicine blood levels and adjustments in dose during pregnancy is very important. It can prevent the medicine level from decreasing too much below the individual's non-pregnant baseline level and helps prevent seizure worsening. Clearance of most of the antiseizure medicines normalizes over the first few weeks to months postpartum.

Labor and Delivery

Most women with epilepsy will have a safe vaginal delivery without sei-zure occurrence. Only a small fraction of women with epilepsy will have seizures during labor or in the first few days after delivery. The presence of epilepsy and use of antiseizure medicines do not limit the options available to women for their type of delivery or plan for use of pain control measures.

Postpartum Care

Most infants of women with epilepsy can successfully breastfeed with-out complications. For most antiseizure medicines, the concentrations in breast milk are considerably less than those in the mother's blood and what the fetus was exposed to in the womb. The benefits of breastfeeding are believed to outweigh the small risk of the antiseizure medicines. Women should discuss the decision to breastfeed with all doctors, including obste-trician, neurologist/epilepsy specialist, and baby's pediatrician. Not all doctors are well informed about antiseizure medicines and breastfeeding, and they may provide the mother with different information.

The newborn and its inevitable sleep-disruption can be a time of sei-zure worsening and may even provoke seizure recurrence for women with previously controlled seizures. Extra precautions should be taken during this time. If a particular woman is likely to drop objects she is holding, but remains upright during her seizures, such as with myoclonic seizures or many complex partial seizures, then she should use a harness when car-rying the baby. If she is likely to fall, then a stroller within the house is an even better option. Changing diapers and clothes are best performed on the floor, rather than on an elevated changing table. Bathing of the baby should never be performed alone, as a brief lapse in attention can result in a fatal drowning. The new mother should also avoid tub baths without another adult around and/or the door locked. The important role that sleep-deprivation plays in worsening seizures needs to be consid-ered, especially if the mother is breastfeeding, as sleep-deprivation may be unavoidable. The possibility of other adults sharing the burden of night-time feedings with formula or harvested breastmilk should be considered, and the mother should attempt to make up any missed sleep during the infant's daytime naps.

In summary, although women with epilepsy on antiseizure medicines can have increased risks during pregnancy, these risks can be considerably reduced with effective birth control and planning prior to pregnancy, choosing antiseizure medicines with known information about low risk for birth defects and adverse neurodevelopmental consequences, beginning supplemental folic acid prior to and continuing during pregnancy, careful management of antiseizure medicine dosing during pregnancy and the postpartum period, and close communication and well-coordinated care with the obstetrics team.

FREQUENTLY ASKED QUESTIONS

Q   **How can pregnancy affect my seizures?**

Most women will not see a change in their seizures. It is important to take your antiseizure medicine as prescribed by your doctor and not to miss any doses. Even if you take all your doses of medicine during pregnancy, the concentrations of seizure medicines in your bloodstream may change or decrease, putting you at greater risk for seizures. Your physician will need to check blood levels of your medicine more often, and they may need to adjust your dose. The first two months after delivery are another important time when your hormones and your body chemistry may change, affecting levels of your antiseizure medicine. Check with your doctor about dose adjustments or extra lab work that may be necessary.

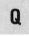 **Q**   **I have received conflicting information about the safety of medicines during pregnancy and breastfeeding. What should I believe?**

This is a difficult question. The risks of antiseizure medicines during pregnancy and breastfeeding are often exaggerated, even by physicians. The Internet is a great source of information, but not all the information is reviewed for scientific accuracy. Similarly, your pharmacist can provide you information from the *Physicians' Desk Reference* (PDR), which is essentially a compiled set of package inserts that represent limited information in many cases. Many articles and books are typically 1–2 years behind the available research information. The references on the websites listed in the checklist at the end of this chapter include some of the most reputable and current sources of information. Please remember that none of these sources take into account your individual situation and the severity of the illness. It is important to discuss this with the doctor prescribing your antiseizure medicine.

Q **I just found out that I am pregnant and I am taking anti-seizure medicines. What should I do?**

First, don't panic! The risks of antiseizure medicines are relatively modest, and exposure has already occurred. If you were to stop your medicine(s) suddenly, your seizures could be longer and more severe than any that you have experienced before. This puts you and your pregnancy at much higher risk than the medicines you are taking. Do let the doctor prescribing your medicine know right away to make sure your dose, your medicine regimen, and your supplemental vitamins are ideal for pregnancy. Also, establish care by an obstetrician early in your pregnancy for close follow-up during pregnancy, including planning for a detailed, structural ultrasound. Some obstetricians may choose to perform ultrasounds more frequently than once.

Q **Should I stop my antiseizure medicine before I get pregnant?**

This is a complicated decision. Pregnancy without antiseizure medicines may lessen some of the possible risks to the baby in very specific cases.

Discuss with your doctor whether you are a candidate to come off medicines if you have not had seizures for several years. Most adult women cannot come off antiseizure medicines safely, and the danger of seizures to both the mother and the child is a serious one. Seizures can result in falls or in lack of oxygen for the baby. They can increase the risk of miscarriage or stillbirths. For most women with epilepsy, staying on medicine poses less risk to their own health and the health of their babies than discontinuing medicine. In most cases, a single antiseizure medicine at the lowest possible dose that provides seizure control is the best option.

The North American Antiepileptic Drug Pregnancy Registry

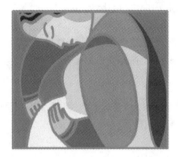

If you are pregnant, and take antiepileptic drugs (AEDs), please call TOLL FREE (1-888) 233-2334 or contact them through the following website: http://www.aedpregnancyregistry.org/.

What is the purpose of the Registry?

At present, we lack complete information about the relative safety of specific antiseizure medicines, also known as antiepileptic drugs (AEDs), during pregnancy. Pregnant women, who are taking seizure medicines, can enroll in the Registry over the telephone. This will help them find answers to their questions. As more women register and report the outcome of their pregnancy, the researchers of this Registry will be able to identify the safest medicines for seizures during pregnancy.

When should I call the Registry?

As early in your pregnancy as possible. It is best to enroll during your first trimester, but you can still participate if you are already in your second or third trimester.

How do I register?

By calling toll free (1-888) 233-2334.

There are only 3 telephone interviews:

1. The first call is the longest and can take up to 12 minutes.
2. The registry will then call you when you are 7 months pregnant (this is only a 5-minute call).
3. The registry will call you again after your baby is born (this is only a 5-minute call).

Your identity will remain confidential!

Checklist for Women with Epilepsy
Planning or During a Pregnancy

Pre-Conception (Prior to Pregnancy)

- In addition to your seizure medication(s), you should be taking the following medications daily, as suggested by your doctor:
  1. Multivitamins or prenatal vitamins
  2. Folic acid 0.4–5 mg(s)
- Discuss with your doctor that you are planning a pregnancy. Tell him/her you want to transition to the best medicine regimen for the safety of you and your developing child.
- Additional resources: Epilepsy Foundation brochures, and websites:
  - http://www.epilepsy.com
  - http://www.aedpregnancyregistry.org

Pregnancy

- For the duration of your pregnancy, you should be taking the following medications daily, as prescribed by your doctor:
  1. Multivitamins or prenatal vitamins
  2. Folic acid 0.4–5 mg(s)
- The level of antiseizure medicine in your blood may decrease during pregnancy. It is recommended that you discuss with your doctor regular monitoring of your drug levels during pregnancy.
- The dose of your antiseizure medicines may be changed based on the results of your lab tests, the worsening of your seizures, or the side effects of the medicine.
- It is very important not to miss any doses. If you have problems with vomiting within 30 minutes of taking your antiseizure medicine, ask your doctor if you should repeat the dose.

- Plan on good prenatal care with your obstetrics team. This will include a detailed, structural ultrasound at 16–20 weeks gestation.
- Choose a pediatrician at least 1 month prior to your due date and discuss your plans for breastfeeding.
- Discuss a birth plan with both your obstetrician and the doctor who is prescribing your antiseizure medicine.

Day of Delivery

- Take a copy of your birth plan from your seizure doctor to the hospital. Notify your seizure doctor of your delivery to help manage any complications of changes in your seizures or in the effects of your medicine.
- Take your antiseizure medicines as directed. Do not miss any doses in the hospital during labor, delivery, or postpartum.
- Bring an extra supply of your antiseizure medicine with you to the hospital.
- Following delivery, you may be asked to decrease your antiseizure medicine.

***If your seizures get worse during your pregnancy, please call your doctor. If you have a convulsive seizure, you should contact your obstetrician. You may need to go to the Emergency Room.

CHAPTER 10

Sleep and Epilepsy

- Patients with epilepsy are at higher risk for sleep disorders than the general population.
- Lack of sleep can cause seizures and make epilepsy more difficult to treat.
- Some seizures are more likely to occur during sleep.
- Sudden unexpected death in epilepsy (SUDEP) is more likely to occur during sleep.

Successful treatment of sleep disorders may decrease seizure frequency and reduce risk for SUDEP.

Sleep and epilepsy have a strong relationship. It has long been appreciated that sleep deprivation can lead to seizure, but also that sleep itself can provoke seizure. Sleep is essential and should occur nightly as a part of a restorative process for the body. The amount of sleep one needs varies by age and can be impacted by lifestyle factors and illness. Some people can experience seizures only in relation to sleep, either during sleep, as one falls asleep, or as one wakes from sleep. Sleep fragmentation or reduced number of hours asleep can result in an increase in seizures. Sleep disorders, such as obstructive sleep apnea, insomnia, or restless leg syndrome can cause too little sleep and non-refreshing sleep. People with epilepsy who also have a sleep disorder are at risk for poor seizure control. In fact, it has been found that patients with epilepsy are at higher risk for sleep disorders, which may contribute negatively to their epilepsy care. It is critical to evaluate all patients with epilepsy for symptoms of a sleep disorder. If present, it is important to determine the correct diagnosis and start an effective treatment for the sleep disorder, as part of an epilepsy care plan.

Physiology of Sleep

Sleep Basics

Sleep is frequently viewed as a temporary state of inactivity where the body and mind shut down. However, it is quite the opposite, as sleep actively contributes to growth and development, restoration, as well as learning and memory consolidation. Sleep is a dynamic state for the brain, as it cycles through the different stages of sleep every 90–120 minutes (Figure 10.1).

The *sleep-wake cycle* is a tightly regulated process dependent on two processes: the homeostatic sleep drive and the circadian rhythm. The *homeostatic sleep drive* is the body's natural desire toward falling asleep. This process is dependent on the brain to signal the need to return to sleep. This starts in the morning, and the signal becomes stronger as the day goes on.

The *circadian rhythm* is our body's day/night clock that cycles over about 24 hours. It is controlled by a part of the brain called the *suprachiasmatic nucleus*. The homeostatic sleep drive and the circadian rhythm are influenced by a person's genetics, but they are also influenced by exposure to things like stress, medications, napping, or exercise.

During the day, the homeostatic sleep drive promotes the need to fall asleep as the day goes on. This desire to sleep, however, is countered by the circadian rhythms' drive to maintain wakefulness. Generally, the homeostatic drive and circadian rhythm are relatively balanced during the day, resulting in being able to stay awake and function normally. During the early evening hours, as the day becomes darker, the circadian rhythm reduces wakefulness stimulation and begins to promote the need to sleep by producing melatonin. *Melatonin* is a hormone that promotes sleepiness, which is produced in the brain (pineal gland) in response to the eye's perception of decreasing daylight. Now both the homeostatic sleep and the circadian rhythm are directed toward sleep promotion, resulting in unopposed sleepiness (Figure 10.1). Pictorially, this point marks the greatest

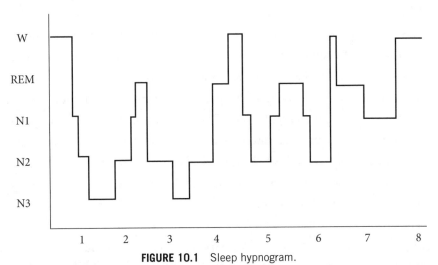

FIGURE 10.1 Sleep hypnogram.
A sleep hypnogram is a way of showing how a person sleeps in the night and how much time is spent in each stage of sleep. Typically, the hypnogram will show that a person cycles through the different stages of Non-REM and REM sleep every 90–120 minutes.

difference between the homeostatic drive to sleep and the circadian drive for arousal. It is considered the *sleep gate*, as it is the entrance to falling asleep. During nighttime sleep, the need for sleep is replenished and the homeostatic sleep drive is rapidly reduced. On the other hand, the circadian-regulated melatonin production continues and helps maintain sleep until the early morning. Once melatonin production stops, the circadian rhythm again increases its wake-promoting activity again. A person will then awaken once the circadian drive for arousal is greater than the drive for sleep.

Although the sleep-wake cycle is tightly regulated by the interaction of the circadian rhythm and homeostatic sleep drive, it can be influenced by external factors. It is not uncommon for sleep disruption to occur due to these variables and, therefore, it should be considered when discussing sleep. Lifestyle factors, such as meal times, naps, stress, and exercise can serve as cues that may shift either the circadian rhythm or reduce sleep inertia. In addition, willful behavior, such as resistance to sleep, can result in sleep-wake schedule changes as well.

There are four stages of sleep, which include rapid eye movement (REM) sleep, non-REM 1 (N1), non-REM 2 (N2), and non-REM 3 (N3). These sleep stages are characterized by findings on an electroencephalogram (EEG), the same brain wave test that evaluates for seizure. *Stage N1* is considered a transitional or light sleep, and it is characterized by slowing of the wake EEG waveforms. Stage N1 generally accounts for about 2 percent to 5 percent of the total night's sleep. *Stage N2* is a deeper stage of sleep and is characterized again by a slower frequency waveform. However, Stage N2 becomes more synchronized and is marked by the presence of specific sleep waveforms, rhythmic sleep spindles, and sharply contoured waveforms, called vertex waves and K-complexes. This is the most abundant stage of sleep and accounts for 45 percent to 55 percent of the total night's sleep. *Stage N3* sleep is also known as *slow-wave sleep (SWS)* because of the high voltage, very slow waveforms present during this stage of sleep. Slow-wave sleep generally occurs more in the first third of the night and accounts for from 5 percent to 15 percent of the total night's sleep. Slow-wave sleep is considered the restorative form of sleep, as time spent in stage N3 increases when there is prior sleep deprivation or sleep debt. REM sleep is characterized by EEG findings of low-voltage, mixed frequency waveform with evidence of complete loss of muscle tone and rapid eye movements, hence the name. It accounts for about 20 percent to 25 percent of total sleep time. It occurs in 4 to 5 episodes throughout the night with progressive lengthening of time spent in REM throughout the night.

Sleep duration varies across the ages. In infancy, there is only broadly REM and non-REM sleep, or active and quiet sleep, without further differentiation. Sleep architecture evolves with age, and distinct stages of sleep that are similar to adults develop by approximately 1 year. Hours of sleep per day and time spent in each stage of sleep also continue to evolve. In the elderly, there is a decrease of time spent in stage N3, with a compensatory increase in the time spent in stage N1 and N2. Also, time spent awake increases with older age due to a prolonged time to fall asleep, as well as an increase in the number and duration of overnight arousals.

The amount of sleep needed is an age-dependent factor that likely represents a developmental phenomenon of growth and brain maturation (Table 10.1). The newborn (ages 0–3 months) generally requires 14 to 17 hours in the course of a 24-hour day, which is broken down between shorter daytime naps and a longer nocturnal slumber. Infants (ages 4 to 11 months) should have between 12 to 15 hours, toddlers (ages 1 to 2 years) 11 to 14 hours, and pre-school age children 10–13 hours of sleep, with a progressive reduction in daytime napping time and increase in consolidated time spent asleep overnight. Most children should be without a need for a daytime nap by age 5. There continues to be a decrease in sleep need over time with school-age children (ages 6 to 13 years) requiring about 9 to 11 hours, teenagers (ages 14 to 17 years) requiring 8 to 10 hours, adults (ages 18 to 64 years) requiring 7 to 8 hours and the elderly (age > 65 years) only requiring 7 to 8 hours, but they may need as little as 5 to 6 hours of sleep.

TABLE 10.1   Sleep Hours by Age

Stage	Age	Average Sleep Need (hours)	Minimum Sleep Need (hours)	Maximum Sleep need (hours)	Distribution of Sleep over 24 hours
Newborn	0–3 months	14–17	11–13	18–19	Several short day naps (minutes up to 1–2 hours) Long night sleep (several hours at a time with waking for feeding)
Infant	4–11 months	12–15	10–11	16–18	Several short day naps (minutes up to 1–2 hour; Reduced number and length of naps) Long night sleep (waking for feeding; increased time between feedings; may sleep entire night)
Toddler	1–2 years	11–14	9–10	15–16	1–2 day naps (Reduced number and length of naps) Long night sleep (may sleep entire night, but waking 1–2x for feeding can be normal)
Preschool	3–5 years	10–13	8–9	14	Decreased to no day naps (occasional napping still normal) Consolidated night time sleep
Pre-Teen	6-13 years	9-10	7-8	12	Consolidated night time sleep
Teenager	14-17 years	8-10	7	11	Consolidated night time sleep (may have delayed sleep onset)*
Young Adult	18-25 years	7-9	6	10-11	Consolidated night time sleep
Adult	26-64 years	7-9	6	10	Consolidated night time sleep
Elderly	>/= 65 years	7-8	5-6	9	Consolidated night time sleep (may have early sleep onset)*

* Delayed and Early onset sleep may be a normal biologic shift in circadian rhythm

Why Do We Sleep?

Sleep is an essential physiologic process with its necessity being best demonstrated in the setting of sleep deprivation, evidenced by symptoms of fatigue, poor concentration, impaired memory, and overall poor performance, as well as an increased risk for illness and even death. The exact details of why we sleep continues to be researched, however, the working theories include beneficial effects on energy utilization, learning and memory, growth, development and restoration.

Sleep and Epilepsy

Sleep, especially NREM sleep, can activate the electrical charges in the brain that can result in seizures (Table 10.2) and this may be related to the intense neuronal synchrony that occurs among different parts of the brain. On the other hand, sleep deprivation can also result in an increase in sei-

TABLE 10.2 Effects of Sleep Stages on Epilepsy

Sleep Stage	Protective Effect	Provoking Effect	Risk of Seizure*
N1			↑↑↑
N2		Synchronization of EEG Activation of IEDs Generalization of IEDS Increased likelihood of seizure	↑↑↑↑↑
N3			↑↑
REM	Desynchronization of EEG Suppression of IEDs Decreased likelihood of seizures	More localized IEDs	↑↓

* ↑—increase risk; ↑↓—equivocal to protective risk; IED—interictal discharges; EEG—electroencephalogram

zure activity seen both clinically and on EEG. In fact, research has shown that up to 45 percent of people with epilepsy have seizures that occur either predominantly or exclusively during sleep or due to sleep deprivation. This is why EEGs are frequently performed after sleep deprivation, and they try to capture sleep and wakefulness. In addition, seizures can follow the circadian rhythm (Table 10.3), resulting in a subset of sleep-related epilepsies. Healthy sleep can be compromised by nocturnal seizures, but it may also be affected by the medications used to treat seizures. It is important to examine sleep in patients with epilepsy, as this is a high-risk period of time for experiencing sudden unexpected death in epilepsy (SUDEP).

TABLE 10.3   Circadian Influence on Seizures

Wakefulness	Arousal from Sleep	During Sleep
Absence Epilepsy Clonic Seizure Atonic Seizure Myoclonic Seizure Temporal Lobe Seizures	Juvenile Myoclonic Epilepsy Infantile Spasms (West Syndrome) Generalized Tonic-Clonic Seizures Tonic Seizures	BECTS* Frontal Lobe Seizures (including ADNFLE*) Landau Kleffner Syndrome Lennox Gastaut Syndrome ESES* Parietal Lobe Seizures Benign Occipital Epilepsy

*ADNFLE—autosomal dominant nocturnal frontal lobe epilepsy; BECTS—benign epilepsy with centrotemporal spikes (aka, benign Rolandic epilepsy); ESES—electrical status epilepticus in slow-wave sleep

Sleep-Related Epilepsies

Infantile Spasms (West Syndrome)

Infantile spasms is a catastrophic epilepsy syndrome that usually develops between the ages of 2 months and 2 years with clinical features of epileptic flexor and/or extensor spasms of the body and a specific EEG finding called *hypsarrythmia.* It may also be termed *West Syndrome* if it consists of the triad of epileptic flexor/extensor spasms of the body, intellectual disability, and the finding of hypsarrythmia on EEG. These spasms or tonic seizures tend to cluster on awakening in the morning. Additionally, at the onset of the disorder, the finding of hypsarrythmia on EEG first develops in NREM sleep.

Benign Occipital Lobe Epilepsy

Benign occipital lobe epilepsy (BOLE) (aka Panayiotopoulos Syndrome) is an epilepsy syndrome that generally occurs in children between ages 2 and 6 years, with remission generally occurring within 2 years from onset. Hallmark features of this syndrome include prolonged periods of eye deviation and autonomic (i.e., temperature, heart rate, respiration, blood pressure) instability. Seizures include one-sided (hemiconvulsive) seizure or generalized tonic-clonic seizures in sleep, with vomiting on awakening. EEG performed in-between seizure episodes show spikes in the occipital region. EEG performed during a seizure show the seizure activity in the occipital region during sleep.

Electrical Status Epilepticus in Slow-Wave Sleep

Electrical status epilepticus in slow-wave sleep (ESES) is an interesting epilepsy syndrome with sleep-specific EEG abnormalities, described as prolonged epileptiform activity occurring during the majority of the non-REM sleep. This syndrome typically begins around ages 4 to 5 years in children with evidence of developmental regression, primarily affecting language. There may also be symptoms of cognitive decline and mental retardation. The seizure activity seen on EEG becomes nearly continuous during NREM sleep and can even obscure the distinction between sleep stages. Clinically seizures may be partial or generalized events, occurring more in sleep.

Landau-Kleffner Syndrome

Landau-Kleffner syndrome (LKS) (aka acquired epileptic aphasia) is a pediatric epilepsy syndrome with clinical similarity to ESES. It affects children, typically beginning around ages 3 to 8 years, and results in language regression and/or *verbal auditory agnosia,* the inability to identify sounds. Clinical seizure may not be a significant feature seen in these patients, as only about 70 percent may have clinical seizure and up to a third may only have an isolated clinical seizure. Sleep is an activating state for EEG abnormalities in these patients and, at times, the abnormality is seen only in sleep recordings. It may even have continuous spike-and-wave activity during sleep, as is seen in ESES.

Benign Epilepsy with Centro-Temporal Spikes

Benign epilepsy with centro-temporal spikes (BECTS) (aka benign rolandic epilepsy) is the most common focal onset epilepsy syndrome in children and is predominantly symptomatic during sleep. In fact, more than half of children with BECTS have seizures exclusively during sleep. Typically, BECTS presents between 3 and 13 years old, with partial seizure described as paraesthesias, and tonic or clonic activity of the lower face, associated with drooling and dysarthria, generally occurring during sleep. EEG abnormalities are increased during sleep. It is called *benign* because most patients grow out of the epilepsy syndrome by age 13 years.

Lennox-Gastaut Syndrome

Lennox-Gastaut syndrome (LGS) is a seizure disorder that generally starts in childhood and has several different types of seizures. The most common findings in the syndrome are tonic seizures, a finding on the EEG called slow spike and wave, and cognitive impairment. Tonic seizures in LGS are frequently triggered by sleep. These seizures may occur frequently throughout the night with an increase in frequency during lighter sleep (Non-REM) sleep, but they stop during deep (REM) sleep.

Autosomal Dominant Nocturnal Frontal Lobe Epilepsy

Autosomal dominant nocturnal frontal lobe epilepsy (ADNFLE) is an inheritable epilepsy syndrome with onset in adolescence or young adulthood, generally with a family history of nocturnal seizure. Seizure descriptions may include sudden awakenings with abnormal movements, complex behaviors, or even sleep-related violent behavior. These frequently may be misidentified as a parasomnia (see the section on parasomnias). This can be further complicated by the fact that about one-third of these patients can also have non-REM parasomnia, such as sleep walking, sleep talking, or confusional arousals.

Anti-Epileptic Therapies and Sleep

Excessive daytime sleepiness (EDS) is common in patients with epilepsy, affecting about half of the patients, and it is frequently attributed to antiepileptic medication. *EDS* is a medical term used to describe feeling too tired during the day and can have a negative impact on mood, focusing, and ability to feel able to function normally. EDS can be a side effect of antiepileptic drugs (AEDs) that is frequently related to the dosing, but it may also be related to disruption of the normal sleep pattern due to the medications' effects on sleep staging and co-morbid sleep disorders. For instance, some AEDs may improve sleep by decreasing the time to fall asleep and number of nocturnal awakenings, but others, such as phenytoin, can increase awakenings and disturb sleep quality. AEDs can also alter the time spent in various sleep stages. For instance, benzodiazepines can increase NREM sleep and shorten REM sleep, while gabapentin and pregablin can increase stage N3 specifically.

In addition, therapeutic interventions may also negatively impact co-morbid sleep disorders. For instance, benzodiazepines and barbiturates have sedating properties that may cause relaxation of muscles, including muscles in the airway. This may cause more episodes of breathing difficulty and, therefore, worse sleep apnea. Insomnia symptoms can be the result of treatment with felbamate or lamotrigine. Vagus nerve stimulation, which may be used to treat AED-resistant epilepsies, can worsen the severity of obstructive sleep apnea.

Sudden Unexpected Death in Epilepsy

Sudden unexpected death in epilepsy (SUDEP) is defined as a death that occurs in an individual with epilepsy that occurs suddenly and unexpected, and there is no history or evidence of trauma, drowning, anatomic, or toxicologic cause. It is estimated to account for up to 15 percent of deaths in adult patients and up to 4 percent of deaths in children with epilepsy. The exact cause is unknown. However, it is observed that sleep appears to represent a significant risk, as many of these deaths occur during sleep, mainly in the prone (lying on abdomen) position. Unfortunately, there are no known effective strategies for preventing SUDEP. However, it is suggested that one should optimize sleep quality and treat any co-morbid sleep disorder to reduce arousal frequency and autonomic instability, possibly impacting the likelihood of nocturnal seizures and autonomic changes associated with them.

Approach to Sleep in Epilepsy

Sleep Disorders in Epilepsy

Nearly half of patients with epilepsy have frequent or chronic complaints of excessive daytime sleepiness, with probably more having episodic symptoms that they may not have addressed. Seizures and frequent inter-ictal discharges can disrupt sleep architecture, resulting in non-restorative sleep.

Additionally, patients with epilepsy are also higher risk for co-morbid sleep disorders than the general population (Table 10.4), including obstructive sleep apnea, restless leg syndrome, parasomnias, and insomnia, which may also contribute to symptoms of non-restorative sleep and excessive daytime sleepiness. Disrupted sleep may also be a contributory factor to the

TABLE 10.4 Sleep Disorders and Symptoms in Epilepsy

Sleep Disorder	Symptoms	Evaluation Tools
Sleep Apnea Obstructive Central	Snoring Apnea (stopping of breathing) Restless sleep Bedwetting Open mouth breathing Excessive daytime sleepiness	Polysomnography
Insomnia	Excessive daytime sleepiness Difficulty falling asleep or staying asleep Shortened sleep duration (even if sleep opportunity allows)	Sleep Diary Actigraphy
Circadian Rhythm Disorder	Excessive daytime sleepiness Later or earlier bedtime than desired Appropriate sleep duration (if sleep opportunity allows)	Sleep Diary Actigraphy
Periodic Limb Movement Disorder RLS	Excessive daytime sleepiness Occur in the early part of the night, but can be throughout the night Series of >4 in any sleep stage, up to hundreds per hour Most to every night Discomfort in early evening (RLS)	Clinical History +/– Polysomnography
Narcolepsy	Excessive daytime sleepiness Fragmented sleep Sleep paralysis Sleep-related hallucinations Cataplexy	Polysomnography Multiple Sleep Latency Test

(continued on next page)

TABLE 10.4 Sleep Disorders and Symptoms in Epilepsy (*continued*)

Sleep Disorder	Symptoms	Evaluation Tools

Parasomnias
NREM
  Sleepwalking
  Sleep talking
  Confusional
    arousal
  Sleep terrors
	Excessive daytime sleepiness first half of the night, mainly during N3
	Frequency varies, 1–3 episodes per night Onset frequently in childhood
	+ family history
	Non-violent
		Clinical History
		+/– Polysomnography

REM RBD	Excessive daytime sleepiness Second half of night during REM sleep Frequency varies, 1–2 episodes per night Can be violent	Clinical History +/– Polysomnography

prolonged recovery time that some patients experience following seizures. Optimizing the identification and treatment of both sleep disorders and epilepsy is important for improved patient care and outcomes.

Insomnia is a complicated condition that may represent either difficulty falling asleep, staying asleep, or both, and results in a decreased number of hours of sleep and a sense of sleeplessness in the night and daytime sleepiness. In addition, symptoms of insomnia can be short term (acute), long term, or recurring (chronic), and they may even be a result of co-morbid epilepsy. It is not uncommon for patients who have epilepsy to have symptoms of insomnia due to fear of sleeping because of nocturnal seizures or concerns of SUDEP.

Obstructive sleep apnea (OSA) is a sleep-related breathing disorder that occurs because of transient episodes of breathing difficulty because of obstruction in the upper airway. In adults, this is commonly related to body habitus, including overweight, large neck size, and large breasts, which act as a force against breathing easily. In children, it is more commonly related to enlarged tonsils, adenoids, or a small jaw or flattened nasal bridge/facial features, which physically reduce the size of the airway. In both cases, the patients have a greater risk for obstruction during sleep because of a more relaxed airway that is more prone to episodes of closure. Individuals who have obstructive sleep apnea commonly have the following signs and symptoms: snoring, open mouth breathing, episodes of stopping breathing (apnea), episodes of difficulty breathing (hypopnea), frequent arousals during sleep. There may also be symptoms of increased nocturnal urination or bedwetting, morning headache, restless sleep, morning thirst, excessive daytime sleepiness, and cognitive slowing.

Periodic limb movement disorders (PLMD) are repetitive movements, typically in the lower extremities, that occur about every 20 to 40 seconds during sleep. Individuals with PLMD frequently have movements, described as brief muscle twitches, jerking movements, or an upward flexing of the feet that may cluster into episodes that last from minutes to several hours. It is not uncommon for sleep to be disrupted because of arousals associated with these events. Restless leg syndrome (RLS) is a category of periodic limb movement disorders. Individuals with RLS have evidence of PLMD, but they also have an uncomfortable sensation in the calves or thighs, as they attempt to fall asleep or during an episode of arousal.

Parasomnias are disorders of arousal that are characterized by abnormal or unusual behavior during sleep. There are NREM and REM parasomnias (Table 10.4). NREM parasomnias typically occur when a patient has an arousal during slow-wave sleep (stage N3) and REM parasomnias occur when the arousal comes out of REM sleep. Typically, NREM parasomnias are more common during childhood and become less frequent with age. On the other hand, REM parasomnias are more common in the adult population and can worsen with aging. The most commonly discussed REM parasomnia is *REM behavior disorder* (RBD), which is characterized by increased tone, activity, and even dream enactment behavior during REM sleep. This is a period of sleep marked by vivid dreaming and normally identified by loss of tone and no movement. *Dream enactment behavior* can result in large movements, such as jumping out of the bed, and even violent acts like punching and kicking, mimicking activity experienced in the dream. Therefore, this is a condition that can potentially pose harm for the individual with the disorder and his bed partner.

How to Screen for Sleep Disorders?

A comprehensive sleep assessment should be performed in all patients with epilepsy. This may be completed by the treating neurologist or by a sleep specialist who is part of a multi-disciplinary epilepsy treatment team. Initially, the physician should evaluate for complaints regarding sleep or wakefulness, such as complaints of excessive daytime sleepiness, snoring, or difficulty falling or staying asleep. It is common to use validated questionnaires, such as the Epworth Sleepiness Scale, STOP-BANG, or the Pittsburgh Sleep Quality Index to screen patients. There are also epilepsy-specific screening tools, such as the frontal lobe epilepsy and parasomnia (FLEP) scale that may be used.

A detailed sleep-wake history should then be performed in all patients to determine if there are features concerning for a sleep disorder. Patients should also be re-evaluated for sleep-wake symptoms annually, at minimum. If there is suggestion of a sleep disorder, the physician may require the patient to maintain a sleep diary, wear a sleep-tracking device called an *actigraphy,* or have a polysomnography (PSG) performed. Time to sleep and wake up on weekdays and weekends must always be ascertained because of poor sleep hygiene on weekends, which can worsen seizure frequency.

A *polysomnography* is a sleep study and is most commonly used to evaluate patients who are high risk for sleep apnea. However, it is also used to evaluate for other types of sleep disorders. A typical in-lab sleep study uses a limited EEG to record brain waves to stage sleep, a nasal cannula device to evaluate breathing through the nose and mouth, a pulse oximeter on the finger to measure oxygen levels, a belt around the chest and abdomen to evaluate breathing, and leads to evaluate heart rate and rhythm, eyes leads, and leg movements during the study. If there is concern for seizure, extra EEG leads and body leads may be used to better assess brain activity and body movements.

Patients with symptoms of significant daytime sleepiness may be evaluated with additional testing, such as a *multiple sleep latency test* (MSLT) or the *maintenance of wakefulness test* (MWT). Multiple sleep latency testing occurs on the day following an overnight polysomnography. The goal of the MSLT is to evaluate the severity of sleepiness by evaluating the likelihood and time taken for a patient to fall asleep again and evaluate if they will enter REM sleep after a full night's rest. The patient has 4 to 5 opportunities to nap, with each opportunity lasting 20 minutes and separated by 2 hours.

On the other hand, the MWT evaluates the ability to stay awake, and generally is used to determine if interventions for daytime sleepiness are successful by determining if an individual is able to stay awake for a defined period of time. The test consists of 4 trials, each lasting about 40 minutes, with a 2-hour break between each trial. For each trial, the patient will sit quietly in bed in a dimly lit room with their back and head supported by a pillow. Then the patient tries to stay awake for as long as they can while maintaining that position.

Sleep Interventions

Insomnia

The treatment of insomnia should always include sleep hygiene education (Tables 10.5a and b), regular sleep scheduling, and cognitive behavioral therapy (CBT-I). Cognitive behavioral therapy is a safe and highly effective method of treating insomnia by targeting bad sleep habits and problematic sleep schedules, as well as a patient's approach to sleep and views on insomnia. The result is generally the development of a skill set to help combat insomnia. CBT-I has been shown to be more effective than any of the leading sedatives or hypnotics for long-term insomnia treatment. At times, a physician may also prescribe sedative or hypnotic medications to help

TABLE 10.5a   Sleep Hygiene: a) for Adults b) for Children

Sleep Hygiene Tips for Adults
• Sleep only as much as you need to feel refreshed during the following day. Restricting time in bed helps consolidate and deepen sleep. Too much time in bed is bad for sleep.
• Get up at the same time each day, 7 days a week. A regular wake time in the morning leads to regular times of sleep onset, and helps to set your "biological clock."
• Exercise regularly. Schedule exercise times, so they do not occur within 3 hours of when you intend to go to bed. Exercise makes it easier to initiate and deepen sleep.
• Make sure your bedroom is comfortable and free from light and noise. A comfortable, noise-free sleep environment will reduce the chance that you will wake up during the night. Noise that does not awaken you may also disturb the quality of your sleep.
• Make sure that your bedroom is at a comfortable temperature during the night. Excessively warm or cold sleep environments may disturb sleep.
• Eat regular meals and do not go to bed hungry. Hunger may disturb sleep. A light snack at bedtime (especially carbohydrates) may help sleep, but avoid greasy or "heavy" foods.
• Avoid excessive liquids in the evening. Reducing liquid intake will minimize the need for nighttime trips to the bathroom.
• Cut down on all caffeine products. Caffeinated beverages and foods (coffee, tea, cola, chocolate) can cause difficulty falling and staying asleep, as well as shallow sleep.
• Avoid alcohol, especially in the evening. Although alcohol can help people fall asleep more easily, it causes awakenings later in the night.
• Smoking may disturb sleep. Nicotine is a stimulant.
• Don't take your problems to bed. Plan some time earlier in the day for working on your problems or planning the next day's activities. Worrying interferes with sleep.
• Train yourself to use the bedroom only for sleep and sex. This will help condition your brain to see bed as the place for sleeping. Do _not_ read, watch TV, use electronics/phone, or eat in bed.
• Do not **try** to fall asleep. This only makes the problem worse. Instead, turn on the light, leave the bedroom, and do something different, like reading a book. Don't engage in stimulating activity. Return to bed only when you are sleepy.
• Put the clock under the bed or turn it so that you can't see it. Clock watching may lead to frustration, anger, and worry, which interfere with sleep.
• Avoid naps. Staying awake during the day helps you to fall asleep at night.

TABLE 10.5b   Sleep Hygiene: a) for Adults b) for Children

Sleep Hygiene Tips for Children

- Sleep only as much as you need to feel refreshed during the following day. Restricting your time in bed helps to consolidate and deepen your sleep (see sleep hours for age).

- Get up at the same time each day, 7 days a week. A regular wake time in the morning leads to regular times of sleep onset, and helps to set your "biological clock."

- Exercise regularly. Exercise more than 3 hours before bedtime. Exercise makes it easier to initiate and deepen sleep.

- Make sure your bedroom is comfortable and free from light and noise. A comfortable, noise-free sleep environment will reduce the likelihood that you will wake up during the night.

- Make the bedroom a safe, inviting place to sleep. Play time or reading earlier in the day out of the bed, but in the room, makes the association that the child's bedroom is an inviting, safe place to sleep.

- The bed is only for sleeping. This will help condition your brain to see bed as the place for sleeping. Do *not* read, watch TV, play with tablets or phone, or eat in bed.

- Make sure that your bedroom is at a comfortable temperature during the night. Excessively warm or cold sleep environments may disturb sleep. Be sure to dress the child appropriately for the temperature.

- Eat regular meals and do not go to bed hungry. Hunger may disturb sleep. A light snack at bedtime (especially carbohydrates) may help sleep, but avoid greasy or "heavy" foods.

- Avoid excessive liquids in the evening. Reducing liquid intake will minimize the need for nighttime trips to the bathroom and wetting the bed.

- Cut down on all caffeine products. Caffeinated beverages and foods (coffee, tea, cola, chocolate, energy drinks) can cause difficulty falling asleep, awakenings during the night, and shallow sleep.

- Don't take your problems to bed. Take time to discuss worries with your child earlier in the day and create strategies to reduce worry. Worrying may interfere with initiating sleep and produce shallow sleep.

- Do not *try* to fall asleep. This only makes the problem worse. Instead, turn on the light, leave the bedroom, and do something different, like reading a book. Don't engage in stimulating activity. Return to bed only when you are sleepy.

- Put the clock under the bed or turn it so that you can't see it. Clock watching may lead to frustration, anger, and worry, which interfere with sleep.

- Avoid naps. Staying awake during the day helps you to fall asleep at night (see sleep hours by age for age appropriate napping).

a patient fall or stay asleep. These medications include benzodiazepines, anti-depressants, melatonin, melatonin-receptor agonists, and non-benzo-diazepine receptor agonists. Caution needs to be exercised when prescribing these medications, however, as some may lower the seizure threshold or worsen other sleep disorders, such as RLS or OSA.

Sleep Disordered Breathing

The gold standard treatment for adults with obstructive sleep apnea is with a *continuous positive airway pressure* (CPAP) device. In children, surgical intervention, with removal of the adenoids and tonsils, is considered first, as adenotonsillar enlargement is a common cause. Patients with genetic syndromes and epilepsy may have craniofacial disproportion (e.g., small jaw, pushed back jaw, high arched palate) or hypotonia, which may contribute to breathing difficulty. If craniofacial disproportion is present, greater benefit may come from surgical intervention to correct the disproportion. Patients with *hypotonia* may have a significant sleep positioning component to their breathing difficulty (i.e., worse when sleeping on their back). If the severity of sleep apnea is mild, then alternative treatment options, such as oral appliances for repositioning of the airway, surgery to improve airway dynamics, sleep positioning, and weight loss should be considered. Treatment is considered appropriate if it reduces the frequency of episodes of breathing difficulty to fewer than 5 events per hour.

Central sleep apnea is generally treated with either a positive airway pressure device, supplemental oxygen, or in some cases, both. However, patients with epilepsy, especially those with temporal lobe seizures, who have findings of predominant or isolated central sleep apnea, should have a critical evaluation of the episodes to ensure that this does not represent seizures. Additionally, when central apnea is predominant, there should be consideration for evaluating the health of the heart, lungs, and kidneys, as well as other medications the patient may be taking that may contribute to development of central apneas.

Periodic Limb Movement Disorder and Restless Leg Syndrome

Periodic limb movement disorder can occur *incidentally* (without identified cause) or as a result of some medications. Bloodwork (iron and ferritin levels) is frequently obtained in patients who have RLS/PLMD, as low *ferritin* (a protein related to iron) or iron can contribute to symptoms. If ferritin level is less than 50 mcg/L, iron supplementation is frequently recommended for at least 3 months, if no contraindications to its use exist. If iron supplementation is not optimal, either due to contraindication or lack of efficacy, then use of a medication called gabapentin may be considered. When a medication is suspected to be the precipitating factor causing PLMS/RLS (like the use of an antidepressant) it should be considered to remove the offending medication if possible.

Excessive Daytime Sleepiness (EDS)

As discussed previously, the cause of EDS can be due to many things. If symptoms of EDS persist even after thorough evaluation and optimized management of contributing factors, then consideration for a medication that increases the ability to stay awake, such as modafinil, armodafinil, and alternative stimulants, should be considered. Although there is a theoretical risk for decreased seizure threshold with use of these medications, in reality, they are used successfully in patients with epilepsy to improve sleepiness, resulting in improved quality of life, without worsening seizures.

In conclusion, sleep and epilepsy clearly have an intimate relationship that should be considered in the care of patients with epilepsy. Excessive daytime sleepiness and poor sleep are not acceptable norms for patients with epilepsy and contribute to poor quality of life and increased risk for poor seizure control. Patients and caregivers should include sleep as a part of their conversations with their epilepsy provider and, if necessary, they should encourage that they be evaluated by a sleep specialist.

CHAPTER 11

Epilepsy in Special Populations

- Fainting is the most frequent cause of loss of consciousness in a person, especially in the elderly.
- Strokes are the most common cause of new-onset seizures in the elderly, accounting for about 40 percent to 50 percent of new-onset epilepsy in this age group.
- Selecting an AED for an elderly patient is even more important than for a child since life-long treatment may be needed.
- Seizures are a common and sometimes devastating complication of brain tumors, and meticulous attention to their diagnosis and treatment is critical.
- Several older AEDs, such as carbamazepine, phenobarbital, phenytoin, and primidone, are most commonly associated with osteoporosis.

This chapter addresses a few special conditions and situations, such as seizures in the elderly, special problems in patients with brain tumors, and the effects of some antiepileptic drugs (AEDs) on bone health.

Seizures and Epilepsy in the Elderly

As life expectancy continues to increase, it is harder and harder to define who is an elder. Two hundred years ago, a 40-year-old was considered old; nowadays, a 60-year-old is still looked upon as relatively young (Figure 11.1).

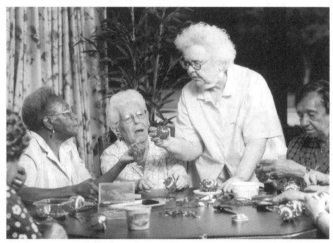

FIGURE 11.1 Elderly patients are able to remain active much longer.

For most working definitions, *elderly* is someone older than 65 years. As we get older, the possibility of having seizures increases with each passing decade. Those older than 85 have more than three times that chance for having a seizure than do 70 year olds. Because this is the most rapidly growing segment of our population, new-onset epilepsy in the elderly is a very important issue. It is also important because the elderly react differently to drugs used to treat seizures, and the causes of seizures and epilepsy in the elderly are different from those in children and young adults.

Seizures and Epilepsy Types in the Elderly

As with any person experiencing a seizure, the first questions that should be addressed are whether the patient indeed had an epileptic seizure and, if so, whether the seizure was provoked. As we have seen in other chapters, it is important to be sure that a seizure is not confused with fainting or *syncope*. Fainting is the most frequent cause of loss of consciousness in a person, especially in the elderly. Many individuals in this age group have conditions affecting the heart or blood pressure and, thus, are prone to faint. True seizures, however, can also be caused by chemical and electrolyte disturbances (e.g., low blood sugar or low salt), certain medications, medication withdrawal (e.g., Valium or lorazepam), or substance abuse (e.g., alcohol, drugs). Although these are truly seizures, they typically do not require AED treatment and are considered *provoked* seizures.

If a seizure is unprovoked, and it is clear that we are dealing with epilepsy, then it's important to classify the seizure type to determine what type of treatment is needed. As we know by now, epileptic seizures can be due to an identified or suspected cause, such as a tumor or stroke. The cause may be identified by *imaging* (brain scans), such as *magnetic resonance imaging* (MRI) or *computed tomography* (CT). Some seizures have a suspected cause that cannot be definitively identified (i.e., imaging is inconclusive). Most elderly patients with new-onset epilepsy have either an identified cause or a clear lesion found on scans that can be blamed as the cause of seizures. However, in the largest study of the elderly (the Veterans Administration Cooperative Study), 25 percent of the patients had seizures of unknown cause.

Generalized seizures most often have a genetic cause and start before age 18 years. Therefore, new-onset seizures in the elderly are *focal seizures,* with either loss of awareness or without loss of awareness, and they may turn into possible convulsions. This is the case for most people in this group. However, patients with apparent new-onset *absence seizures* in the elderly (episodes of staring and loss of attention) are actually focal seizures with loss of awareness. Finding the correct diagnosis can be a challenging problem.

Causes of Epilepsy in the Elderly

Strokes are the most common cause of new-onset seizures in the elderly, accounting for about 40 percent to 50 percent of new-onset epilepsy in this age group. In some instances, the patient may have evidence of a stroke (e.g., weakness of a limb) before the first seizure, while in others, the seizure may be the first and only sign of a stroke. Furthermore, in a few number of cases, patients may have a seizure, and when investigated with a brain scan, a stroke can be found.

Other causes of seizures in the elderly include brain tumors, head trauma, and Alzheimer's disease. In particular, patients with Alzheimer's disease have a greater chance for seizures as the disorder progresses. Identification of the cause of new-onset seizures in the elderly is important because it can help to focus treatment. For example, if the seizures are found to be the first indication of an unrecognized disorder such as small tumor, treatment may be life-saving. Unfortunately, even using the newer methods of diagnosis, in as many as 30 percent to 40 percent of older patients, new-onset seizures do not have an apparent cause.

Diagnostic Testing

Once an unprovoked seizure has been diagnosed in a given patient, the physician must look for a cause. As with children and adults, we rely on imaging and the electroencephalogram (EEG) to find the source of the seizures. MRI is the best test to look for a lesion in the brain. As described in Chapter 2, an MRI will find tumors, scar tissue, malformations, and evidence of strokes. The EEG can confirm the diagnosis of epilepsy by showing areas of the brain that are irritable and the location of the seizure focus.

Treatment

New-onset seizures in the elderly have a high chance of recurring because they typically arise from a *lesion* (abnormality) in the brain. Thus, the risk is high for seizures recurring even after a single unprovoked seizure in an elderly patient. Because of that, it is common to begin treatment after the first seizure in an elderly patient. The high risk for recurrence is a key difference of new seizures in the elderly, as opposed to seizures in younger adults or children. However, even if the risk is high, the chances for adequate control are very good with current drugs.

Selecting an AED for an elderly patient is even more important than for a child since life-long treatment will be likely needed. Physician selection of an initial drug for an elderly patient must take into consideration how well the patient will tolerate the drug and its potential side effects, as well as how effective the drug will be at stopping seizures. In studies of patients with new-onset epileptic seizures, those seizures that are readily controlled are often controlled with relatively modest dosages.

Because most new seizures in the elderly are typically focal seizures with or without secondary generalization, almost all commonly used AEDs, both first- and second-generation, work well for focal seizures (see Chapters 3 and 4). An important study (VA trial 428) evaluated AED treatment of new-onset seizures in the elderly. This trial assessed how well the drugs worked and how well they were tolerated by the patient. The three drugs studied were gabapentin (Neurontin), lamotrigine (Lamictal), and carbamazepine (Tegretol). Carbamazepine, an older drug, is the most commonly used AED worldwide for the treatment of focal seizures. Gabapentin and lamotrigine are AEDs of a newer generation, with good safety records. The trial showed no significant difference in how well each drug controlled seizures. Carbamazepine, however, was associated with significantly more *dropouts* (people stopping the medication) due to side effects (27 percent) compared with gabapentin (17 percent) or lamotrigine (10 percent). These results suggest that the newer drugs should be considered in initial treatment of the elderly because they are better tolerated.

An obvious question that arises is whether any of the newer AEDs are better than older AEDs for decreasing or stopping seizures. More than a dozen new oral AEDs have been introduced in the United States since

1993. Unfortunately, only very few studies have compared the newer AEDs with the old AEDs. In each of these studies, no significant differences have been shown on how effective the drugs are at treating seizures. Therefore, at present, the decision regarding AED selection should focus on safety and side effects.

Initial treatment should use only one drug (*monotherapy*). The American Academy of Neurology (AAN) and the American Epilepsy Society (AES), two very important medical societies in the United States, have issued guidelines for the treatment of new-onset and difficult epilepsy using newer AEDs. The guidelines support the use of gabapentin (Neurontin), lamotrigine (Lamictal), topiramate (Topamax), and oxcarbazepine (Trileptal) as starting treatment for focal or mixed seizures, even though formal U.S. Food and Drug Administration (FDA) approval does not exist yet for some of them.

Elderly patients are more sensitive to adverse side effects in general, and these effects may occur at lower drug doses. Side effects such as unsteadiness, tremor, and sleepiness are common, but often difficult to pinpoint in elderly patients with memory problems. Elderly patients typically are taking other medications for health problems other than seizures. One study found that elderly patients treated with AEDs were also taking an average of five other medications. These *co-medications* increase the risk for drug interactions with AEDs, which may create new health problems.

Use of Antiepileptic Drugs in the Elderly

For details on AEDs, see Chapters 3 and 4. Here we only highlight the most important points regarding AEDs and their use in the elderly.

Phenobarbital and Primidone

Phenobarbital and primidone (which is converted to phenobarbital by the liver) are sedatives. In general, these are not a good choice as initial treatment for elderly patients.

Phenytoin (Dilantin)

Phenytoin (Dilantin) is one of the most widely prescribed AEDs in the United States. Phenytoin has several potentially severe disadvantages for the elderly, including an increased risk for *osteoporosis* (brittle bones) and possibly dyslipidemia (high bad cholesterol). In addition, the metabolism of phenytoin is very peculiar: it's extremely difficult to find the proper effective dose, and it's very easy to overdose. Since phenytoin is cleared by the liver, many other drugs will affect it and can be affected by its use. These factors have made many physicians stop prescribing phenytoin (Dilantin) in the elderly.

Carbamazepine (Tegretol)

Worldwide, carbamazepine is the most commonly used AED to treat focal seizures. Carbamazepine (Tegretol) does not pose the same problems as phenytoin, but it is metabolized by the liver and, thus, makes potential drug interactions a significant problem. For example, fluoxetine (Prozac) and even grapefruit juice can significantly increase carbamazepine blood levels to toxic levels. Lower sodium concentrations in blood (a condition known as *hyponatremia*) can be produced by carbamazepine, a side effect that is more common in the elderly. Sedation and osteoporosis are also important side effects that are of concern in the elderly.

Valproic Acid (Valproate, Depakote)

Valproate is commonly used in Europe as an AED. Although rare, liver toxicity can occur. *Tremor* of the hands is a common side effect, and since many elderly patients may already have tremor, it can make it worse. Valproate has less interactions with other drugs, and it does not induce osteoporosis. For that reason, it can be a good choice for some patients. However, because of its side effects, it is not the first choice for most patients.

Gabapentin (Neurontin)

Gabapentin is one of the newer generation AEDs and has potential advantages over some of the older drugs. First, it is extremely safe, has very few side effects, and needs very little monitoring, which makes this drug an attractive choice for the elderly patient. Although it is not a powerful drug, it can work fairly well for the older patient, since seizures in the elderly are easier to control than in younger patients. It is, however, a sedative, which can be a problem for patients already compromised by memory problems. Gabapentin may occasionally cause swelling of the extremities or weight gain.

Levetiracetam (Keppra)

Levetiracetam is one of the newer AEDs. It presents no safety concerns and has no interactions with, and is not affected by, other medications. It has an excellent cognitive profile and rarely causes toxicity. Levetiracetam may be associated with mild irritability and psychiatric side effects, but these are rare and uncommon in the elderly. Levetiracetam is also available for intravenous injection, thus making it a good choice for those unable to drink or eat. Because the drug is metabolized in the kidneys, careful use is warranted in the elderly.

Lamotrigine (Lamictal)

Lamotrigine offers many of the same benefits of gabapentin and levetiracetam. It is well tolerated, has few side effects, and doesn't cause cognitive problems. Several studies showed that lamotrigine is better tolerated than carbamazepine in elderly patients with new-onset seizures. Lamotrigine is approved as a mood stabilizer, and since depression is a common problem in the elderly and in patients with epilepsy, it can have a major beneficial impact on quality of life. Although the most serious side effect is rash, if introduced slowly, the risk of rash is extremely small. The rash is seen most commonly in patients of Chinese ascendency. Lamotrigine is not a sedative and, thus, is a very good choice for elderly patients with cognitive impairment.

Oxcarbazepine (Trileptal)

Oxcarbazepine works very similarly to carbamazepine, but it is better tolerated and has a much lower risk of causing bone marrow problems, such as anemia and low-white cell counts. Drug interactions also are fewer than with carbamazepine. The major concern with oxcarbazepine in the elderly is the increased risk for inducing low sodium levels (*hyponatremia*) in the blood. About 5 percent to 10 percent of people taking oxcarbazepine develop low-sodium levels, and because many elderly patients take diuretics (which tend to reduce sodium levels), the risk is even higher. Because of this, oxcarbazepine should be use with caution in elderly patients.

Topiramate (Topamax) and Zonisamide (Zonegran)

Topiramate and zonisamide have more cognitive side effects than the other AEDs discussed and, thus, are not drugs normally prescribed for elderly patients. When it's necessary to try topiramate and zonisamide, these side effects can be reduced by starting very slowly and using lower doses. Both drugs have few serious side effects, but both can induce kidney stones. Therefore, they are not appropriate in patients with a history of previous kidney stones. Both these AEDs can induce weight loss, which could be either a problem or an advantage, depending on the patient's weight. Zonisamide can be taken once a day, which is an advantage.

Lacosamide (Vimpat)

Lacosamide is one of the newest AEDs. It appears to be very well tolerated with the exception of mild dizziness. It is commonly prescribed for focal seizures, but not commonly for new-onset seizures. It does not appear to interfere with other medications. Because it is available as an intravenous formulation, it can be started rapidly in emergency rooms and hospitals, making it a very useful medication.

Perampanel (Fycompa) and Brivaracetam (Briviact)

These are the latest additions to the number of AEDs available in the market to treat seizures. Perampanel has been recently found to be an effective drug to treat generalized seizures, while brivaracetam works in focal seizures. Perampanel is one of the few AEDs that can be given only once a day. These two medications are not used frequently in the elderly.

Clobazam (Onfi)

Clobazam is a medication that has been available for several years in Europe and for about a decade in the US. It is a useful medication for certain types of syndromes. This medication may cause sedation and is used less in the elderly. However, low doses and slow increases are usually well tolerated.

Brain Tumors and Epilepsy

Seizures are a common and sometimes devastating complication of brain tumors, and meticulous attention to their diagnosis and treatment is critical. The frequency of seizures is common in patients with brain tumors, and is related to tumor location and probably to tumor type. Brain tumors are divided between *primary,* which originate in the brain, and *secondary*, which start elsewhere in the body and migrate to the brain (*metastasis*). Most brain tumors are either gliomas (which may be *malignant,* or cancerous) or meningiomas (which are *benign,* or noncancerous). For primary brain tumors, epilepsy occurs in more than 80 percent of patients with low-grade gliomas, in 30 percent to 60 percent of patients with higher-grade gliomas (more malignant), and in as many as 40 percent of patients with meningiomas. Low grade and *cortical* (in close proximity to the cerebral cortex) tumor location are the main risk factors for epilepsy. Brain tumor patients who have epilepsy are significantly younger than older patients with tumors (without seizures), but it is unclear why this is the case.

As expected, most tumor-associated seizures are initially *focal* (originating from a specific location in the brain), although *generalization* (causing epileptic electrical discharges throughout the brain) may occur so quickly that the focal phase passes unnoticed. Seizure generalization is observed in one-half of the patients at the onset of the disease. Seizures may be the first sign of a brain tumor, although in most patients, other signs, such as headaches or dizziness, are the first signs of a brain tumor. If a patient is diagnosed as having a brain tumor, but does not have seizures, it's unlikely that seizures will develop later in the course of the illness. Because patients with brain tumors often have surgery or radiation treatments, the chance of developing seizures may differ from patient to patient.

Use of AEDs in Brain Tumor

Although the use of AEDs in patients with brain tumors is widespread, it is difficult to know if their use is necessary before seizures occur. Common practice is that, once a patient is diagnosed with a brain tumor, they are placed on an AED. The available evidence suggests, however, that *prophylactic* administration of anticonvulsant medications (medications given to prevent a problem, rather than to treat an existing problem) only reduces the risk of developing seizures by about 25 percent. On the other hand, the side effects associated with AEDs are fairly common and can be serious.

If a patient with a brain tumor develops seizures, then treatment with an AED is necessary. The choice of AED will depend on multiple factors including age, gender, and other drugs being taken. AEDs such as levetiracetam (Keppra), lacosamide (Vimpat), and gabapentin (Neurontin) are good first choices because they pose little risk of interacting with other medications. Unfortunately, despite AED treatment, many patients with

brain tumors continue to have seizures, very often because of drug interactions with chemotherapy and steroid treatments that may change the
amount of AED circulating in the blood. For this reason, careful monitoring of drug levels is often necessary.

Bone Health and Epilepsy

Osteoporosis—a weakening of the bones—is another problem worthy of
special comment. Although more commonly seen in women, both old and
young, osteoporosis can affect men as well. *Estrogen,* a hormone produced
in the bodies of both sexes, is responsible for good bone health. Because
drugs that suppress estrogen are commonly used to treat breast cancer,
osteoporosis is common in breast cancer survivors. And because post-
menopausal women are no longer routinely prescribed estrogen replacement medications, older women are also at increased risk for osteoporosis.

Several older AEDs, such as carbamazepine, phenobarbital, phenytoin,
and primidone, are most commonly associated with osteoporosis. These
drugs increase the metabolism of vitamin D, which is a crucial vitamin that
helps to deposit calcium in the bones and keep them strong. The newer
AEDs have little effect on vitamin D metabolism and, therefore, they don't
pose the same risk of osteoporosis.

Osteoporosis can lead to fractures—in particular, hip fractures—
which are a serious medical problem in the elderly. Death from complications of hip fracture in the elderly can occur in about 20 percent of people.
A recent study estimated that women taking phenytoin had a 30 percent
increased risk for hip fractures over 5 years compared with women not
taking this AED.

Osteoporosis cannot be detected unless bone density scans are done.
Unfortunately, most patients receive a diagnosis of osteoporosis *after* a
bone fracture has taken place. Avoiding AEDs that promote osteoporosis
is recommended in the elderly, in postmenopausal women, and in patients

who are immobile (because immobility increases the chance of osteoporosis bones). If these AEDs must be used, bone mineral density should be measured and monitored, and supplemental vitamin D and calcium should be prescribed. Some physicians also recommend vitamin D and calcium supplements for any patient who is taking medications to treat liver disorders.

FREQUENTLY ASKED QUESTIONS

Q What are common causes of seizures in elderly patients?

Elderly patients have an increased risk for seizures and epilepsy. The most common cause of epilepsy in this group is stroke. Other causes include tumors, trauma, and infections.

Q Which are the best antiepileptic drugs for an elderly individual?

There is no simple answer to this question. Each patient should receive a particular drug, depending on their condition, the number of other drugs that are being taking, and other variables. Certainly, the trend is to use drugs that are not sedative and are easy to use while taking other medications.

Q Should a patient who has been taking phenytoin (Dilantin) for many years also be taking vitamin D and calcium supplements?

Although there are no strict guidelines on the use of vitamin D and calcium for patients with epilepsy, the consensus among many specialists is that vitamin D and calcium may help reverse some of the effects of phenytoin on bone health and, thus, it is recommended.

Q **How many years does an elderly patient need to take an antiepileptic drug after the diagnosis?**

This is a very difficult question. Many patients who develop seizures in adulthood need to take medications for life. This is because, as we know, most seizures in this age group are caused by lesions (strokes, and so forth). Once a lesion is detected, the likelihood of a seizure returning once a patient stops taking the medications is high. In addition, seizures in the elderly carry a higher risk of injury and medical complications.

CHAPTER 12

Living with Epilepsy: Addressing Common Concerns

- Antiepileptic drugs side effects can change a person's overall quality of life.
- People with epilepsy are protected by the Americans with Disabilities Act of 1990.
- Epilepsy can cause you to have alterations in sleep.
- Seizures can interfere with a child's ability to learn at the same pace as other children their age.
- A healthy diet is essential to everyone, especially for people with epilepsy.

Living with epilepsy has challenges. Your work, activities, transportation, education, diet, memory, and even sleep may be different from that of people without epilepsy. This chapter discusses these issues and provides patients with good resources to assist in dealing with them. Whether you are newly diagnosed or have had epilepsy for years, this chapter will address common concerns of both you and your family.

Epilepsy may affect many aspects of a person's life. Although the challenges of living with epilepsy may solidify family ties or allow a more empathetic perspective toward others, many of the effects of epilepsy put limits on an individual's goals and aspirations. Over the past decade, researchers from around the world have attempted to identify the most important concerns of persons living with epilepsy. The most commonly identified areas of concern include transportation, personal independence, social embarrassment, safety, mood, and medication problems (Figure 12.1). To help you talk about your own concerns with your physician, you may want to use the short form shown in Table 12.1.

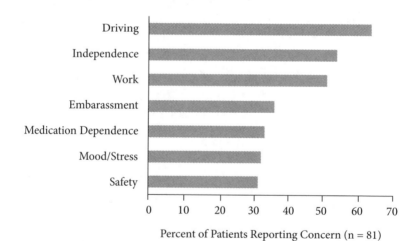

Percent of Patients Reporting Concern (n = 81)

FIGURE 12.1   Concerns listed by more than one-third of patients who have had one or more seizures in the past 6 months.

TABLE 12.1   A "Concerns Form" to Share with Your Physician

EFA Concerns Index

Name_____   Date_____

Patient's ID#_____ Gender_____   Birth Date_____

Instructions:
This questionnaire asks about your concerns of living with epilepsy. Please answer every question by circling the appropriate number (1, 2, 3, 4, or 5).

If you are unsure of an answer to a question, please give your best response. You may write comments in the margin to explain your answer, if needed.

1-13: For each of the PROBLEMS listed below, circle one number for how much they have concerned you during the past 4 weeks on a scale of 1 to 5, where 1 = Not at all concerned and 5 = Extremely concerned.

		Not at all concerned				Extremely concerned
1.	Your legal right or ability to drive	1	2	3	4	5
2.	Fear of being injured during a seizure	1	2	3	4	5
3.	Having to take seizure medications	1	2	3	4	5
4.	Holding down a job	1	2	3	4	5
5.	Getting the work or education you want	1	2	3	4	5
6.	Not being able to do things alone	1	2	3	4	5
7.	Having a seizure unexpectedly	1	2	3	4	5
8.	Being treated unfairly by others	1	2	3	4	5
9.	Being a burden or worry to your family	1	2	3	4	5
10.	Medical costs of your epilepsy	1	2	3	4	5
11.	Effects of your epi-lepsy on your family	1	2	3	4	5

(continued on next page)

TABLE 12.1   A "Concerns Form" to Share with Your Physician (*continued*).

		Not at all concerned				Extremely concerned
12.	Your future	1	2	3	4	5
13.	Lack of other people's understanding of epilepsy	1	2	3	4	5

14-20: During the past 4 weeks, have you...

		None of the time	Some of the time	A good bit of the time	Most of the time	All of the time
14.	Been worried about having another seizure?	1	2	3	4	4
15.	Had problems with medication side effects?	1	2	3	4	5
16.	Felt embarrassed about your seizures?	1	2	3	4	5
17.	Been unable to do things "for fun" that you wanted to do?	1	2	3	4	5
18.	Had problems thinking or remembering?	1	2	3	4	5
19.	Felt nervous, depressed, or "stressed out" because of your seizures?	1	2	3	4	5
20.	Had difficulty obtaining transportation?	1	2	3	4	5

COMMENTS:

_____

_____

In addition to physicians, *advocates* are working through the legal system to improve the overall quality of life for people with epilepsy. The *Americans with Disabilities Act* (ADA) of 1990 is an important piece of legislation that applies to people with epilepsy. This act aims to eliminate discrimination against the more than 43 million Americans with disabilities. It addresses employment, public transportation, housing, education, recreation, health services, and other issues. Persons with epilepsy are entitled to the rights protected under this act. Your disability gives you additional protection from discrimination. For example, if epilepsy prevents you from driving, this act allows you to access certain community resources, such as paratransit vehicles, to transport you when you are unable to drive. For more information on rights for disabled Americans, visit disabilityinfo. gov or disabilityresources.org, and see Chapter 14.

Managing Antiepileptic Drug Side Effects

Antiepileptic drugs (AEDs) are a necessary component of epilepsy treatment. For most people, seizures are decreased and may ultimately stop completely with these medications. These drugs, however, cause undesirable side effects for many people. Some side effects disappear after a few weeks of taking the drug, while others persist. Depending on which drug you are taking, you could experience fatigue, sleepiness, dizziness, weight gain, mood changes, memory changes, abnormal hair growth, or other adverse effects. Some drug side effects are unavoidable. However, in other cases, your doctor can alleviate side effects by changing the medications you take. You should always consult your doctor regarding options for other medications if your side effects are affecting your lifestyle in ways that are unacceptable to you. If your body reacts poorly to one drug, other options may be open to you. The way these drugs interact with your body may be different from the way they behave in another person. You are an individual and your unique needs should be considered.

Experiencing side effects from AEDs generally occurs when a new drug is started or with increasing dosage. You should be aware of the side effects of the particular drug that you are taking. Please refer to Chapters 3 and 4 for more information. Although side effects may decrease with time, there are several methods to help you handle them in your daily life.

Fatigue

Try establishing a normal sleep pattern. Keep the time you go to sleep and the time you wake up the same every day (including weekends).

- Moderate amounts of exercise may help your body to feel less stressed and less tired.
- Make sure you do not let the fatigue keep you from eating healthy foods. Your diet can help lessen fatigue. Try keeping ready-to-eat or easy-to-cook foods handy, so you can eat well even when you do not have the energy to prepare a meal.

Skin Changes (Rash or Sun Sensitivity)

- Avoid extra-hot showers and baths since hot water may irritate your skin further.
- Avoid excessive sun exposure and always wear sunscreen and protective clothing.

Headache

To relieve a headache:

- Try resting in a quiet place with minimal light and noise.
- Place a cold washcloth over your forehead and eyes.

To avoid a headache:

- Observe possible triggers of your headaches and attempt to avoid them. For example, bright lights, certain foods, and caffeine can trigger a headache.

Hair Loss

- Try to avoid or limit the use of certain hair care practices, such as dyeing, straightening, or braiding your hair.
- Attempt to decrease your amount of stress because this can worsen hair loss.

Upset Stomach

- Place crackers by your bedside and eat a few when you wake up in the morning. Sit in your bed for a few minutes after you eat them.
- Try certain stomach-soothing teas, such as ginger, chamomile, or peppermint.
- Slowly sip a carbonated beverage, such as ginger ale or Sprite.
- Avoid spicy, strong smelling, and greasy foods.

Weight Changes

- Establish a regular exercise routine of at least 30 minutes of activity three times a week.
- Avoid eating more food than you usually consume or need to feel satisfied. Try to eat healthy foods on a regular basis.

Memory Difficulties

Try using memory aids:

- Use sticky notes to remind yourself of appointments or things to do. Place the notes where you will see them, such as on the front door or refrigerator.
- Keep an appointment book and to-do list to help keep track of your schedule for the day.
- Use pill boxes with the days of the week to help you remember your daily medications. Use a separate box for morning, afternoon, and night doses. Place the meds in a place where you will see them and remember to take them. For example, place your morning and night meds by your toothbrush, so you will take them when you perform other routine hygiene tasks.
- Use a tape recorder to tell yourself about appointments or things you have to do. Most cellular phones have an option to use your voice to record a memo. When you need to remember some information, you can leave yourself a message on your cell phone. Check your phone daily to listen to your reminders.
- Ask a family member or coworker to remind you of things to do or appointments you must keep.
- Remembering names:
    - Try repeating the person's name to yourself multiple times when you meet them.
    - Try associating the person's name with an image or object that will help you remember it.
- Forgetting where you placed objects:
    - Try to keep things you commonly use in the same place all the time.
    - When you put an object in a new place, take the time to focus on where you put it, so it will be easier to recall its location when you need the item again.

AED side effects change a person's overall quality of life. The ultimate goal of your physician is to stop your seizures. In this process, however, the side effects of the drugs you are prescribed are often overlooked. Of course, you want your seizures stopped, too, but living with intolerable drug side effects is not acceptable. This crucial difference in ideas of what constitutes successful treatment can be a problem, so it is important to be an advocate for yourself. When you visit with your doctor, make sure you have a list of the side effects you are experiencing. The Adverse Events Profile in Table 12.2 will help you to do this. Fill out this table prior to every visit with your doctor.

For further information on AED side effects visit:

- epilepsy.com/epilepsy/medicine_sideeffects.html
- epilepsynse.org.uk/pages/info/leaflets/drug.cfm.

TABLE 12.2   Adverse Events Profile

Adverse Events Profile

During the past 4 weeks, have you had any of the problems or side effects listed below?

For each item, if it has always or often been a problem, circle 4; if it has sometimes been a problem, circle 3; and so on. Please be sure to answer every item.

	Always or often a problem	Sometimes a problem	Rarely a problem	Never a problem
Unsteadiness	4	3	2	1
Tiredness	4	3	2	1
Restlessness	4	3	2	1
Feelings of aggression	4	3	2	1
Nervousness and/or agitation	4	3	2	1
Headache	4	3	2	1
Hair loss	4	3	2	1
Problems with skin, e.g., acne, rash	4	3	2	1

(continued on next page)

TABLE 12.2 Adverse Events Profile (*continued*)

	Always or often a problem	Sometimes a problem	Rarely a problem	Never a problem
Double or blurred vision	4	3	2	1
Upset stomach		4	3	2
Difficulty in concentrating	4	3	2	1
Trouble with mouth or gums	4	3	2	1
Shaky hands	4	3	2	1
Weight gain	4	3	2	1
Dizziness	4	3	2	1
Sleepiness	4	3	2	1
Depression	4	3	2	1
Memory Problems	4	3	2	1
Disturbed sleep	4	3	2	1

Driving Laws

Imagine having a sales job that requires travel throughout the city to negotiate deals on a daily basis. How would you work if you were unable to drive? This is a question facing over a million people with epilepsy in the United States on a daily basis. In a country where most cities lack a good public transportation system, driving a car is a necessity of daily life. Being able to drive gives a person both independence and the ability to be self-sufficient. Both of these characteristics are highly valued in our society. Adults with epilepsy and their family members acknowledge that the most difficult and debilitating aspect of having uncontrolled seizures is the restriction on driving.

Driving regulations for people with seizures vary from state to state (see Chapter 14). Generally, you can expect to be prohibited from driving for 3 to 12 months following a seizure. This is a necessary mandate by the state to keep both you and other people on the roads safe. Accidents can occur if a person has a seizure while driving a car. A recent study reviewing fatal car crashes from 1995 to 1997 revealed that 0.2 percent (86) of the 44,027 deaths involved drivers with epilepsy. Despite this seemingly small fraction of epilepsy-associated automobile fatalities, it is still important to restrict people with active seizures from driving. In most states, it is not required for your physician to report that you have had a seizure. Therefore, it is your responsibility to know your seizure record and follow the laws in your state regarding driving. To find out what your state's laws are regarding driving restrictions after a seizure, visit www.epilepsy.com/epilepsy/rights_driving.

Although alternative modes of transportation are available, locating and utilizing these resources can be frustrating. According to the ADA of 1990, you are eligible for services, such as paratransit systems. These are vehicles that will pick you up and transport you to your required destination for a minimal cost. This service is available in most cities that lack easily accessible public transportation. The United States lacks a central system for dealing with the issue of transportation for people with disabilities. However, the following list of resources may help you to locate available methods of transportation in your area.

- www.ctaa.org/ntrc/accessibility/weblinks.asp
  This website offers links to available transportation for people with disabilities. National, as well as state, programs are listed.

- www.paratransit.net
  This website offers information for paratransit systems in Oregon, California, Alaska, and Washington. Although this will not be helpful to everyone, you can use an Internet search engine to locate a paratransit system in your area.

- www.publictransportation.org/systems
  This site links you to community public transportation in each state.

■ www.tlpa.org/findaride/index.cfm
This is the website of the Taxicab, Limousine, & Paratransit Association (TLPA). It allows you to select both domestic and international locations, and it will give you the transportation options for that area.

■ http://projectaction.easterseals.com/cgi-bin/traveler_search.cgi
This is a database of accessible community transportation for all 50 states and most major cities within each state. The database has all available companies' information in each state.

Alcohol Use

The recreational use of alcohol is common in almost every society. It is present at meals, work functions, and most social gatherings. While having epilepsy should not restrict you from drinking alcohol, your intake should not be excessive. There are no clear guidelines established regarding the amount of alcohol acceptable for persons with epilepsy. It appears that one drink, especially with a meal, is well tolerated by most people. The concern most physicians hold is that excess alcohol can potentially increase your chance of having a seizure. It can also interact with your antiepileptic medicines.

A statement from the National Institute on Alcohol Abuse and Alcoholism (NIAAA) points out that many medications interact with alcohol, which can lead to injury, illness, or even death. It notes that for some AEDs specifically, a definite interaction is known. For instance, acute alcohol consumption increases the risk of reaching toxic blood levels of phenytoin (Dilantin), which can cause an increase in drug side effects. With long-term use of both alcohol and Dilantin, blood levels of the drug decrease, necessitating higher doses of the medication to achieve the desired seizure control. Having epilepsy does not mean you cannot have alcohol, but be sure to discuss the topic with your physician.

Sleep and Seizures

Epilepsy can cause you to have alterations in sleep. You may feel tired all the time and find yourself needing extra naps just to function during the day. You may also find that, despite spending an adequate amount of time in bed at night, you do not feel rested in the morning. These sleep complaints are common and are caused by a number of different factors. Epilepsy itself can cause changes in your natural sleep pattern. Researchers believe that an inadequate amount of sleep, poor sleep hygiene, sleep disorders, AEDs, and interruptions in natural sleep patterns can all cause problems.

Fatigue is a common difficulty for people with epilepsy. It is not normal to experience excessive fatigue. This tiredness interferes with your ability to interact with your surroundings and with other people. If you find that you require frequent naps or an increase in the amount of hours you spend in bed at night, you should notify your physician. This tiredness could be a side effect of one of your drugs. If this is the case, it may be possible to adjust your dose or change your medicine. However, fatigue can also be the result of an underlying sleep disorder. Many people with epilepsy also suffer from an underlying sleep disorder, such as obstructive *sleep apnea* or restless leg syndrome. Both of these disorders can be diagnosed with a sleep study and are treatable conditions. Once treated, your overall quality of sleep should improve, and your daytime fatigue should decrease significantly. Please see Chapter 10.

Employment and Disclosure of Epilepsy

The unemployment rate for people with epilepsy is higher than that of the general population. In a society that values one's ability to work, this fact is particularly distressing to persons with epilepsy. Being able to hold a successful job can give a person a sense of self-worth. Quality-of-life scores are diminished in many people with epilepsy who do not have a job. The reason for this decreased rate of employment is not clear. However, it is likely that someone with seizures may have difficulty working if they are experiencing medication side effects, or if their seizures are not controlled. Another reason may be that it is difficult for a person with epilepsy to overcome the stigma that can be associated with their disorder. Employers and co-workers may not be educated regarding the disorder and may, therefore, have negative attitudes about your ability to work effectively. These reasons may cause you to decide against disclosing your illness in the workplace.

The decision to discuss your illness with your employer and co-workers is challenging. Many people with epilepsy are concerned that they will be discriminated against when applying for a new job or promotion based on their illness. People with epilepsy are protected by the ADA of 1990. Under the Act, it is unlawful for an employer to discriminate against a qualified applicant or employee with a disability. As an applicant you must, however, meet the employer's qualifications for the job, including education, training, experience, and skills.

For more information regarding the ADA and employment visit:

- www.eeoc.gov/facts/jobapplicant.html
  Websites also are available to help you with your decision to disclose your illness:

- www.onestops.info/print.php?article_id=107
  Offer rules for good disclosure of a nonapparent or hidden disability

- www.epilepsyfoundation.org/epilepsyusa/disclosure.cfm
  Discusses issues of disclosure and attitudes regarding epilepsy in the workplace.

- www.epilepsyinstitute.org/faq/main.htm
  Helps you construct multiple scenarios to assist you in disclosing your illness.

Table 12.4, created by the Epilepsy Foundation, can further assist you in your decision.

TABLE 12.4   Disclosing Epilepsy to Your Employer

Time of Disclosure	Advantages	Disadvantages	Issues
On a job application. (If the employer is covered by the ADA or Rehabilitation Act, the request for information is voluntary. If covered by a state law, such questions may be legal.)	Honesty/peace of mind.	Might disqualify you with no opportunity to present yourself and your qualifications. Potential for discrimination.	Do you know what legal protections are in place regarding information requested on a job application? Need to do some basic research before applying for some jobs. Early disclosure may avoid problems once you are hired.
During the interview.	Opportunity to respond briefly and positively in person to specific issues. Can raise issue of accommodations you need, or the fact that your epilepsy won't interfere with your job.	Puts responsibility on you to handle epilepsy issues clearly. Too much talk on the issue may indicate possible problem. Not being evaluated on your abilities.	How comfortable are you with discussing your epilepsy? These are very difficult questions, but they are ones you can be prepared to answer.
After the interview. (When a job is offered, but before you begin work.)	If the disclosure changes the hiring decision and you are sure of your ability, then you may take legal action for discrimination.	Might lead to distrust.	Need to evaluate your seizure condition in light of your job duties. Need to explain how epilepsy will not interfere with your ability to perform the job.

(continued on next page)

TABLE 12.4 Disclosing Epilepsy to Your Employer (*continued*)

Time of Disclosure	Advantages	Disadvantages	Issues
After you start work.	Opportunity to prove yourself on the job before disclosure. Allows you to respond to epilepsy questions with peers at work. If disclosure affects employment status and the condition doesn't affect your ability to perform the job or job safety, you may be protected by law.	Nervousness or fear of having a seizure on the job. Possible employer accusation of falsifying your application. Could change interaction with peers.	The longer you put off disclosing, the harder it becomes. It may be difficult to identify whom to tell.
After a seizure on the job.	Opportunity to prove yourself on the job before disclosure. If disclosure affects employment status and the condition doesn't affect your ability to perform the job or job safety, you may be protected by law.	Possible employer accusation for falsifying your application. Possibility that your co-workers will not know how to react to your seizure.	You should be prepared to answer questions from your employer and co-workers about epilepsy and why you didn't tell them.
Never.	Employer can't respond to your epilepsy unless you have a seizure.	Nervousness or fear of having a seizure on the job.	If you haven't had a seizure for a long time (like over 1 to 2 years) the issue of disclosure becomes less critical.

This page is from the Epilepsy Foundation© website and can be viewed at www.epilepsyfoundation.org/programs/disclosure.cfm.

Exercise

The overall level of activity and fitness in people with epilepsy is decreased in comparison to the general population. Studies show that people with epilepsy participate in fewer sports, have decreased muscle and aerobic strength, and have a higher body mass index compared with people without epilepsy. Another study found that people with at least one seizure a month were half as active as the average population. These statistics are not ideal for a group that already has significant health issues.

The importance of exercise in everyday life cannot be stressed enough. Exercise improves the body's ability to fight disease, overcome fatigue, and maintain a healthy body weight. It can also improve the quality of sleep a person achieves each night. Also, because people with epilepsy may have increased bone fragility (*osteoporosis*), exercise, especially resistance training, can improve your bone health. It can also improve your overall health, and help you to fight your disease and improve your quality of life.

It is common for someone with epilepsy to be advised to refrain from strenuous activity because it may provoke a seizure. You can, however, engage in physical activities that will improve your health without affecting your seizure rate. To avoid exercise-induced seizure triggers, be sure to follow these instructions:

- Always drink plenty of water to keep your body hydrated.
- If you feel you are overexerting yourself, stop the activity and rest.
- Make sure you rest on several days of the week.
- Maintain a healthy diet.
- Ensure that you are getting adequate sleep and are not fatigued.

Prior to starting a new exercise regimen, consult your doctor. Your exercise regimen should include the three main types of exercise: aerobic, resistance training, and stretching. You should attempt to do at least 30 minutes of aerobic exercise three times a week. This could include walking, jogging, or using a stair-climbing machine. You should attempt to do 20 to

30 minutes of resistance training twice a week. This includes using weight machines or resistance bands. The third element of exercise—stretching—should be done at the end of every workout session. Make sure to include all of your major muscle groups when you stretch. Be sure to start exercising at a level that is comfortable for you. You can increase the time and frequency of your workout as your body adjusts. The benefits to your health from exercising far outweigh the potential risks, but if your seizures are not completely controlled, try to avoid the risky exercises listed here:

- Motor sports
- Horseback riding
- Gymnastics
- Ice activities, such as skating or hockey
- Skiing
- Solo water sports, such as sailing or windsurfing
- Water activities, such as swimming, alone

For information on low-, moderate-, and high-risk sports, and on those sports that require a helmet, visit www.epilepsy.ca/eng/content/teens.html.

Safety

It may be frustrating to you, as a person with epilepsy, that everyone seems overly concerned about your safety. Your family and friends may take extra precautions to ensure you avoid activities that could be seizure triggers. They are also concerned that you may experience an epilepsy-related injury. Studies show that it is possible for a person to be injured during a seizure. Common injuries include lacerations, burns, dental trauma, and bone fractures. There is reason for concern, but there are some things you can do to decrease your risk of injury:

Safety 101 Checklist

- Keep all bathroom and bedroom doors unlocked.
- Turn down the hot water temperature in your house.
- Take showers, *not* baths.
- Avoid heights and stay off ladders.
- Don't carry hot pots or pans from the oven or stove—bring your plate to the stove.
- Use microwave cooking as much as possible.
- Place handles to pots and saucepans toward the center of the stove.
- Avoid fireplaces or hot radiators.
- Stay clear of furniture with sharp edges.

Diet

A healthy diet is essential to everyone, especially for people with epilepsy. It is common to experience weight gain with some of your medicines. By watching what you eat, you may be able to avoid this effect. The U.S. Department of Agriculture published a new food pyramid recently that puts an emphasis on whole grains, vegetables, and fruits. It allows for sparing amounts of fats and meats. Refer to the nutrition guide in Figure 12.2 to help you develop a healthy diet.

Several foods and food additives should be avoided by people with epilepsy. Certain foods, such as grapefruit juice, can interact with specific AEDs. Check with your doctor to see if any of these restrictions apply to you. It is a common misconception that some food additives can cause seizures. One example is *aspartame,* an artificial sweetener in many diet drinks. Multiple studies with animals and humans have determined there is no evidence this is true. It is safe to use aspartame. To date, no known foods or food additives trigger seizures in people with epilepsy.

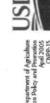

GRAINS Make half your grains whole	VEGETABLES Vary your veggies	FRUITS Focus on fruits	MILK Get your calcium-rich foods	MEAT & BEANS Go lean with protein
Eat at least 3 oz. of whole-grain cereals, breads, crackers, rice, or pasta every day 1 oz. is about 1 slice of bread, about 1 cup of breakfast cereal, or ½ cup of cooked rice, cereal, or pasta	Eat more dark-green veggies like broccoli, spinach, and other dark leafy greens Eat more orange vegetables like carrots and sweetpotatoes Eat more dry beans and peas like pinto beans, kidney beans, and lentils	Eat a variety of fruit Choose fresh, frozen, canned, or dried fruit Go easy on fruit juices	Go low-fat or fat-free when you choose milk, yogurt, and other milk products If you don't or can't consume milk, choose lactose-free products or other calcium sources such as fortified foods and beverages	Choose low-fat or lean meats and poultry Bake it, broil it, or grill it Vary your protein routine – choose more fish, beans, peas, nuts, and seeds

For a 2,000-calorie diet, you need the amounts below from each food group. To find the amounts that are right for you, go to MyPyramid.gov.

| Eat 6 oz. every day | Eat 2½ cups every day | Eat 2 cups every day | Get 3 cups every day;
for kids aged 2 to 8, it's 2 | Eat 5½ oz. every day |

Find your balance between food and physical activity
- Be sure to stay within your daily calorie needs.
- Be physically active for at least 30 minutes most days of the week.
- About 60 minutes a day of physical activity may be needed to prevent weight gain.
- For sustaining weight loss, at least 60 to 90 minutes a day of physical activity may be required.
- Children and teenagers should be physically active for 60 minutes every day, or most days.

Know the limits on fats, sugars, and salt (sodium)
- Make most of your fat sources from fish, nuts, and vegetable oils.
- Limit solid fats like butter, stick margarine, shortening, and lard, as well as foods that contain these.
- Check the Nutrition Facts label to keep saturated fats, trans fats, and sodium low.
- Choose food and beverages low in added sugars. Added sugars contribute calories with few, if any, nutrients.

MyPyramid.gov
STEPS TO A HEALTHIER YOU

USDA

U.S. Department of Agriculture
Center for Nutrition Policy and Promotion
April 2005
CNPP-15

USDA is an equal opportunity provider and employer.

FIGURE 12.2 A healthy-eating guide.

Education Issues for Children

Seizures and the original injury-causing seizures may interfere with a child's ability to learn at the same pace as other children his age. Children can feel isolated and different from their peers as a result. The seizures and some medication side effects can make them miss parts of class, experience extreme fatigue, and have trouble with memory. Government programs and agencies are available to assist your child in receiving the education he deserves.

Students with epilepsy are eligible for special education and related services under the Individuals with Disabilities Education Act (IDEA). This act requires public schools to provide an education in the least restrictive environment that meets each individual child's needs. IDEA requires public school systems to develop appropriate Individualized Education Programs (IEPs) for each child. The specific special education and related services outlined in each IEP reflect the individual needs of each student.

For more information on programs regarding education visit:

- www.nichcy.org. The website for the National Dissemination Center for Children with Disabilities.
- www.pacer.org. The website for the Parent Advocacy Coalition for Educational Rights.
- www.ideapractices.org. The website for the Council of Exceptional Children. This council advocates as the voice and vision of special education.

FREQUENTLY ASKED QUESTIONS

Q   How long do I have to be seizure-free to be able to drive?

The time restriction varies from state to state. In most states, it is 6 months, but it can be up to 1 year. Please ask your doctor about your particular situation and the state law.

Q Can I still drink alcohol?

Alcohol is acceptable to drink in moderation. For example, one glass of wine or one beer with a meal should not affect your medicine. However, each patient is different and you should discuss this with your doctor. Alcohol can interfere with some AEDs and can also affect the metabolism of your liver.

Q Do I have to live with the side effects of my AEDs, such as extreme fatigue or dizziness?

No! Talk to your doctor if you are experiencing side effects that you cannot tolerate. Other drugs are available. Side effects are individual and every patient is different on how they react to medications. It is important for you to tell your doctor about any problems you may have with your medications.

Q Do I have to tell my boss that I have epilepsy?

You are not legally required to tell your employer about your condition. It is your decision to determine if this is necessary.

Q Will my seizures cause permanent or progressive brain damage that will affect things like my speech?

No. In most types of epilepsy, recurrent seizures will not cause progressive trouble with speech or motor function. It depends on many factors—location of seizures, medications, cause of your seizures, and so forth. Some patients do experience changes, while the majority do not.

CHAPTER 13

Cognition and Mood

- In epilepsy, many things can potentially produce adverse effects on cognitive abilities.
- The frequency, duration, and severity of seizures may affect cognition in several ways.
- Several recent studies in humans provide evidence that exposure to valproate during pregnancy poses a special risk to development.
- Attention deficit disorders (ADDs) are the most frequent psychiatric disorder identified in children with epilepsy, although they occur in adults as well.
- Depression and anxiety disorders are common in patients with epilepsy.

Cognition in Epilepsy

Cognition refers to abilities such as intelligence, attention, memory, language, thinking speed, and ability to plan and problem solve. A survey in Europe by the International Bureau for Epilepsy (IBE) found that 44 percent of patients with epilepsy (PWE) complained of difficulty learning, 45 percent of slowed thinking, 59 percent of sedation, and 63 percent felt that their antiepileptic drugs (AEDs) prevented them from achieving activities or goals. A survey in the United States over a decade ago found similar results. Thus, the cognitive side effects of AEDs are clearly a problem for PWE. Most people with epilepsy have normal intelligence, and some even have superior intelligence. However, epilepsy is more common and more likely to be difficult to control in patients with mental retardation. In the general population, many things contribute to a person's cognitive abilities, such as genetic and environmental factors. In PWE, many things can potentially produce adverse effects on cognitive abilities. Table 13.1 lists factors that may affect cognition in PWE.

The cause of seizures may be one of the strongest factors influencing cognitive abilities. For example, if the seizures are due to progressive brain

TABLE 13.1   Factors That May Affect Cognition in People with Epilepsy

Underlying cause of seizures

Brain lesions acquired prior to onset of seizures

Type of seizures

Age at onset of epilepsy

Seizure frequency, duration, and severity

Impairments during and after seizures

Adverse effects of epileptic discharges between seizures

Brain damage from multiple seizures

Psychosocial factors resulting from epilepsy

Hereditary factors

Side effects of treatments for epilepsy, such as surgery or AEDs degeneration, patients will usually develop *dementia*. If the seizures are caused by brain injury (*trauma*), stroke, or tumor, the patient may have specific cognitive deficits. In contrast, if the cause of seizures is *idiopathic* (unknown), patients are more likely to have normal intelligence. Cognitive abilities have also been related to seizure type. For example, patients with *juvenile myoclonic epilepsy* usually have normal intelligence, but children with *infantile spasms* frequently have poor cognitive abilities. Overall, patients are more likely to have cognitive impairment if the first seizures occur at an earlier age.

The frequency, duration, and severity of seizures may affect cognition in several ways. During seizures, patients may lose consciousness or experience confusion. Following a seizure (the *postictal state*), a patient may be very confused or have problems with memory. This effect may last to some degree for minutes, hours, or even days. For example, patients who have had recent *temporal lobe seizures* may have increased problems with memory in the period following a seizure even after their confusion has resolved.

In a person with epilepsy, the abnormal electrical discharges in the brain that occur between seizures (during the interictal state) also may impair cognition, although the exact amount of impairment from these interictal discharges is uncertain. Nevertheless, it is clear that in some patients such EEG discharges may cause very brief, passing reductions in cognitive performance. For example, children are more likely to make errors on a video game during brief runs of interictal EEG discharges. Patients with *focal epilepsy* (seizures begin at one place in the brain) may have chronic dysfunction of the brain in that region. Further, the dysfunction may extend beyond the area of actual seizure onset. For example, *positron emission tomography (PET)* scans can show reduced brain activity between seizures not only in the region of seizure onset (the *focal* region), but also extending to surrounding brain regions. This reduced activity can be reversed if the seizures are stopped. However, repetitive or prolonged seizures may permanently damage the brain.

Hereditary factors can strongly influence intelligence. The *intelligence quotient (IQ)* of a child's mother is the single most important factor in predicting that child's IQ. Other factors, such as the father's IQ, living conditions (*socioeconomic status*), and brain injuries also influence a child's IQ.

Psychosocial factors may affect cognition. For example, poor socioeconomic status or poor access to educational opportunities during childhood can adversely affect cognitive development.

Finally, therapies for epilepsy, such as AEDs or surgery, also may affect cognition. These will be discussed next.

Epilepsy Surgery

In people with epilepsy whose seizures are refractory to AEDs, epilepsy surgery may offer the best hope of freedom from seizures if the onset of seizures can be localized and the damaged area removed without producing new problems. The risk of postoperative cognitive problems depends on the function of the area of the brain that is to be removed (*resected*). For example, if the seizure focus involves language areas of the brain, removal could lead to forms of *aphasia,* such as difficulties with spontaneous speech, understanding words, naming, or reading. Even in this situation, aphasic problems may be reduced by mapping the brain to tailor the resection to avoid critical language areas or by performing a special type of surgical procedure, known as *multiple subpial transections.* Alternatively to brain resection, direct stimulation of the brain near the epileptic focus can be used to control seizures in regions where resections would cause deficits (see RNS below). Fortunately, resective epilepsy surgery frequently does not usually lead to general cognitive decline because the tissue removed at the focus does not function well. Surgery may even result in improved cognition because of the reduction in seizures and need for AEDs.

The most common type of epilepsy surgery is *anterior temporal lobectomy.* The anterior medial temporal lobe has the lowest seizure threshold in the brain and is the most common site for the onset of focal epilepsy.

Surgeons are very experienced in treating that area of the brain. However, anterior temporal lobectomy can result in postoperative cognitive problems. The medial temporal lobes are critical for forming new memories. If both temporal lobes are damaged, then the patient will become *amnestic* (unable to remember events on a day-to-day basis). As long as one temporal lobe remains functional, the patient will not become amnestic, although they might experience some decline in memory. The best candidates for anterior temporal lobectomy have seizures arising from a nonfunctional medial temporal lobe, with the temporal lobe on the opposite side of the brain functioning well. Therefore, the preoperative evaluation must determine if and how much of the temporal lobe to be removed contributes to memory, and if the remaining temporal lobe can support memory.

Luckily, the risks are largely predictable. The occurrence of severe amnesia is extremely rare, and most patients undergoing temporal lobectomy will not suffer significant declines. A major concern in the preoperative evaluation is predicting even a partial decline in memory, especially *verbal memory* (the ability to remember words and names). The risks are greater if the patient's epilepsy started at an older age (not as an infant or young child), or if hippocampal scarring and atrophy are not present. The risk of significant problems is higher if the language-dominant temporal lobe (usually the left side) is involved, and if there is no abnormality on the MRI.

Preoperative assessments done by your doctors will be used to predict what sort of memory problems may occur following surgery. These assessments may include *neuropsychological testing*, the *Wada test*, PET scans, or *functional* magnetic resonance imaging (MRI) scans. Neuropsychological testing involves evaluation of cognitive abilities, such as attention, memory, language, and processing speed. The Wada test is also called the *intracarotid amobarbital test*. To perform the Wada test, the physician threads a very small tube (a *catheter*) up from the big arteries in the leg to the carotid arteries in the neck. A short-acting anesthetic agent, such as amobarbital, is injected. This basically puts one side of the brain to sleep for a few minutes, so that language and memory function can be assessed. The point is to determine which side of the brain controls language and how much each side contributes to memory. New *noninvasive techniques,* such as functional MRI, may soon replace the *invasive* Wada test. The PET scan measures the *metabolism* (activity) of the brain. The finding of *hypometabolism* (low activity) in one medial temporal lobe is consistent with a seizure focus and reduced function on that side.

Vagal Nerve Stimulation and Deep Brain Stimulation

Vagal nerve stimulation (VNS) and *deep brain stimulation* (DBS) of the anterior thalamus can reduce seizures and do not appear to produce any adverse cognitive effects. DBS is not available in the United States at this time, but it may be available soon. Refer to Chapter 6 for more information.

Antiepileptic Drugs

AEDs control seizures by reducing nerve cell irritability, but they can also affect cognition by suppressing nerve cell excitability. In general, the cognitive side effects of AEDs are mild, especially when only one AED is prescribed (*monotherapy*) within the usual therapeutic ranges. The main cognitive side effects of AEDs include slowing of motor and cognitive speed, reduced attention and vigilance (*sedation, somnolence,* and *distractibility*), impaired memory, and difficulty with complex mental functions. Patients treated with multiple AEDs (*polytherapy*), high dosages, or high blood levels of AEDs are at the highest risk of cognitive deficits. However, some patients require high AED dosages or multiple AEDs to obtain seizure control, and these patients may tolerate high dosages or multiple AEDs without significant cognitive side effects. Everyone is different, and everyone responds a little differently to AEDs. In some people, the cognitive effects of AEDs can be severe enough to reduce a patient's perceived quality of life. Table 13.2 identifies the adverse side effects of each of the AEDs you take; it may help you and your doctor determine if you are suffering side effects from your AED.

TABLE 13.2 Adverse Events Profile

During the past 4 weeks, have you had any of the problems or side effects listed below?

For each item, if it has always or often been a problem, circle 4; if it has sometimes been a problem, circle 3; and so on. Please be sure to answer every item.

	Always or often a problem	Sometimes a problem	Rarely a problem	Never a problem
Unsteadiness	4	3	2	1
Tiredness	4	3	2	1
Restlessness	4	3	2	1
Feelings of aggression	4	3	2	1
Nervousness and/or agitation	4	3	2	1
Headache	4	3	2	1
Hair loss	4	3	2	1
Problems with skin, e.g., acne, rash	4	3	2	1
Double or blurred vision	4	3	2	1
Upset stomach	4	3	2	1
Difficulty in concentration	4	3	2	1
Trouble with mouth or gums	4	3	2	1
Shaky hands	4	3	2	1
Weight gain	4	3	2	1
Dizziness	4	3	2	1
Sleepiness	4	3	2	1
Depression	4	3	2	1
Memory problems	4	3	2	1
Disturbed sleep	4	3	2	1

Older AEDs

Carbamazepine (Tegretol, Carbatrol), phenytoin (Dilantin), valproate (Depakote), phenobarbital, and benzodiazepines are the "traditional" AEDs that have been used to treat epilepsy for many years. Cognitive side effects associated with these drugs in monotherapy are generally moderate, but they may be a problem for some. The cognitive effects of carbamazepine, phenytoin, and valproate appear to be very similar. In contrast, phenobarbital produces greater cognitive deficits than these other traditional AEDs.

Newer AEDs

Several, but not all, of the newer AEDs appear to have fewer cognitive effects than the older AEDs. However, not all of the newer AEDs have been tested adequately for their cognitive effects. Gabapentin (Neurontin), lacosamide (Vimpat), lamotrigine (Lamictal), and levetiracetam (Keppra) have few cognitive side effects and have been shown to have significantly fewer cognitive effects than traditional AEDs like carbamazepine. Perampanel (Fycompa) has been shown to have low cognitive side effects compared to placebo.

Gabapentin, lamotrigine, and some traditional AEDs have demonstrated fewer cognitive side effects than topiramate (Topamax). Both traditional AEDs and topiramate can reduce verbal memory by 10 percent to 20 percent, but gabapentin, lamotrigine, and levetiracetam do not appear to noticeably or adversely affect this type of memory in most people. The cognitive effects of topiramate are increased if it is started rapidly, increased to high dosages, or used in polytherapy. These effects are also seen with other AEDs, but are more dramatic with topiramate. Nevertheless, topiramate is tolerated well in some patients, especially at lower dosages. Because other factors contribute to the choice of AED—such as effectiveness in controlling seizures and other effects (e.g., migraine treatment or weight loss)—topiramate may be the AED of choice for some patients.

Oxcarbazepine (Trileptal) is better tolerated than several traditional AEDs, but it has not been shown to have fewer cognitive effects than traditional AEDs in the few studies that directly assessed its cognitive effects. Zonisamide (Zonogran) has pharmacological properties similar to topiramate, and zonisamide can cause cognitive side effects, but these are not as well delineated as topiramate. Not all of newer AEDs available in the United States have been tested for cognitive side effects, especially in populations at special risk, such as children and the elderly.

Cognitive Effects of AEDs in Children and the Elderly

Children and the elderly are at special risk to suffer cognitive side effects from AEDs. The elderly are more susceptible to the cognitive effects of AEDs because they metabolize drugs differently and because drugs are more likely to impair their brain function. Children are potentially more susceptible because even modest effects of AEDs on attention and learning may be very important during early brain development. Unfortunately, there are few studies that have examined the cognitive effects of AEDs in both these age groups.

Several AEDs have been shown to cause greater cognitive side effects in the elderly. Benzodiazepines (Valium or diazepam) can impair cognitive abilities in the elderly and increase the risk of falling and hip fracture, presumably due to its effect on coordination. The cognitive side effects of carbamazepine, phenobarbital, phenytoin, and primidone (Mysoline) have been shown to be greater in elderly epileptic patients. Gabapentin and lamotrigine have been found to be better tolerated than carbamazepine in the elderly, primarily due to fewer side effects affecting the brain (cognitive problems, sedation, and dizziness). However, very few studies have directly compared the effects of different AEDs in the elderly.

Our information on the cognitive side effects of AEDs in children is limited, especially given the potential consequences. Overall, the cognitive

effects of carbamazepine, lamotrigine, levetiracetam, oxcarbazepine, phenobarbital, phenytoin, topiramate, and valproate appear to be similar in
children to the effects seen in adults. The most marked adverse effects are
seen with phenobarbital and topiramate, and no significant cognitive effects
for lamotrigine and levetiracetam. Phenobarbital has been shown to cause
adverse cognitive effects compared to *placebo* (a sugar pill) in children with
febrile convulsions. Other studies have demonstrated greater adverse cognitive effects for phenobarbital compared to valproate. In a study of children with absence epilepsy, ethosuximide (Zarontin), and lamotrigine had
fewer cognitive side effects than valproate. In a study of adolescents with
epilepsy, perampanel exhibited few adverse cognitive effects. In addition,
children may be at increased risk for long-term cognitive effects because of
the possible additive effects of prolonged AED exposure on brain development (*neurodevelopment*). Since no adequate long-term studies have been
done, the risks of AEDs in children remain uncertain.

Exposure of the Fetus to AEDs

Concerns have been raised about the cognitive risk of AEDs in the fetus
and in *neonates* (newborns). Experiments using newborn rats have shown
that several older AEDs and phenobarbital cause long-term problems in
cognition. Similar animal studies have found that phenytoin, phenobarbital, diazepam, clonazepam, and vigabatrin produce widespread loss of
nerve cells in the brain. Carbamazepine, lamotrigine, levetiracetam, and
topiramate in monotherapy do not produce these adverse effects in the
newborn rat brain. However, carbamazepine, lamotrigine, and topiramate
can enhance nerve cell death when given with one of the AEDs that does
it in monotherapy. In contrast, levetiracetam does not. Unfortunately, the
many other existing AEDs have not been tested in this way.

These studies raise concern that similar effects may occur in newborn
humans since the developmental state of the neonatal rat brain is similar
to the human fetal brain in the last few months of pregnancy. Thus, AED

exposure in pregnant women may pose a risk for loss of brain cells in the unborn child. Furthermore, the animal models suggest that impaired function in the surviving nerve cells may be even more important as the cause of impaired cognitive abilities in the animal. However, results in animals and in humans can differ as our information in humans is less complete and less certain.

Several recent studies in humans provide evidence that exposure to valproate during pregnancy poses the greatest risks for both congenital malformation and impaired cognition in the child. A few studies have also suggested a risk for phenobarbital exposure during pregnancy. In contrast, a few studies have suggested no increased cognitive risks exist for carbamazepine, lamotrigine, and levetiracetam.

It's important to remember, however, that many AEDs have not been studied in humans or animals, and much more information is needed for physicians to better advise women with epilepsy who want to become pregnant. Despite the increased risks, *the majority of children born to epileptic women taking AEDs are normal.*

Women with epilepsy should not stop or decrease their AEDs without talking with their physician. The risks of the AED must be balanced against the risk of seizures. Women with epilepsy are at increased risk to die during pregnancy, primarily due to seizures—many of which occurred because the woman stopped or reduced her AED without talking with her physician.

Summary

Patients with epilepsy frequently suffer from cognitive problems (see Table 13.1). Because epilepsy is caused by multiple diseases, the cognitive abilities of patients with epilepsy vary greatly. AEDs are the main treatment for epilepsy. The main concern in choosing an appropriate AED and dosage is control of seizures. However, another important concern is the effect of the AED on cognition, because adverse effects are common and may impair a patient's quality of life. Risk factors include polypharmacy and higher AED dosages or blood levels. Some AEDs pose an increased risk of cognitive side effects (phenobarbital). Several of the newer AEDs (such as lamotrigine and levetiracetam) have been shown to have fewer cognitive effects than the traditional older AEDs. Our understanding of the cognitive effects of AEDs on children and the elderly is limited. Fetal valproate exposure can adversely affect the child, but the risks of many AEDs have not been assessed.

In patients who fail to achieve seizure control with AEDs, epilepsy surgery may offer their best hope of seizure freedom. Most patients can undergo epilepsy surgery without suffering new cognitive problems, but some risk exists (such as verbal memory decline after left temporal lobectomy). Studies done before the operation can largely define this risk and, thus, help patients and their physicians make a decision based on the relative potential benefits and risks of the surgery. Neurostimulation therapies for epilepsy do not appear to pose any cognitive risks.

Common Psychiatric Disorders in Epilepsy

For a long time, physicians have been aware of the fact that people with epilepsy are likely to experience various types of psychiatric disorders more frequently than the general population, as shown in Table 13.3. *Depression, anxiety disorders*, and *attention deficit disorders* (ADD) are the three most frequent psychiatric disorders identified in PWE people with epilepsy. We'll take a closer look at these three problems here.

A common question asked by patients and physicians alike is to what degree is epilepsy the cause of these psychiatric disorders. It's important to remember that seizure disorders are only one of many causes. Studies have suggested that several causes can contribute to the development of these three psychiatric disorders in people with epilepsy. We will explain this point in greater detail in the following. However, we are far from having a complete understanding of *all* the causes of these psychiatric disorders in epilepsy.

TABLE 13.3   Prevalence Rates of Psychiatric Disorders in Epilepsy and the General Population

Psychiatric Disorder	Prevalence Rates	
	Epilepsy	General Population
Depression	11–50%	5–17%
Anxiety Disorders Generalized Anxiety Disorders Panic Disorder	15–25%	5–7%
	5–21%	0.5–3%
Attention Deficit Disorder (ADD)	12–37%	4–12%

In general, these three psychiatric disorders are more likely to be identified among people whose seizures are not well controlled. Unfortunately, patients are very often reluctant to let their doctor know about the presence of psychiatric symptoms, and consequently, they go untreated. This can have serious consequences on quality of life. Failure to seek treatment stems from various reasons, the two most frequent being: (1) a fear of being labeled "crazy" and (2) incorrectly believing that psychiatric symptoms are "part of the epilepsy" and don't need special treatment.

Patients often say: "Wouldn't you be depressed or feel anxious if you were having epileptic seizures?" The fact is that, more often than not, these three psychiatric disorders are *not* due to a reaction to having epilepsy. Therefore, any patient with psychiatric symptoms should be evaluated to determine the need for treatment. The good news is that today, effective treatment is available for depression, anxiety, and ADD in people with epilepsy, which we review in the following.

Frequency

Table 13.3 compares the frequency of all three psychiatric disorders between people with epilepsy and the general population. Notice the higher frequencies among PWE. This does not mean that everyone with epilepsy will have these psychiatric problems. Also, people with milder forms of epilepsy are less likely to have psychiatric problems, or will have only mild symptoms. For example, the frequency of depression ranges from 10 percent to 50 percent among people with epilepsy; the lower percentages reflect the frequency of depressive disorders among patients with milder forms of epilepsy. This is also true for the other two disorders.

Depressive and anxiety disorders are the most frequently identified psychiatric disorders in adults with epilepsy, while ADD is the most frequent psychiatric disorder of children with epilepsy. This does not mean that depressive and anxiety disorders do not occur in children, or that ADD only occurs in children. In fact, all these disorders can occur both in adults and children, but their frequency has yet to be determined in these age groups.

Psychiatric Symptoms Related to Epilepsy

People with poorly controlled seizures may experience a *cluster* (or group) of psychiatric symptoms related in time to the occurrence of a seizure. Psychiatric symptoms can precede a seizure by a few hours to up to three days. We call these *preictal* symptoms. Psychiatric symptoms can also occur within a period of five days *after* a seizure, in which case we refer to them as *postictal* symptoms. Psychiatric symptoms may be the only or principal type of symptoms of the actual seizure. We call these *ictal* psychiatric symptoms. Symptoms that occur independently of seizures are called *interictal* psychiatric symptoms.

Studies have shown that preictal and postictal psychiatric symptoms can include a wide variety of symptoms of depression (for example, feeling sad, being unable to enjoy things, losing all hope, feeling helpless, crying constantly, and feeling guilty without a reason, wanting to be dead), symptoms of anxiety (for example, worrying about everything without any apparent reason, feeling restlessness, inability to sleep, problems with concentration), as well as behavioral symptoms (for example, irritability, impulsive and aggressive behavior, and hyperactivity). In the case of children, parents often report that they can predict when their child will have a seizure because they become more irritable and cranky, display hyperactive behavior, and become more impulsive. Their behavior returns to "normal" after the seizure.

The studies have shown that postictal symptoms of depression, anxiety, and irritability can occur in up to 40 percent to 45 percent of people with poorly controlled seizures after more than 50 percent of their seizures. This means that these symptoms are a habitual occurrence. Often, these three types of psychiatric symptoms occur in the same patient. In contrast to preictal symptoms, patients often fail to make the connection between the occurrence of the seizure and their postictal symptoms. This is because in the majority of cases, these symptoms do not occur the same day of the seizure, but rather one or two days later. Postictal symptoms of depression, anxiety, and behavior disturbances have been found to last from a few hours to several days, with an average duration of 24 hours. Clearly, the occurrence of pre- and postictal psychiatric symptoms can cause as much or more distress than the actual seizure to patients and family members alike!

As previously stated, ictal psychiatric symptoms are those that are the *only* or *principal* symptoms of the actual seizure. They may occur in *simple partial seizures* and in some types of *temporal* or *frontal lobe epilepsies*. These symptoms are also known as *auras* (in which patients do not lose awareness of their surroundings) in some types of temporal or frontal lobe epilepsy. Studies have shown that ictal feelings of fear or ictal panic are the most frequently identified type of ictal psychiatric symptom, followed by ictal symptoms of depression. Often, auras are followed by a *complex partial seizure* or a convulsion, hence, the nature of these ictal psychiatric symptoms cannot be confused with a psychiatric disorder. On the other hand, patients experiencing only auras consisting of ictal panic can be erroneously diagnosed as suffering from panic attacks.

Depressive Disorders

Interictal depressive disorders are the most frequent psychiatric disorders in people with epilepsy. The most frequent types of depressive disorders include *major depression* and *dysthymic disorder.* The difference between major depression and dysthymic disorder is based largely on severity, persistence, and duration of symptoms.

Symptoms in both disorders may include combinations of depressed mood, inability to find any pleasure in any activity, feelings of worthlessness and guilt (without any apparent reason), feelings of helplessness and hopelessness, decreased ability to concentrate, recurrent thoughts of death, and problems with appetite resulting in weight loss or gain, changes in sleep causing insomnia or excessive sleep, slow thinking, agitation, and fatigue.

The diagnosis of a major depressive episode requires *at least 2 weeks* of either a depressed mood or inability to find pleasure accompanied by four or more of the additional symptoms listed occurring *every day* and lasting *the majority* of the day.

In contrast, dysthymic disorder is a more chronic but less intense situation, with symptoms present more days than not *for at least 2 years.*

People who have experienced one major depressive episode have a 50 percent chance of having more episodes. Those who have had two episodes have a 70 percent chance, and those who have experienced more than two episodes are likely to have recurrent major depressive episodes, unless they take medication to prevent it.

In addition, up to 50 percent of depressed people with epilepsy have an *atypical presentation* (unusual form) of their particular depressive disorder, one not usually seen in the general population. These atypical characteristics include the fact that their symptoms are recurrent but not continuous, with symptom-free periods that may last several days in duration. In addition, these patients report more apparent and frequent symptoms of irritability, poor frustration tolerance, and physical symptoms.

Studies have also shown that a large percentage of people with epilepsy and depression can also experience symptoms of anxiety or a full anxiety disorder and vice versa. This means that if your doctor is doing an evaluation to establish the presence of a depressive disorder, they also must evaluate you to inquire about the presence of symptoms of anxiety.

You should be aware of a disease called *manic-depressive illness* or *bipolar disorder* since it can present with major depressive episodes and it can occur in people with epilepsy more frequently than in the general population. Indeed, a recent study showed that 12 percent of people with epilepsy had experienced symptoms of this condition at some point in their life. In bipolar disorder, the patient experiences recurrent major depressive episodes, followed by *manic* or *hypomanic* episodes. A manic episode consists of at least four of the following symptoms for a minimal period of at least two 2 weeks: (1) inflated self-esteem or grandiosity; (2) decreased need for sleep; (3) more talkative than usual or pressured speech; (4) flight of ideas or racing thoughts; (5) distractibility; or (6) excessive involvement in pleasurable activities that have a high potential for painful consequences (i.e., unrestricted buying sprees, sexual indiscretions, and so forth). The difference between manic and hypomanic episodes is also based on severity. A diagnosis of a hypomanic episode is reached after 4 days of a distinct and persistently elevated expansive or irritable mood associated with at least 3 of the previously listed symptoms.

Depressive Disorders in Children with Epilepsy

Recognition of depressive disorders may be difficult in children, both those with and without epilepsy, as they do not verbalize the "typical" symptoms of depression, such as "I am sad" or "I feel there is no hope for me." Instead, children tend to act out, become irritable or impulsive, and often display aggressive behavior at home and in school. They exhibit problems with concentration in school and have motor restlessness, which often leads physicians to make an erroneous diagnosis of ADD. The following should help parents and physicians suspect the possibility of a depressive disorder in a child who has (1) a family history of depression or alcoholism in a first-degree relative, such as a parent or sibling; (2) problems with sleep, presenting as either difficulty falling asleep and waking up in the middle of the night, or excessive sleeping during the day; (3) changes in appetite, presenting either as loss of appetite or excessive eating; (4) a tendency to withdraw from friends; (5) an avoidance or loss of interest in habitual or new recreational activities; and (6) a tendency of symptoms to recur with or without any apparent external reason following symptom-free intervals.

As in adults, depressive disorders in children can often be associated with anxiety disorders or symptoms of anxiety. In the section on anxiety disorders, we describe the symptoms of anxiety that are more typical of children.

Recognizing Depression in Epilepsy

It's important to recognize and treat depressive disorders or clusters of depressive symptoms early, because they may have a negative effect on quality of life in people with epilepsy. In fact, in people with persistent seizures, the presence of depression has a *worse* impact on their quality of life than the actual seizures themselves!

In addition, people with epilepsy have a greater risk of attempting or committing suicide than the general population. Clearly, an untreated depressive disorder can contribute to such higher suicidal risk.

Possible Causes of Depression in Epilepsy

Many things can contribute to depression in epilepsy. They include:

- A reaction to the multiple obstacles that people with epilepsy have to face, such as having to give up driving privileges (at least temporarily) and increased dependency on others for transportation.

- The stigma associated with having seizures in our society and the discrimination that often takes place at work and by peers, and the need to take daily medication, to name a few.

- Changes in the brain, consisting primarily of chemical and electrical changes caused by the actual seizure disorder. In addition, some of the areas of the brain that are affected by the epilepsy and the depressive disorder (in people without epilepsy) may be the same. For example, patients with temporal or frontal lobe epilepsy are more likely to experience depressive disorders. By the same token, people without epilepsy who suffer from major depression also may show abnormalities in their temporal and frontal lobes.

- A genetic predisposition. People with a family history of depression, especially in first-degree relatives (parents, siblings), may be at greater risk of experiencing depression associated with their epilepsy. It is important that you inform your doctor about a history of depression in your parents and close relatives, as certain AEDs can facilitate the development of depression in patients with this type of family history. For example, if your mother suffered from depression, and you are started on a medication like phenobarbital, you are more likely to experience a depressive disorder.

- An *iatrogenic process*. This is the occurrence of psychiatric complications directly related to the actual treatment of the seizure disorder with either antiepileptic medication or brain surgery (such as removal of the anterior part of the temporal lobe in patients with temporal lobe epilepsy). Table 13.4 shows the AEDs that have been found to often cause *more frequent* symptoms of depression or depressive disorders. When an AED causes symptoms of depression, lowering its dose may be enough to get rid of these symptoms. However, very often it is necessary to change the AED. On the other hand, in some patients with recurrent major

TABLE 13.4 AED Antiepileptic Drugs That Are More Likely to Cause Psychiatric Symptoms as Adverse Events

Symptoms of Depression/Anxiety	Behavioral Symptoms
Phenobarbital	Phenobarbital
Primidone (Mysoline®)	Primidone
Clonazepam (Klonopin®)	Clonazepam and other benzodiazepines
Felabamate (Felbamate®)	Valproic acid (at high doses)
Topiramate (Topamax®)	Topiramate
Levetiracetam (Keppra®)	Levetiracetam
Zonisamide (Zonegran®)	Gabapentin (in mentally retarded children)
	Lamotrigine (in mentally retarded children)
	Fycompa

depressive disorders or manic depressive illness, some AEDs, like carbamazepine (Tegretol), valproic acid (Depakote), and lamotrigine (Lamictal) can be very effective in preventing their recurrence. Stopping these AEDs in some people can actually cause psychiatric symptoms.

Treatment of Depression

Depressive disorders can be successfully treated with *antidepressants*. In addition, certain types of *psychotherapy* (or talk therapy), specifically *cognitive behavior therapy* (CBT), may be very effective in helping patients come out of a depressive episode. At times, a combination of antidepressant medication and CBT is recommended.

Because many physicians are afraid that antidepressant medication can worsen seizures, some have been reluctant to recommend this type of treatment. Nevertheless, studies have shown that the use of antidepressants known as *selective serotonin-reuptake inhibitors* (SSRIs) are safe in people with epilepsy and do not worsen seizures. There is no reason to withhold this type of treatment, above all in people with epilepsy who are experienc-

TABLE 13.5 Efficacy of SSRIs and SNRIs in Primary Depression and Anxiety Disorders

Antidepressant Drug	Depression	Panic Disorder	Generalized Anxiety
Paroxetine*	+	+	+
Sertraline*	+	+	
Fluoxetine*	+	+	
Citalopram*	+		
Escitalopram*	+	+	+

ing a major depressive episode. SSRIs are also helpful in suppressing the symptoms of anxiety that very often accompany depressive episodes. Table 13.5 lists the most frequently used SSRIs in people with epilepsy.

Antidepressant medication can be used safely in children and adolescents with depressive disorders and epilepsy. If this is necessary, however, they should be administered under the supervision of a child psychiatrist and not by the child's pediatrician.

As with any medication, SSRIs can potentially cause side effects. These include gastrointestinal symptoms (nausea, abdominal cramps, diarrhea, and heartburn), sedation or insomnia, and symptoms of sexual dysfunction (problems with erection or ejaculation). If any side effect occurs, inform your doctor. She may lower the dose and, if the symptoms do not disappear, change to another type of SSRI. You should not stop these medications abruptly, however, as you may experience some temporary nausea, headache, and flu-like symptoms.

Anxiety Disorders

As shown in Table 13.3, anxiety disorders are the second most common psychiatric disorder in people with epilepsy and they very often occur together with depressive disorders. The classification of anxiety disorders includes eight different types, of which *generalized anxiety disorder* and *panic disorder* are the two most frequent, both in the general population and in people with epilepsy. The other six disorders (agoraphobia without panic disorder, obsessive-compulsive disorder, social phobia, specific phobia, posttraumatic stress disorder, and acute stress disorder) may occur in people with epilepsy, but with a much lower frequency. This will not be reviewed here.

In people with epilepsy, interictal panic and generalized anxiety disorders can be identical to those seen in the general population. Generalized anxiety disorder consists of constant uncontrollable worry on a daily basis, *of at least 6 months* duration, that is associated with at least three of the following six symptoms: restlessness, easy fatigability, decreased concentration, irritability, muscle tension, and sleep disturbances.

Panic disorder consists of recurrent panic attacks that are defined as "a discrete period" of intense fear or discomfort, in which 4 or more of the following symptoms developed abruptly and reached a peak within 10 minutes: (1) fear of losing control or going crazy; (2) fear of dying; (3) palpitations or accelerated heart rate; (4) sweating; (5) trembling or shaking; (6) sensation of shortness of breath; (7) feeling of choking; (8) chest pain or discomfort; (9) nausea or discomfort in the abdomen; (10) feeling dizzy, unsteady, or faint; (11) feeling detached from oneself; (12) feelings of pins and needles; and (13) chills or hot flushes. It is not unusual for patients with panic disorders to avoid leaving the house or being left alone for fear of having a panic attack. When this happens, the patient is considered to have panic disorder with *agoraphobia*.

Patients with panic disorder may go through a period of several weeks to months with frequent panic attacks, and then be free of panic attacks for prolonged periods. Also, panic attacks are not unusual when a patient is in the middle of a major depressive episode.

Ictal Panic and Its Differences with Interictal Panic Attacks

A feeling of panic can be the only expression of an aura or simple partial seizure. At times, patients with ictal panic have been erroneously diagnosed as having panic attacks. Taking a careful history of the event may avoid making such errors. The principal differences are: (1) ictal panics are short episodes lasting less than 30 seconds, while panic attacks last *at least* 10 to 20 minutes; (2) the intensity of the panic sensation is much less severe in ictal panic than in that of panic attacks and rarely do patients feel as if they are dying or going crazy; (3) the episodes of ictal fear are identical each time they occur, while this is not necessarily the case in panic attacks; and (4) patients with ictal fear may become confused or lose awareness of their surroundings if the seizure evolves to a complex partial seizure, however, this does not happen in panic attacks.

Anxiety Disorders in Children with Epilepsy

In children, symptoms of anxiety usually are apparent primarily in the form of *separation anxiety disorder*, which consists of the following symptoms: (1) fear (to the point of reaching a panic state) of staying alone in a room; (2) fear of going to bed alone or in a dark room; (3) constant worry about the whereabouts and welfare of their parents; (4) fear of something bad happening that may result in a separation from their parents; and (5) complaints of a variety of physical symptoms such as headaches, stomach aches, and so forth.

In its most severe form, separation anxiety can result in the child refusing to go to school. This is known as *school phobia*. When this happens, the child may wake up early in the morning complaining about a variety of physical symptoms to avoid going to school, along with a long list of complaints. However, the child can verbalize multiple other reasons why they should stay at home. When school phobia occurs, immediate intervention by a child psychiatrist is advised, because the problem may become long-lasting.

The suspected causes of anxiety disorders in epilepsy are similar to the causes listed for depressive disorders.

Treatment of Anxiety Disorders in Epilepsy

As in the case of depressive disorders, treatment of anxiety includes the use of medication, CBT or other form of talk therapy, or a combination of both.

The same type of SSRI antidepressants listed for the treatment of depression are also very useful in the management of generalized anxiety disorder and panic disorder, at similar doses (see Table 13.5). In addition, *benzodiazepines* have been used for a very long time to treat anxiety disorders. The benzodiazepines include clonazepam and lorazepam, but these should only be given for a few weeks, as their efficacy may only last for a short time before fading.

Attention Deficit Disorders

ADDs are the most frequent psychiatric disorder identified in children with epilepsy, although they occur in adults as well. ADD can be divided into three principal categories: ADD predominantly with inattention, ADD predominantly with motor hyperactivity, and ADD with prominent presence of *both* inattention and motor hyperactivity. This last form is called *attention deficit hyperactivity disorder* (ADHD). The principal symptoms of interictal ADHD include motor hyperactivity, impulsive behavior, poor frustration tolerance, short attention span, and distractibility, which results in an inability to get organized in activities. Failure to concentrate makes learning difficult, and the child may lead teachers to complain that the child is not listening, appears forgetful, and frequently loses things.

In the absence of motor hyperactivity and impulsive behavior, the child experiences all the problems derived from poor concentration, but no or fewer behavioral problems. With the exception of very severe forms of ADHD, symptoms listed previously often improve when the child is placed in a structured and quiet environment without too many things around them that may "over-stimulate" or distract them. It is not infrequent for children with ADHD often to have associated learning disabilities and, therefore, they should be evaluated with neuropsychological tests to identify their presence.

ADD in Adolescents and Adults with Epilepsy

Typically, when children with ADHD enter adolescence, their motor hyperactivity improves significantly, but they may be left with problems of inattention, impulsive behavior, and poor frustration tolerance. Adults with ADD complain primarily of difficulty concentrating, which results in problems with getting organized at their work and finishing their tasks, and may lead to constant job changes. In addition, they notice a propensity for being irritable and having a poor frustration tolerance.

ADHD can vary in severity from very mild to very severe. When mild in severity, the symptoms may only be manifested as the child enters junior high school or high school, where there is less structure and classes become more complex on their academic demands.

Suspected Causes of ADHD in Epilepsy

The suspected causes of ADHD in epilepsy include:

- Changes in the brain resulting in chemical and electrical changes caused by the epilepsy, or changes in the brain caused by the injury to the brain that caused the epilepsy. ADHD can be seen in all types of epilepsy, but more frequently in children with temporal and frontal lobe epilepsy. ADD can be seen frequently in children and adolescents who suffer from absence seizures and juvenile myoclonic epilepsy.
- A genetic predisposition. ADD can be inherited from one generation to the other.
- Iatrogenic causes. The antiepileptic medications that can cause symptoms of ADD are listed in Table 13.5.

Treatment of ADD

The treatment of ADD in patients with epilepsy includes medication and, in some cases, behavior and family therapy. Among the medications, drugs known as *central nervous system stimulants,* are the most frequently used, and they are considered safe in children and adults with epilepsy. These include methylphenidate (Ritalin®) and dextroamphetamine (Adderall®). Up until recently, the effect of these medications was of short duration, from 3 to 4 hours, which required the need to take repeated doses. Children were required to get their midday dose from the school nurse, which often can be very distressing and a cause of poor compliance. In the last decade, these medications have become available in formulations where the effect can last up to 12 hours. These formulations known as *extended-release* formulations are now favored over the older ones.

Some physicians fear that the use of these medications can worsen seizures, but this is not true. Most pediatric neurologists and epileptologists believe that these drugs can be used safely in patients with epilepsy, and treatment should not be withheld because of such concerns.

The most frequent adverse events of central nervous system stimulants include decreased appetite, insomnia, abdominal pain, dry mouth, headaches, and nervousness. Approximately 10 percent of children with ADD may not be able to tolerate these drugs, becoming more irritable and moody instead. In these cases, the medication must be discontinued at once. In such cases, another type of medication can be considered.

In addition to drug treatments, behavior therapy can be very helpful in training patients to develop strategies to control their impulsivity and poor frustration tolerance. Family therapy is often necessary to teach parents how to deal with these children.

Summary

Patients with epilepsy are at a greater risk of experiencing depressive, anxiety, and attention deficit disorders than the general population. Early recognition of these psychiatric disorders is extremely important, as they can have a very negative impact on the quality of life of these patients. While there may be an identifiable association between the seizure disorder and the development of any of these three psychiatric disorders, there are several causes of these psychiatric disorders in people with epilepsy.. They include a reaction to facing the obstacles of a life with seizures, changes in the brain resulting from the seizure disorder, a genetic predisposition, and side effects caused by AEDs. Nevertheless, we are not yet able to identify all the causes of these psychiatric disorders in epilepsy. People with epilepsy and any of these three psychiatric disorders need to be evaluated for treatment, which is available and safe, and includes the use of medication, psychotherapy, or a combination of both of the two treatment modalities.

FREQUENTLY ASKED QUESTIONS

Q **Can AEDs impair my job performance?**

Most people taking AEDs can perform their job without problems, but AEDs can impair job performance in some people. Your risk may be increased if your job requires rapid motor responses, rapid processing of information, vigilance, or learning. Your risk may also be increased if you are taking multiple AEDs, higher dosages of AEDs with higher blood levels, or certain AEDs (such as topiramate or older AEDs, especially phenobarbital). If you have a concern, discuss it with your doctor.

Q **I am worried about cognitive problems. What should I do, and what should I expect of my doctor?**

Talk with your doctor and let them know exactly what problems you are experiencing and how these problems are affecting your life. Factors that you and your doctor should consider as possibly contributing to your problem are listed in Table 13.1. If you are unsure if your AED(s) could be contributing to your problems, fill out the Adverse Events Profile in Table

13.2. If your total score is greater than 45, AED toxicity may be adversely impacting you. Your doctor may consider altering your AED treatment to reduce the dose, reduce the number of AEDs, or change to an AED with less cognitive side effects. Of course, these changes must take into account seizure control. Your doctor may also consider evaluations such as blood tests (AED blood levels, serum B_{12} level, thyroid tests), MRI, electroencephalogram (EEG), or formal neuropsychological testing to detect abnormalities and direct your treatment.

Be aware that the underlying brain disorder that leads to epilepsy may also affect cognition. In fact, the size of the effect of the pre-existing brain disorder on cognition is usually larger than the effect of AEDs. However, the effect of AEDs can be significant, and AED effects can potentially be altered. Also, be aware that your mood can markedly affect your perception of your cognitive performance. In several studies, a patient's perception of their own cognitive abilities was more related to depressed mood than their actual cognitive performance. Further, depression can actually affect your attention and memory. Thus, your doctor may consider assessment and possible treatment for depression.

Q I am worried about cognitive problems in my child with epilepsy. What should I do?

Many of the issues that you and your doctor should consider are the same as those discussed in Question 2, which also concern this problem in the adult patient. However, this issue is complicated in children because their cognitive abilities are changing as they grow and because children may not be able to express their problems like an adult. School performance is an important factor that should be monitored. If you are concerned about your child's abilities, talk with your doctor. Your child may be eligible for Early Intervention Services. The Early Intervention Program for Infants and Toddlers with Disabilities of the Individuals with Disabilities Education Act (IDEA) (Part C) is available in all 50 states and 7 territories of the United States. This program provides speech/language, occupational, and physical therapies to any child under the age of 3 who has a disability or significant delays in development. If your child has reached 3 years, they may be eligible for similar services through the Preschool Special Education Program in your local school district. Eligibility is determined by assessing your child's five skill areas: adaptive development, cognition, communication, physical development (gross and fine motor), and social/emotional development. Similar programs and therapies may also be available privately in your area.

> **Q** **I have suffered from epilepsy for several years, and my doctor has never asked me whether I was experiencing any symptoms of depression. Does that mean I do not have depression or I do not need to worry about ever suffering from this disorder?**

The answer to this question is a definite No! Unfortunately, doctors may not inquire about the presence of depression or anxiety symptoms unless you appear sad and distressed in during your medical visit or you verbalize symptoms of depression. Also, some doctors erroneously assume that experiencing symptoms of depression and anxiety is a "normal" reaction to having epilepsy and, hence, such symptoms do not require special treatment. Yet, as we discussed previously, several causes may influence the development of depressive disorders, some of which may require an intervention. For example, if you are experiencing depressive symptoms caused by the AED that you are taking, you may be able to get rid of your symptoms by having your doctor lower the dose or changing your medication. The important point to remember is that depression in people with epilepsy can disrupt their lives significantly, and the presence of symptoms of depression merits an evaluation to establish the need and type of treatment.

> **Q** **Can depressive and anxiety disorders interfere with my job performance?**

Absolutely! Depressive disorders can affect your job performance by interfering with your ability to think and to relate to others. For example, if you were to have a major depressive episode, you would experience slowing of your thinking and, you would have difficulty concentrating and problems with remembering things. Because major depression causes irritability and poor frustration tolerance, you may end up arguing a lot with your coworkers and superiors, which could get you in trouble, and you could potentially lose your job. If you are also experiencing symptoms of anxiety, you would have difficulty concentrating in your job because of the constant worries and restlessness that would get in the way of your performance.

CHAPTER 14

Taking Control Over Your Epilepsy

- Managing a life with epilepsy is a multi-faceted process, ranging from establishing a good doctor-patient relationship to knowing how the law affects your ability to live independently.
- Numerous national laws protect the patient's rights to privacy, access to personal health information, health insurance coverage, and more.
- The American Disabilities Act (ADA) protects people with epilepsy against workplace discrimination.
- Driving with epilepsy is regulated by each state, with varying requirements for the time you must be seizure-free before driving legally.

Living with and managing a health condition like epilepsy often means working together with numerous parties to receive the healthcare you need. From physicians and insurance companies to various state and federal agencies, you may be asked to share a lot of personal information and to navigate complicated bureaucratic systems. It can be confusing, but it's possible to take control of your health and your life if you're equipped with the information and tools to do so. In this chapter, we'll review ways in which you can establish a mutually beneficial relationship with your doctor, which laws establish certain rights for patients, and what resources are available to help you receive the best healthcare. We'll also look at what roadblocks you may face along the way and what you need to know to inform your choices moving forward. Certainly, a life with epilepsy can be challenging. But it's in your power to take control of your condition and your life.

The Doctor-Patient Relationship

The doctor-patient interaction is a special relationship that asks something from both parties to make it work. Entrusted with their patients' health and quality of life, doctors take on the responsibility of providing the best care, while following the highest standards of professional ethics. In order to do so, however, patients are asked to divulge intimate details that can go beyond their condition, such as deeply personal information about their sexual history; their family health history; whether they drink, smoke, and do drugs (and how often); details about their mental and emotional health; and so forth. This exchange of information and care between doctors and patients creates a special bond. So sacred is this trust, that many patients tell their doctors things about themselves they would never tell anyone else, trusting that their doctors will safeguard this information and use it to help provide the best care.

The first step in establishing this relationship, though, begins with the patient.

As mentioned in detail later in this chapter, the patient has certain responsibilities to help improve their health care. Since most medical care takes place in a medical office, there are certain things in your power to make your doctor's visits as successful as possible. The first is to tell your story as accurately as you can. The following are some pointers to keep in mind.

Tips for Sharing Your Story with Your Doctor

- **Use everyday language.** How would you tell a trusted friend about your health? Use the same approach with your doctor, and use your own words to tell your story. For example, telling your doctor that after a seizure, you feel "confused and sleepy" perfectly fine. Don't feel pressured to use medical words, even if other doctors may have used them with you.

- **Be honest.** If you are asked a question that you can't answer, say so. Don't make up an answer to say what you think the doctor wants to hear. To provide you the best care, it's more helpful for your doctor to have less information in some cases than to have false information.

- **Bring detailed notes.** If your story is complicated, don't be afraid to write it down before your visit. If you keep a seizure diary or something like it, this can provide a lot of insight as well.

- **Bring your medications with you in their prescription bottles.** For people with epilepsy, bring a list of antiseizure medications you've tried in the past and how your seizures responded, the maximum doses you took, and whether you had any side effects from the medications.

- **Bring a list of your other physicians.** Your new doctor will benefit from having the information of who has cared for you in the past, as well as to whom you want your records sent. This can include your primary care physician, other epilepsy specialists, and so forth. It's best if you can provide the complete addresses and phone numbers of the doctors' offices.

- **Bring a copy of your medical records.** If you've been seen by other specialists, had any surgeries related to your condition, or had any testing done, try to bring copies of these records with you to your visit. Having them will better inform your doctor of your condition and treatment history.

- **Bring a trusted friend or family member who is familiar with your condition.** If you can't describe what happens when you have a seizure, if possible, bring along someone who has seen your seizures.

- **Bring a list of questions you want answered.** You may be doing a lot of the talking, but this is also the opportune time to ask questions about your health, medications, treatment options, and so forth. Don't be afraid to write down your questions. Alternatively, you can also record the conversation on your phone or a tape recorder, or you can ask someone else to sit in to take notes for you.

Your Doctor's Responsibilities to You

As this is a relationship between two parties, your doctor also has certain responsibilities to uphold at your office visit. Ultimately, it's your doctor's ability and willingness to fulfill these responsibilities that will help you decide whether they are the best person to lead your healthcare plan. Here are some questions to consider when making this very important decision.

A Checklist for Your Doctor's Visit(s)

- **Is your doctor greeting you by name?** Your doctor is someone who will come to deeply know some aspects of your life—maybe more so than some of your closest friends and family members.

Knowing your name is simply a small indication that they recognize you as more than just a patient, but rather as a person with a life outside their office.

- **Is your doctor listening attentively when you talk?** Remember that you know your health story better than anyone else. It's important that your doctor is willing to listen to you share your story, listen to your concerns, and answer your questions to the best of their ability. It's also pertinent that they believe you when you tell them how you feel, both in terms of how your condition is affecting you and otherwise.

- **Is your doctor explaining your diagnosis thoroughly?** There are different types of epilepsy, and the first step in leading a seizure-free life is to understand your diagnosis. Consider whether your doctor is taking the time to explain more than what the diagnosis is called. You should be able to leave the office visit and explain your diagnosis to someone else, whether it's another health professional or a friend.

- **Is your doctor giving you options to consider for diagnostic testing and treatment?** Your doctor should recognize that their role is to provide you with a set of sound medical choices and let you decide which one is best for your health. After all, it is *your life, and you need to be able to make informed decisions about it.*

- **If you're prescribed a medication, is your doctor telling you about some of the side effects and explaining whether there are any drug interactions you should watch out for?** While you'll have the opportunity to talk to your pharmacist about these things, your doctor should be the first person to discuss side effects, risk factors, and other important details about any drug you're prescribed.

- **Is your doctor giving you some idea about the likelihood of success in controlling your seizures and which treatments may provide the best chance of seizure control?** Similarly, they should provide detailed explanations about the risks and benefits of epilepsy surgery or implanted devices if those are being considered for treatment options.

■ **Is your doctor trying to answer your questions in terms you can understand?** Lastly, don't forget that your interactions with your doctor should feel casual and personable. You should both speak in everyday language, using terms that are easy to understand. The goal for your visit is to be able to leave and remember what you talked about, which is much harder to do if your doctor speaks mostly in medical jargon.

Keep in mind that most doctors take care of about 2,000 patients, so your doctor may not be able to spend as much time as either of you would like during your office visit. On average, doctors allot 60 minutes for visits with new patients and 30 minutes for returning patients. When asking questions or expressing your concerns, be sure to cover the most important ones first. If your problem is complicated, expect that it may take several visits to cover most of the questions you have. Be sure to ask your doctor the best method of communication outside of the office if you have questions after your visit. For example, many doctor's offices use an online patient portal, on which you can request prescription refills, message your doctor, and pay bills. If you call into the office, it's likely a nurse on your doctor's staff will field your questions and return your calls. Unless you're experiencing serious side effects or have a very pressing question about your medication, prescription-related questions are often best handled through the phone or online patient portal.

Another rule of thumb: If you're seeing a specialist for your epilepsy care, try to call them for issues related to your epilepsy, and contact your primary care doctor for more general problems such as colds and refills of medications for other medical problems, such as high blood pressure. If you do call for refills, have your pharmacy's name and phone number ready before you call, as well as a pen and paper handy in case you're given new directions during the phone call.

Additional Considerations for a Successful Doctor's Visit

Ultimately, both patients and doctors should treat each other with courtesy and respect. It's the only way to establish a trusting and productive doctor-patient relationship that results in the highest quality of care. It's also good to keep in mind that everyone has different ways of communicating, through words and body language, and miscommunication can occur, even in the doctor's office. For example, it's common for people to "size each other up," by judging whether the one person is making (or avoiding) eye contact, whether they are standing or sitting, by how they are dressed, and in many other nonverbal ways. It's likely you've met someone and come away feeling strongly positive or negative feelings about them, subconsciously basing your judgment on their mannerisms. Maybe they reminded you of someone you liked or disliked? These unconscious strong feelings are driven by hidden positive and negative bias everyone has based on individual upbringings; sets of ideals for beauty, race, sex, and social standing; and many other factors. Psychiatrists use the term *transference* to refer to these powerful emotions that patients have toward their doctors and *counter-transference* for the feelings that doctors have for their patients. No matter who you are, these feelings are universally experienced. By reflecting on these feelings, though, it's possible to prevent yourself from making snap judgments about strangers and new acquaintances. In the case of establishing a new doctor-patient relationship, acknowledging the presence of transference can help you make a sound decision about whether your doctor is the right fit for you without involving biases in the mix. Practicing "The Golden Rule" will serve you well in this circumstance. As you expect your doctor to see you as a real person with a real life, you should do the same for them. Try to put yourself in your doctor's shoes when you sense a conflict. Ask yourself these questions before forming a negative opinion: Are you making a reasonable request? Are you misunderstanding your doctor, or do you suspect they are misunderstanding you? Does your dissatisfaction stem from the prognosis, or do you feel unheard? Is your doctor rushing you out or is your appointment running long?

In the end, you are responsible for your healthcare. Don't forget that while your doctor is a source of information, it's up to you to choose the treatment option that's best for you. Therefore, listen with an open mind. Don't be afraid to speak up. Ask questions when you don't understand something. Only you know your own thoughts, so don't be afraid to express them. Lastly, take the time to reflect on your options, but don't be paralyzed by indecision. By channeling your inner courage, you can always make changes if you don't like how things are going. Whether that means having additional testing, trying a new medication, considering epilepsy surgery, volunteering for a drug or device trial, or seeking out a new doctor, it's ultimately in your hands.

Your Rights as a Patient

In March 1998, President Bill Clinton's Advisory Commission on Consumer Protection and Quality in the Health Care Industry issued a report titled, "Quality First: Better Health Care for All Americans," which contained the Consumer Bill of Rights and Responsibilities. The Commission listed 7 sets of rights and 1 set of responsibilities. The following includes a summary of the bill of rights.

The Consumer Bill of Rights

1. **Information Disclosure.** Patients have the right to receive accurate, easily understood information to help them in making informed decisions about their doctors and other providers, hospitals and medical offices, and health plans.
2. **Choice of Providers and Plans.** Patients have the right to a choice of health care providers that is sufficient to assure access to appropriate high-quality healthcare including giving patients with serious medical conditions and chronic illnesses access to specialists.

3. **Access to Emergency Services.** Patients have the right to access emergency health services when and where the need arises. Health plans should pay for services when patients go to any emergency department with acute serious symptoms, "including severe pain" that "prudent laypersons" could reasonably expect that would place their health at risk if they did not seek medical care.

4. **Participation in Treatment Decisions.** Patients have the right to fully participate in all decisions related to their healthcare. Consumers who are unable to fully participate in treatment decisions have the right to be represented by parents, guardians, family members, or others. Additionally, provider contracts should not contain any so-called "gag clauses" that restrict health professionals' ability to discuss and advise patients on medically necessary treatment options.

5. **Respect and Nondiscrimination.** Patients have the right to considerate, respectful care from all members of the healthcare industry at all times and under all circumstances. Patients must not be discriminated against in the marketing or enrollment or in the provision of health care services, consistent with the benefits covered in their policy and/or as required by law, based on race, ethnicity, national origin, religion, sex, age, current or anticipated mental or physical disability, sexual orientation, genetic information, or source of payment.

6. **Confidentiality of Health Information.** Patients have the right to communicate with healthcare providers in confidence and to have the confidentiality of their individually identifiable health care information protected. Patients also have the right to review and copy their own medical records and request amendments to their records.

7. **Complaints and Appeals.** Patients have the right to a fair and efficient process for resolving differences with their health plans, healthcare providers, and the institutions that serve them, includ-

ing a rigorous system of internal review and an independent system of external review.

8. **Consumer Responsibilities.** In a healthcare system that affords patients' rights and protections, patients must also take greater responsibility for maintaining good health. Greater involvement in their healthcare increases the likelihood of patients achieving the best outcomes and helps support quality improvement in a cost-conscious manner. According to the report, patient's responsibilities include:

    ■ Take responsibility for maximizing healthy habits, such as exercising, not smoking, and eating a healthy diet.

    ■ Become involved in specific health care decisions.

    ■ Work collaboratively with health care providers in developing and carrying out agreed-upon treatment plans.

    ■ Disclose relevant information and clearly communicate wants and needs.

    ■ Use the health plan's internal complaint and appeal processes to address concerns that may arise.

    ■ Avoid knowingly spreading disease.

    ■ Recognize the reality of risks and limits of the science of medical care and the human fallibility of the health care professional.

    ■ Be aware of a health care provider's obligation to be reasonably efficient and equitable in providing care to other patients and the community.

    ■ Become knowledgeable about their health plan coverage and health plan options (when available) including all covered benefits, limitations, and exclusions, rules regarding use of network providers, coverage and referral rules, appropriate processes to secure additional information, and the process to appeal coverage decisions.

    ■ Show respect for other patients and health workers.

- Make a good-faith effort to meet financial obligations.
- Abide by administrative and operational procedures of health plans, health care providers, and Government health benefit programs.
- Report wrongdoing and fraud to appropriate resources or legal authorities.

The Health Insurance Portability and Accountability Act

When the *Health Insurance Portability and Accountability Act* (HIPAA) was enacted by Congress on August 21, 1996, and signed into law by President Bill Clinton, the HIPAA Privacy Rule created for the first time, national standards to protect individuals' medical records and other personal health information. The Privacy Rule came into effect in stages beginning on April 14, 2003. While most of this section deals with the privacy aspects of the law, there are other sections to the law that are relevant to patients' privacy and protection. For example, one section protects workers and their families from losing health insurance coverage when they change or lose jobs. Another section establishes national standards for identification of healthcare providers, employers, hospitals, and health insurance plans, and it regulates how electronic transmission of healthcare information can occur so that security and privacy of the data is protected. The HIPAA Act also spells out how your personal health information can be released and to whom it can be released. In general, the law gives patients more control over their data than ever before. In short, knowing your rights under HIPAA is a vital part of being in control of your healthcare.

Your Rights Under HIPAA

There are many ways that HIPAA affects patients. These are some of the most important protections granted to you by law:

1. **The right to obtain and make corrections to your health records.** Under HIPAA, you can always ask for a copy of your medical records and other personal health information from your healthcare provider. You also have the right to examine the information and request changes if the information is wrong or if you think the information is missing or incomplete. If you believe something is wrong (a test result, for example) and the hospital believes it's correct, you still have the right to have this disagreement noted in your file.

2. **The right to know how your health information is shared.** The law allows your health information to be used for specific purposes that aren't directly related to your healthcare like ensuring doctors are providing good care, reporting when the flu is in your area, and other reasons related to public health. HIPAA also sets up rules for safeguarding the privacy of your medical records and details the penalties that can be imposed if privacy is not maintained. For example, your health information cannot be shared with your employer or for marketing or advertising purposes without your written permission. Most often, you will receive a notice detailing how your information may be shared on your first visit to the doctor, but you can ask for a copy of this information at any time.

3. **The right to limit the release of some aspects of your health records.** Under HIPAA, you can request that your information not be shared with certain people, groups, or companies. For example, you can ask your doctor not to share you information with other doctors or nurses at the hospital or clinic. If, however, your request impedes with your doctor's ability to provide good care, they may not have to agree to your request. You also have the right to ask your doctor not to share what care you receive or what medications you take with your health insurance company if you pay for the drugs and/or treatment fully out-of-pocket.

4. **The right to be reached somewhere else than home.** By law, you
    can make reasonable requests to be contacted where and how you
    choose. For example, if you prefer to be called at the office, it's
    your right to ask the doctor's office to reach you there.

How HIPAA Applies to Minors

HIPAA generally allows parents and guardians to have access to the medical records of their minor children as long as there are no other laws covering the release of the information. Examples of when parents would not
have access:

- If the court has ordered the child to undergo some medical treatment.
- If the minor consents to care that does not require parental
  approval.
- If the parent agrees that the minor could have a confidential relationship with the provider.

Even in these situations, there may be some state laws or other rules
that would allow parents access to some of the information. On the other
hand, the minor's privacy may be protected in certain circumstances, for
example, if the provider believes that the child might be subject to domestic violence or abuse if the information became known to the parent. The
HIPAA Privacy Rule does not change the rules regarding a child's ability to
be treated without parental consent.

The details of the national standards can be found at the Health and
Human Services Office of Civil Rights website (hhs.gov/ocr/hipaa).

The Patient Protection and Affordable Care Act (PPACA)

On March 23, 2010, the PPACA, also known as the *Affordable Care Act*
(ACA) or "Obamacare," was enacted into law. Full implementation of the

law took place on January 1, 2014. The ACA aimed to provide more health-care coverage for more citizens by making healthcare more affordable for everyone, expanding the Medicaid program, and creating new protections for those with health conditions. The law also established new rules by which insurance companies had to comply.

Your Rights Under ACA

Receiving coverage for necessary testing, medications, and treatments starts with a good insurance plan. These are some of the protections granted to you by the ACA:

1. **Health insurance companies must provide coverage for those with pre-existing conditions, including pregnancy.** Prior to the enactment of the ACA, it was common to be turned away by health insurance companies for living with a health condition. Not only cannot they discriminate based on this factor under ACA, insurance companies cannot charge you more for coverage or refuse to pay for essential health benefits for any pre-existing conditions. Once your plan begins, your insurance company cannot deny you coverage or raise your rates based only on your health. If you're pregnant, your pregnancy and childbirth are also covered from the day your plan starts.

2. **Most private health plans and all Marketplace health plans must cover preventative services at no cost to you.** This rule applies even if you haven't met your yearly deductible, but the services must be provided by a doctor or healthcare profes-sional in your plan's network. There are three sets of preventative services: for all adults, for women, and for children. Examples of these services include flu shots, immunization vaccines, certain screening tests, well-woman visits, and even some counseling vis-its. For a full list of these services, visit the healthcare.gov website (healthcare.gov/coverage/preventative-care-benefits).

3. **Insurance policies that cover children must allow young adults to stay on their parents' plans until age 26.** The law applies even if the child no longer lives with their parents and/or is not a dependent on their tax return. As expected, this regulation is particularly helpful for those whose health conditions may pose a barrier to achieving financial stability and independence by allowing them to have access to essential healthcare services and insurance coverage.

4. **All Marketplace plans must cover certain essential health benefits.** When you buy a plan in the newly established health insurance Marketplace, you can rest assured that certain services have guaranteed coverage by your plan. These include:
   - Ambulatory patient services
   - Emergency services
   - Hospitalization
   - Pregnancy, maternity, and newborn care
   - Birth control coverage
   - Breastfeeding coverage
   - Mental health and substance use disorder services
   - Prescription drugs
   - Rehabilitative and habilitative services and devices
   - Laboratory services
   - Preventative/wellness services and chronic disease management
   - Pediatric services, including oral and vision care

There are exceptions to these requirements that you should be mindful of. For example, "grandfathered plans," or plans purchased before March 23, 2010, are not required to provide certain benefits and protections. Additionally, if your employer is a religious institution or a religious non-profit organization, it may not have to offer health plans that cover contraceptive methods and counseling, requiring you to pay for them out-of-pocket. Marketplace plans do not consider vision and dental care as essential benefits, and whether your plan includes them can vary by state. The healthcare.gov website has more information on the requirements and exceptions that apply to the ACA.

Dealing with Your Insurance Company

Another area in which the informed patient should be well-versed is basic health insurance terminology, as well as common blockades you may encounter with your insurance provider and how to navigate around them. Conflicts with your insurance company can range between annoying back-and-forths, during which you must obtain multiple authorizations before your plan will cover a certain test or medication, to unlawful situations, in which your insurance provider refuses to cover a necessary treatment by citing innocuous fine print. In these situations, the relationship begins with a dispute. One side says one thing, while the other claims something else. You can increase your chances of successfully fighting back against an unfair decision by first educating yourself on the basics. Here's a brief overview to get you started.

The Basics of Health Insurance Plans

1. **You can buy a plan from your employer or from the Marketplace.** Insurance companies generally sell policies to employers, who then provide various plan options to their employees and their families. The employer may cover a portion of the premium or, in some cases, 100 percent of the premium, offering it to employees at no cost to them. But not every job has an option to purchase the employer's insurance. For people in this circumstance and those who are self-employed or unemployed, you can purchase a plan from the health insurance Marketplace, as we discussed earlier in this chapter.

2. **You must purchase a health insurance policy during Open Enrollment.** This is the yearly period of time when you can sign up for a new plan or switch plans. Certain "life events" like getting married, having a baby, losing your job, or starting a new job can qualify you for a Special Enrollment Period. The other exception to this rule is applying for Medicaid or the *Children's Health Insurance Program* (CHIP), which you can do at any time of the year.

3. **Every policy is a contract that serves as an agreement that certain medical services will be paid for and others will not.** The services that the policy will pay for are called *covered benefits*. A covered benefit may be fully paid by the policy, or only a portion may be paid with the expectation that you will be responsible for paying the remaining amount. The amount that you pay for your covered benefits before your insurance company begins to pay is called a *deductible*. Many policies have a number of fixed deductibles for which you might be required to pay $5, $10, $50 or more for certain services. Other policies may require you to pay a certain percentage of the total charge for the same services. It's common for policies to have a mixture of both types of deductibles.

4. **There are multiple types of insurance plans.** What model your policy follows will determine a number of things, such as your ability to see a specialist without a referral from your primary care physician, your options to see a doctor out-of-network, how much you pay upfront and for out-of-pocket costs, and so forth. The most common models are: *Health management organizations* (HMOs), *preferred provider organizations* (PPOs), *exclusive provider organizations* (EPOs), and *point-of service plans* (POS). Certain aspects of these models can make a difference in receiving specialized healthcare, as with epilepsy management, so it's important to do your research before purchasing a plan.

5. **You have the right to appeal a denied claim.** If your insurance provider refuses to pay a claim or ends your coverage, it must tell you why. The insurance company must also tell you how to dispute the decision. There are two ways to appeal the decision: by internal appeal or external appeal. Visit the healthcare.gov website for more information about each process (healthcare.gov/appeal-insurance-company-decision/appeals).

If your appeal is unsuccessful, you may consider obtaining a lawyer and filing a lawsuit against your insurance provider if you believe it has acted unlawfully in your case. Of course, this is the worst-case scenario, and it can be very costly and time-consuming. To avoid the added stress and expense, it's first advised that you exhaust your options to appeal the decision by the methods mentioned earlier.

If your doctor does not give you a referral to the specialist you would like to see, you have some options. Fortunately, HMO plans all have appeals processes for its members. You have the right to petition the HMO for a referral. If you are unsuccessful in getting the referral you want, call the HMO central administration office, and ask to speak to the person who handles appeals for referrals. You may need to fill out some forms. You need to be assertive and explain clearly why you want to be referred and to whom. If you have epilepsy, you should not accept anything less than "no seizures, no side effects" until you have gotten a thorough evaluation by a specialist, including diagnostic tests such as a video EEG monitoring of your typical seizures and appropriate diagnostic tests, such as a high quality MRI. If you are turned down by the appeals board, do not hesitate to ask your employer or your union to help you with your appeal. After all, your employer is paying a lot of money for your health care and the company deserves to get its money's worth for the premiums it pays. If all else fails, you can appeal to the state insurance commissioner.

Successfully Achieving Self-Management

An important element of achieving good health is to feel that you are in charge of your destiny and to take steps to do those things that are important to controlling your health. When you take steps to positively influence your health, called *self-management*, you'll find that your self-esteem will improve and you'll feel more confident in your abilities to navigate the world around you. One tricky area of self-management is feeling that the care you're getting may not be the best for you. Perhaps you continue to have seizures, despite doing everything your doctor has recommended. Maybe you feel your doctor isn't really listening to your concerns or answering your questions fully. The goal of epilepsy treatment is to be free of seizures and free of side effects. If you continue to have seizures, despite working with your doctor for many months, or if you have side effects from medications that interfere with doing the things that you want to do, you should consider trying a new approach. What next steps you take will depend on whether you're generally unhappy with your doctor or with the treatment.

Trying a New Treatment

If you are comfortable with and trust your doctor, but are discontent with your treatment regimen, the first step is to talk to your doctor about whether it's time to try something different. Ask about diagnostic tests that might be done, such as epilepsy video EEG monitoring, which can provide your doctor with a clearer understanding about why you're still having seizures. This can also help your doctor determine whether you could be a candidate for epilepsy surgery. Ask about new medications that have recently become available and treatments, such as surgery, that might help you achieve seizure freedom. Every patient's case is different, but you'll benefit from learning what percentage of patients achieve seizure reduction or seizure freedom from certain treatments. Informed with real data, you can make an educated decision about what's right for you. Lastly, don't be afraid to talk to your doctor about alternative therapies, such as holistic or homeopathic treatments. Ask them about cannabis-based medications you could try. Even if your doctor isn't an expert on these therapies and can't officially prescribe them to you as part of your regimen, it's wise to have an open discussion about the various treatment options you're interested in learning about. At the very least, your doctor may be able to point you to additional resources or give you an idea of how much or little research has been conducted on various alternative therapies.

Seeking a Second Opinion

If you have a condition like epilepsy, the goal is to achieve seizure freedom with little to no side effects from the treatment. If you work with your *primary care physician* (PCP) and you continue to have seizures or serious side effects from medications, request a referral to see a neurologist who specializes in epilepsy. If you are referred to a general neurologist, give that doctor a reasonable amount of time—six months is standard—to get your seizures under control. If you continue to have seizures or side effects, then ask your PCP to send you to an epilepsy specialist, also known as an *epileptologist*. Most epilepsy specialists practice in epilepsy centers with other specialists and offer special services, such as epilepsy surgery, and opportunities to volunteer for clinical trials that are researching new medications or devices. Additionally, epilepsy centers have social workers, nurses, and psychologists who also specialize in epilepsy care and may provide you with the support you need. Some online resources that have databases of epilepsy specialists include:

- Epilepsy Foundation (epilepsy.com)
- The American Epilepsy Society (aesnet.org)
- The National Association of Epilepsy Centers (naec-epilepsy.org)

Remember, if you feel discontent with your doctor's prognosis, treatment recommendations, or you simply don't feel comfortable seeing them for your care, you're free to find another healthcare provider for a second opinion. Don't feel guilty about going to another physician. Even most doctors will advise getting a second opinion, so that you feel confident about your healthcare choices.

One word of caution, though: Many insurance plans will not pay for a "second opinion" visit, except as a prerequisite to certain elective procedures, such as epilepsy surgery. Another roadblock to getting a second opinion can be that your current doctor is unwilling to give you a referral. To work around both of these issues, you can simply book a consultation, which is the same as seeing a doctor as a new patient. Be sure to bring all your medical records with you to your first visit with them, and/or ask your current doctor's office to send them over. As discussed earlier in the chapter, you'll be asked to sign a consent form to release your information in compliance with HIPAA guidelines.

Getting Your Medications

Anticonvulsant drugs are the mainstay of treatment for people with epilepsy. There are now more than two dozen major drugs to treat people with epilepsy and a number of minor ones, as well. Anticonvulsant drugs vary considerably in price, ranging from pennies a tablet to more than $20 a tablet for some of the newest medications. All insurance plans have many policies on prescription drug coverage. While there are many thousands of different drug benefits, we'll address a few of the most common ones in the following section.

The Basics of Prescription Drug Benefits

Most insurance plans will have a list of drugs that are covered under the policy, called a *formulary* or *drug list*. The drug formulary is typically divided into two or three tiers of drugs for prescription medications. A typical three-tier plan may charge you $10 per prescription for drugs on a *preferred drug list*, such as first-line generic medications. (The $10 is called your *copayment*, or *copay*). Here's more information about the different formulary tiers in a three-tier drug list:

1. **The first-tier drugs are called *first-line drugs* or *first-line treat-ment*.** These have been shown to be helpful for large numbers of patients or conditions, have good safety track record, and have the lowest cost.

2. **The *second-tier drugs* are called *second-line drugs* or *alternative first-line treatment*.** These drugs have more limited uses, more side effects or safety issues, and/or a higher cost than the first-tier drugs. In a three-tier prescription benefit, these drugs may have a copay of $15 to $30 or more. Like first-line drugs, these are usually prescribed on their own, but your doctor may also try a combination of second-line treatment to control your seizures.

3. **The *third-tier drugs* are called *adjunctive treatment* or *add-on treatment*.** These drugs may be particularly difficult to use because of their side effects or interactions with other drugs. Third-tier drugs are the most expensive and may have a fixed copay, such as $50. Alternatively, you may have to pay a percent-age of the total cost of the prescription, which could range from 10 percent to 50 percent or more of the total cost.

Your drug benefits policy will also likely outline how you will receive your medication. For example, many policies will cover medication home delivery, while others will require you to pick up your prescriptions at a brick-and-mortar location. The policy will also have guidelines about how much medication you can get at once. For example, your doctor may be able to write you a prescription for a 90-day supply of a certain drug or a 30-day supply in other cases. Your copay will also be determined by your policy. Remember, your doctor is bound to follow the rules of the contract strictly and cannot legally write you a prescription for more medication than is allowed by your policy.

The Medicare Prescription Drug, Improvement, and Modernization Act

Some people with epilepsy do not have prescription drug coverage benefits. Until recently, this was the case for Medicare beneficiaries. The *Medicare Prescription Drug, Improvement, and Modernization Act* (MMA) of 2003 added the Medicare Prescription Drug Plan, also referred to as *Medicare Part D*, a new optional prescription drug benefit to help people afford expensive medications. This add-on coverage is available to anyone with Medicare, but if you choose not to get Medicare drug coverage when you first become eligible, you may have to pay a late enrollment penalty. The other way to get prescription drug coverage with Medicare is by choosing a Medicare Advantage Plan (like an HMO or PPO) that offers drug coverage. You can also call the Medicare hotline at 1-800-MEDICARE (1-800-633-4227).

The Medicare prescription drug benefit has a complicated formula that can vary based on a number of factors, such as the type of plan you pick, what drugs you take, whether you go to an in-network pharmacy, whether your drugs are on your plan's formulary, and whether you get *Extra Help*, a Medicare program that helps people with limited income to pay for Medicare prescription drug program costs. The following is a summary of the costs associated with a Medicare drug plan:

- **Monthly premium.** This is a monthly fee you'll pay for your drug benefits. The cost will vary by plan. For example, if you enroll in Medicare Part B, you'll pay a premium for the Medicare Part B and a premium for your drug benefits. But if you have a plan that includes Medicare prescription drug coverage, your premium may include an amount for drug coverage.
- **Yearly deductible.** This is the amount you must pay annually for your prescriptions before your drug plan begins to pay. Deductibles vary between Medicare drug plans. Some may not have a deductible, but no Medicare drug plan may have a deductible that exceeds $415 in 2019.

- **Copayments or coinsurance.** This is the amount you'll pay for your prescriptions. It will either be a *copay*, the set amount for all drugs on a tier, or a *coinsurance*, a percentage of the drug cost.
- **Coverage gap costs.** Most Medicare plans have a *coverage gap*, or what's also called the "donut hole," which mean there's a temporary limit on what your drug plan will cover for drugs. The coverage gap only begins after you and your drug plan have spent a certain amount on covered drugs, so it won't apply to everyone who has a Medicare drug plan. In 2019, the coverage gap begins after you and your drug plan have spent $3,820 on covered drugs. Because this amount can change every year, be sure to find out whether the coverage gap applies to you, and, if so, what your drug coverage limit is. Once you're in the coverage gap, you'll pay a percentage of the plan's cost for the prescription drugs.

There may also be associated costs if you get Extra Help or enrolled in Medicare Part D late. However, these will vary by case.

Anticonvulsants as a Protected Drug Class

Since the MMA was enacted in 2003, the *Centers for Medicare and Medicaid Services* (CMS), the federal agency that administers Medicare, has instated changes to help provide more drug coverage at lower costs for more people. In July 2008, CMS implemented that Part D formularies must include drug categories and classes that include all disease states to ensure that the plan's drug list provides access to "an acceptable range of Part D drug choices." The Part D sponsors that adopt the formulary model developed in 2004 by the United States Pharmacopoeia for their own drug lists qualify for approval by CMS. More information about USP's formulary model and its updates are on the USP website (usp.org/health-quality-safety/usp-medi-care-model-guidelines).

For part D plan sponsors that adopt alternative classification systems, their approval is at least partially based on how similar their formulary model is to the USP model or that of other commonly used models, such as the *American Hospital Formulary Service* (AHFS) Pharmalogic-Therapeutic Classification. More information about that model can be found on the AHFS website (ahfsdruginformation.com/ahfs-pharmacologic-therapeutic -classification). In either case, the CMS maintains that every Part D plan must also abide by the following guidelines:

1. **Each drug category or class must include at least two drugs.** The exception to this rule is in the case that two drugs aren't available, or two drugs are available, but one is clinically superior to the other.

2. **The two drugs must be chemically different.** That means the two drugs can't be the same drug in different doses, or the brand name and generic version of the same drug. Additionally, the plan should cover multiple doses and strengths of the two drugs.

3. **Drug lists must include "all or substantially all drugs" in the six protected drug classes, including anticonvulsants.** CMS instated this policy in hopes that Medicare beneficiaries who were reliant on certain drugs wouldn't be discouraged from enrolling in certain Part D plans. Additionally, making more drugs available for people who depend on them helps mitigate the risks and complications associated with altering or interrupting necessary treatment. For those with epilepsy, this is especially important because medications are not interchangeable. Switching or coming off a medication can lead to breakthrough seizures, increased seizure activity, and other, more serious risks.

One important exception is that the *Medicare Modernization Act* (MMA) prohibits reimbursement for controlled substances. Several anticonvulsant drugs are classified as Schedule IV Controlled Substances and will not be covered in Medicare Part D. The non-covered drugs are phenobarbital, diazepam (Valium, Diastat), lorazepam (Ativan), clonazepam (Klonopin), midazolam (Versed), clobazam (Onfi), and clorazepate

(Tranxene). All these drugs are available as inexpensive generic drugs with the exception of the Diastat formulation of diazepam.

Since 2008, there have been numerous proposals to make changes to Medicare's protected drug classes policy. In May 2018, the *U.S. Department of Health and Human Services* (HHS) released a report titled, "American Patients First: The Trump Administration Blueprint to Lower Drug Prices and Out-of-Pocket Costs." In November 2018, CMS proposed policies that were met with strong disapproval from organizations like the Epilepsy Foundation, the American Academy of Family Physicians, the American Cancer Society Action Network, the Diabetes Patient Advocacy Coalition, The Medicare Rights Center, and many more. The organizations said that while they supported some of the proposed rules, such as prohibiting "gag clauses," so pharmacists can tell their patients about more affordable ways to get their medications, the report's recommendations would largely hurt Part D beneficiaries. For example, the proposed changes would weaken protections for the protected drug classes, allowing plans to exclude protected class drugs from their formularies. The ability to implement broader use of prior authorization and step therapy would additionally create more hurdles for patients to get their medications, ultimately delaying or interrupting treatment, and contributing to further risks and costs, as a result. For more information about these proposed changes to Medicare Part D and other advocacy efforts by the Epilepsy Foundation, visit the organization's website (advocacy.epilepsy.com).

Living an Independent Life with Epilepsy

Undoubtedly, living with a seizure disorder can be disruptive to one's everyday activities. The ability to hold a full-time job and drive a car are arguably two of the most impacted. In both cases, the government has established protections against discrimination, as well as put guidelines in place for getting and retaining a driver's license. It's possible to live with self-confidence and independence. Next, we'll review some important legal rights you have in the workplace and what you need to know in order to drive with epilepsy.

Working with Epilepsy

Patients with epilepsy are well aware of the difficulties that they face when trying to get or keep a job. According to the Epilepsy Foundation, the unemployment rate for people with uncontrolled seizures has been estimated to be five times higher than the national average, at up to 50 percent, according to some studies. How much of this is due to discrimination is difficult to determine because even though there are laws that protect individuals from being discriminated against due to their disabilities, it can be difficult for a person to prove that discrimination has occurred. Knowing how the laws protect you, however, is the first step in guarding your rights to equal opportunities.

Americans with Disabilities Act

Signed into law in 1990, The *Americans with Disabilities Act* (ADA) was the first civil rights law of its kind to prohibit discrimination against people with disabilities in all areas of public life including work, school, transportation, and all public and private places that are open to the public. The ADA was amended in 2008 and became effective as the *American with Disabilities Act Amendments Act* (ADAA) on January 1, 2009. Title I of the ADA prohibits employers with 15 or more employees, including state and local governments, employment agencies, and labor organizations from discriminating in employment against qualified individuals with disabilities. Title II of the ADA prohibits state and local governments from discriminating against qualified individuals with disabilities in programs, activities, and services. The ADA is primarily enforced by the *Equal Employment Opportunity Commission* (EEOC), an independent federal agency that has the authority to investigate discrimination charges lodged against employers who are covered by the law. In the following paragraph, we've outlined what you should know specifically about how the ADA applies to people with epilepsy.

Your Rights Under the ADA

1. **Epilepsy is explicitly recognized as a disability.** Reflecting the new changes in the ADAA, there is no question whether people with epilepsy are protected by the terms of the ADA. This applies even for those who have achieved seizure reduction or total seizure freedom from medication, surgery, or other treatments. Any individual with any history of epilepsy, including someone who has been misdiagnosed with epilepsy, is protected by the ADA.

2. **When considering you for a job, an employer cannot ask you if you have epilepsy.** It is not legal for employers to ask about any medical condition, if you've undergone any treatments (or what types), and whether you've applied/received any workers' compensation. The employer is also not legally allowed to ask if you've ever been injured on the job or ask you to take a medical examination as part of the application process.

3. **If you voluntarily disclose you have epilepsy, an employer cannot ask you for details before making a job offer.** The ADA prohibits employers from asking follow-up questions about your seizures, your treatment, or your prognosis. The exception to this rule is that if the employer "reasonably believes that [you] will require an accommodation to perform the job because of [your] epilepsy or treatment." Here is an example scenario provided by the EEOC:

   "An individual applies to be a clerk for a law firm, a job that sometimes requires going out to purchase office supplies, and picking up and delivering documents. When the interviewer explains that clerks typically walk, take a taxi, or occasionally use the company car to run errands, the applicant discloses that she does not have a driver's license due to epilepsy and, therefore, would have to use some other form of transportation to run errands if she could not walk or take a taxi. Because there is no reason to believe that the applicant will need an accommodation to do the job, the interviewer may not ask the applicant follow-up questions about her epilepsy, such as when she was diagnosed, whether her license was suspended because she had a seizure, or whether anyone else in her family has epilepsy."

4. **If you're made a job offer, an employer may not single you out for a medical examination.** Some questions about your health and a required medical examination are permissible at this stage, however, but only if all job applicants are asked to do the same. Upon learning that you have epilepsy, the employer may ask some follow-up questions like whether you take any medications, whether you still have seizures (and if so, what type), how long it takes you to recover from a seizure, and/or whether you'll need assistance if you have a seizure at work. The employer may also ask you to submit documentation from your doctor that answers questions "designed to assess the applicant's ability to perform the job's functions safely."

5. **An employer may not withdraw a conditional job offer if you're able to perform the essential functions of the job with or without reasonable accommodations.** As long as you do not pose a direct threat to yourself or others that can't be eliminated or reduced through the reasonable accommodations, it is unlawful for an employer to rescind a job offer based on your epilepsy. Here's another example scenario from the EEOC:

"An experienced chef receives an offer from a hotel resort. During the post-offer medical examination, he discloses that he has had epilepsy for 10 years. When the doctor expresses concern about the applicant's ability to work around stoves and use sharp utensils, the applicant explains that his seizures are controlled by medication and offers to bring information from his neurologist to answer the doctor's concerns. He also points out that he has worked as a chef for 7 years without incident. Because there is no evidence that the applicant will pose a significant risk of substantial harm while performing the duties of a chef, the employer may not withdraw the job offer."

6. An employer must maintain confidentiality about your medical condition. It is not legal for your employer to share details related to your health information during the application process or after you're hired by anyone. Even if you have a seizure at work, your employer may not tell your colleagues that you have epilepsy. Additionally, your employer may not share details about any reasonable accommodations made for you, such as why you're allowed more breaks or why you've been absent from work. There are some exceptions to this rule, which include:

    ■   The employer has to tell your supervisor(s)/manager(s) in order to provide reasonable accommodations or to meet your work restrictions.

    ■   The employer has to tell first aid and/or safety personnel if you might need emergency treatment or other assistance in case you have a seizure at work.

    ■   The employer has to tell people investigating ADA compliance or similar state and local laws.

    ■   The employer has to provide supplementary information for workers' compensation claims or insurance claims.

Reasonable Accommodations

Of course, it goes without saying that the person applying for a job must have the necessary education, skills, or other functions to do the job. Such a person is called a *qualified individual* in the ADA. However, as mentioned earlier, the employer and the employee both have to make reasonable accommodations if the disability interferes with performing essential features of the job, unless the accommodation poses an "undue burden" or "undue hardship," defined as a significant expense or difficulty, to the employer. What qualifies as an undue burden depends on a number of factors, such as the nature and cost of the accommodation requested, the size of the company, and so forth. It's important to note that the employer is not required to substantially change the job requirements. The accommodation must be tailored to the individual and should be seen as a give-and-take between the employer and the employee, both working in good faith to find an acceptable accommodation that permits the employee to perform the essential features of the job. Sometimes, the patient's physician can play an important role in finding acceptable accommodations. There are three separate categories of reasonable accommodations:

1. **Modifications to the job application process that enables disabled individuals to be considered for the job they qualify for.** For example, if you're experiencing memory problems due to complications from your medications or seizures, and you're asked to submit materials for your application, you may request that your employer send a written request with specific directions.

2. **Modifications or adjustments to the work environment that enables the disabled individual to perform the essential job functions.** For example, if you need a rubber mat around your desk to help safeguard you in case you have a seizure and fall, this is a reasonable accommodation.

3. **Modifications or adjustments that allow the disabled individual to enjoy equal benefits and privileges of other similarly situated employees without disabilities.** For example, if you still experience seizures, you may request the ability to take a break after having a seizure at work and/or to rest in a private area.

If you're having problems meeting job demands, it's smart to be proactive and raise the issue with your employer, rather than wait until disciplinary action is taken. If you and your employer are having difficulty arriving at a satisfactory accommodation, the *Job Accommodation Network* (JAN) may be helpful. You can find more information on the JAN website (askjan.org). For additional details about your rights as an individual with epilepsy under the ADA, you can visit the EEOC website (eeoc.gov/laws/types/epilepsy.cfm).

The Rehabilitation Act of 1973

Replacing the Vocational Rehabilitation Act, the *Rehabilitation Act* (Rehab Act) prohibits discrimination on the basis of disability in programs conducted by federal agencies, in programs receiving federal financial assistance, in federal employment, and in the employment practices of federal contractors. It also requires federal electronic and information technology to be accessible to people with disabilities, including employees and members of the public. Some other protections from discrimination are found in Section 188 of the *Workforce Investment Act* of 1998 (WIA).

The Fair Labor Standards Act of 1938

Signed into law during the years following the Great Depression, the *Fair Labor Standards Act* (FLSA) established the federal minimum wage and overtime pay requirements. However, this law allowed employers to pay workers with disabilities less than the federal minimum wage, or subminimum wages, upon receiving a certificate from the *Wage and Hour Division*

(WHD), the federal agency that oversaw labor standards. Of course, since there have been sweeping changes made to expand rights and protections to those with disabilities, employers fulfill all the following requirements in order to pay a disabled worker less than the federal minimum wage:

1. The worker's disability reduces their ability to do the job.
2. The employer must tell the disabled worker that they are being paid less than the minimum wage.
3. The worker's pay must be based on the amount other employers pay their employees and the worker's ability to do the job.
4. If the worker is providing services for the federal government, the contract may require that they be paid at least an hourly rate, according to the law.

For more information about how the FLSA may affect you, you can visit the website of The United States Department of Labor (dol.gov/whd/regs/compliance/hrg.htm).

What to Do if You've Been Discriminated Against

If you feel that you have been discriminated against at work based on your disability status, you can file a *Charge of Discrimination*, a signed statement saying that an employer, union, or labor organization engaged in employment discrimination, with the EEOC. For all laws enforced by the EEOC, except the Equal Pay Act, you must file a Charge of Discrimination before filing a job discrimination lawsuit against your employer. Here's what you need to know in order to file a Charge of Discrimination:

1. **There are strict time limits.** In general, you must file your complaint within 180 days of when the discrimination took place. This deadline may be extended to 300 days in some cases.
2. **You can file online, in person, or by mail.** Use the EEOC's Public Portal to file a Charge of Discrimination online or to schedule an in-person appointment at your local EEOC agency.

Offices also commonly have walk-in appointments, but check in advance if that's an option. If you want to file your charge through mail, you'll need to include a number of documents, including: when the discrimination took place, a short description of the actions you believe were discriminatory, some personal information, and more. For a full list of what to mail in, visit the EEOC website on filing a Charge of Discrimination (eeoc.gov/employees/howtofile.cfm). Although you cannot file a Charge of Discrimination over the phone, you can speak with a representative for more information and begin the process by calling this number: 1-800-669-4000.

3. **Your case can be resolved in multiple ways.** Within 10 days of filing your charge, the EEOC will send a notice to your employer about the complaint. In some cases, you'll be offered an opportunity to take part in mediation, in which an EEOC mediator will help you and your employer reach a voluntary settlement. If mediation isn't an option, or it doesn't resolve your issue, the EEOC will investigate it formally. This may involve requesting more information, holding interviews, and more. The EEOC reports an average of 10 months to complete an investigation, whereas mediation can help resolve your case faster, typically in less than 3 months.

4. **You must request a Notice of Right to Sue.** Generally, you must allow the EEOC 180 days to resolve your case with some exceptions. If the EEOC is unable to determine whether discrimination occurred or it's unable to reach a voluntary settlement with your employer, but it decides not to file a lawsuit, the EEOC will send you a Notice of Right to Sue. You must have this before you file a lawsuit against your employer for discrimination based on disability under the ADA.

The Epilepsy Foundation also has the Jeanne A. Carpenter Legal Defense Fund to help people who feel they've been discriminated against.

The organization has a list of lawyers across the country who can help you with your problem, as well as information on the type of help that they can provide. You can find more information and contact details online.

Unfortunately, some recent Supreme Court rulings have made it more difficult to claim discrimination under the ADA. The Court has ruled that you must prove the disability to be "substantially limiting" and that a condition that is controlled by medication does not qualify for ADA protection unless substantial disability continues to exist. For example, a woman with epilepsy may have found that medication fully controls her seizures, but the side effects of the medication may slow her thinking to the point that she may have difficulty working at the same rate as other employees. She may ask for accommodation under the ADA in these circumstances.

Seizures and Short-term Disability from Work

Patients often come to the clinic or call after having had a seizure and want to have a letter to return to work. This can put physicians in a dilemma about when a patient can return to work and what kind of job restrictions are necessary to protect the patient and their coworkers if another seizure occurs. If the patient's job involves driving, then the rules are clear-cut and the patient will not be able to work at their usual duties until driving privileges are restored. Unless suitable alternative work can be arranged, this can mean an extended time off work or lifelong loss of job duties for commercial drivers, as detailed in previous sections of this chapter. For people with sedentary jobs, a breakthrough seizures may not pose much of a problem at all. However, there are many people, particularly those in manufacturing or construction fields, where breakthrough seizures produce major problems in deciding when it's safe to return to work. If alternative duties that can be safely performed even if the patient has another seizure, then the patient can promptly return to work. If not, a common approach that many physicians use is to take the driving regulations for their state and use the time that a license is suspended to be a suitable proxy for the time needed to be off work. The reasoning behind such actions is that if the state has determined the seizure-free period is sufficiently safe for driving, then it's considered aptly safe to return to most jobs as well. Most employers also feel comfortable with this approach.

Driving with Epilepsy

With the exception of residents of a few large cities, where public transportation is well-developed and commonly used, driving a car is the primary mode of travel for most Americans. Thus, for people with epilepsy, being unable to drive is one of the greatest frustrations they face. Not only is it inconvenient, it also reinforces the notion that they are not independent adults. It affects their ability to work, socialize, and manage their health. Because having a seizure while driving can be very dangerous for the driver, the passengers, and others on the road, each state sets its own regulations about driving if you have a history of seizures. These guidelines include: the period of time you must be seizure-free in order to have a driver's license, whether your doctor must submit an evaluation to the state of your ability to drive, and whether the state requires periodic medical updates about your condition and how frequently. Fortunately, only a few states require physicians to report patients who have had seizures to the state Department of Motor Vehicles (DMV). Most states make additional restrictions for driving commercial vehicles. In addition, the *Federal Motor Carrier Safety Administration* (FMCSA) has issued recommendations for medical examiners to determine a driver's medical qualifications for driving vehicles for interstate commerce. These guidelines are spelled out in Section 391.41 of the *Federal Motor Carrier Safety Regulations* (FMCSRs) and can be found on the FMCSA website (fmcsa.dot.gov/rules-regulations/administration/medical.html). This regulation is advisory for medical personnel doing certification examinations for interstate commercial driver's licenses. These regulations are considered the minimum restrictions since examiners may hold a driver to a higher standard. Section 391.41(b)(8) deals with epilepsy. In this section, it states that a driver with a clinical diagnosis of epilepsy and recurrent seizures of any cause or who is taking antiseizure medication should never be certified. A driver who has had a single unprovoked seizure or episode of fainting may be certified, but only if the driver is not taking medications and has been free of seizures **off medication** for 5 years following the single seizure. For people with multiple seizures, the driver must be free of seizures for 10 years **off medication** from the last seizure to qualify to drive. Fever seizures of childhood are not disqualifying. All questionable spells require a waiting period of 6 months off medication, followed by a complete neurological examination to be cleared to drive. For people with acute provoked seizures, such as a seizure caused by a drug reaction or an acute metabolic disturbance, the individual must wait until they have fully recovered, have no residual complications, and are not taking antiseizure medication.

The Epilepsy Foundation keeps track of the regulations for each state and posts them on its website (epilspy.com/drivinglaws). The following table includes the most up-to-date driving regulations by state.

Driving Regulations by State

	Required Seizure-Free Period	Ability to Appeal DMV if Denied License?	Doctors to Report Epilepsy?	Required Period Medical Updates After License Is Issued
Alabama	No set period	Yes	Yes	Annually
Alaska	6 months	Yes	No	At DMV's discretion
Arizona	3 months, with exceptions	Yes	No	At DMV's discretion
Arkansas	1 year, with exceptions	Yes	No	At DMV's discretion
California	3 or 6 months, with exceptions	Yes	Yes	At DMV's discretion

	Required Seizure-Free Period	Ability to Appeal DMV if Denied License?	Doctors to Report Epilepsy?	Required Period Medical Updates After License Is Issued
Colorado	No set period	Yes	No	At DMV's discretion
Connecticut	No set period	Yes	No	At DMV's discretion
Delaware	No set period	Yes	Yes	Annually
District of Columbia	1 year	Yes	No	Annually, until seizure-free for 5 years
Florida	6 months (or less, at the physician's discretion)	Yes	No	At Medical Review Board's discretion
Georgia	6 months	Yes	No	At Medical Review Board's discretion
Hawaii	6 months, with exceptions	Yes	No	At DMV's discretion
Idaho	No set period	Yes	No	At DMV's discretion
Illinois	No set period	Yes	No	At Medical Review Board's discretion
Indiana	No set period	Yes	No	At Medical Review Board's discretion
Iowa	6 months, with doctor's statement	Yes	No	After first 6 months, and then at renewal
Kansas	6 months, with exceptions	Yes	No	Annually, until seizure-free for 3 years
Kentucky	3 months or longer	Yes	No	On renewal

	Required Seizure-Free Period	Ability to Appeal DMV if Denied License?	Doctors to Report Epilepsy?	Required Period Medical Updates After License Is Issued
Louisiana	No set period (based on doctor's recommendation)	Yes	No	At DMV'S discretion
Maine	3 months or 2 years (based on medical prognosis)	Yes	No	At DMV'S discretion
Maryland	3 months, with exceptions	Yes	No	At DMV'S discretion
Massachusetts	6 months, with exceptions	Yes	No	At DMV'S discretion
Michigan	6 months, with exceptions	Yes	No	At DMV'S discretion
Minnesota	3 months, with doctor's recommendation	Yes	No	As frequently as once every 6 months, depending on the circumstance
Mississippi	6 months	Yes	No	At Medical Advisory Board's discretion
Missouri	6 months, with doctor's recommendation	No	No	At DMV's discretion
Montana	No set period (based on doctor's recommendation)	Yes	No	At DMV's discretion
Nebraska	No set period	Yes	No	None
Nevada	3 months, with exceptions	Yes	Yes	Annually for 3 years
New Hampshire	1 year, or less at DMV's discretion	Yes	No	None

	Required Seizure-Free Period	Ability to Appeal DMV if Denied License?	Doctors to Report Epilepsy?	Required Period Medical Updates After License Is Issued
New Jersey	6 months	Yes	Yes	Every 6 months for 2 years, and then annually
New Mexico	6 months	Yes	Yes	Every 6 months for 2 years, and then annually
New York	1 year, or less at DMV's discretion	Yes	No	At DMV's discretion
North Carolina	6 months	Yes	No	At DMV's discretion
North Dakota	6 months; restricted license available after 3 months	Yes	No	Annually for at least 3 years
Ohio	No set period	Yes	No	At DMV's discretion
Oklahoma	6 months, with exceptions	Yes	No	At Department of Public Safety's discretion
Oregon	3 months or longer	Yes	Yes	At DMV's discretion
Pennsylvania	6 months, with exceptions	Yes	Yes	At Medical Advisory Board's discretion
Rhode Island	18 months, or less at DMV's discretion	Yes	No	At DMV's discretion
South Carolina	6 months	Yes	No	At 6 months, and then annually for 3 years
South Dakota	6 to 12 months, with doctor's recommendation	Yes	No	Every 6 months until seizure-free for 1 year

	Required Seizure-Free Period	Ability to Appeal DMV if Denied License?	Doctors to Report Epilepsy?	Required Period Medical Updates After License Is Issued
Tennessee	6 to 12 months, with exceptions	Yes	No	At Medical Review Board's discretion
Texas	3 months, with exceptions	Yes	No	At Medical Advisory Board's discretion
Utah	3 months, with exceptions	Yes	No	At Medical Advisory Board's discretion
Vermont	No set period	Yes	No	At Medical Advisory Board's discretion
Virginia	6 months, with exceptions	Yes	No	At Medical Advisory Board's discretion
Washington	6 months, with exceptions	Yes	No	At Medical Advisory Board's discretion
West Virginia	6 months	Yes	No	At Medical Advisory Board's discretion
Wisconsin	3 months, with doctor's recommendation	Yes	No	At Medical Advisory Board's discretion
Wyoming	No set period	Yes	No	At Medical Advisory Board's discretion

Patient Resources

Pharmaceutical and Medical Device Companies: Medications, Websites, and Contact Information

AbbVie, Inc. (Depacon, Depakote)
- Homepage: www.abbvie.com, www.depakote.com
- Contact: 1-800-255-5162

Teva Pharmaceuticals Industries Ltd. (Gabitril)
- Homepage: www.tevausa.com, www.gabitril.com
- Contact: 1-800-896-5855

LivaNova, PLC (Vagus Nerve Stimulation Therapy)
- Homepage: www.us.livanova.cyberonics.com/home
- Contact: 1-888-867-7846 (United States)

GlaxoSmithKline LLC (Lamictal)
- Homepage: www.gsk.com
- Contact: 1-888-825-5249

Novartis Pharmaceuticals Corporation (Tegretol, Trileptal)
- Homepage: www.pharma.us.novartis.com
- Contact: 1-862-778-2100

Janssen Pharmaceuticals, Inc. (Topamax)
- Homepage: www.janssenpharmaceuticalsinc.com, www.topamax.com
- Contact: 1-800-526-7736

Pfizer, Inc. (Cerebyx, Dilantin, Neurontin, Zarontin, Lyrica)
- Homepage: www.pfizer.com, www.dilantin.com, www.lyrica.com
- Contact: 1-800-879-3477

Genentech, Inc. (Klonopin)
- Homepage: www.genentech.com
- Contact: 877-436-3683

Sanofi-Aventis (Mebaral)
- Homepage: www.sanofi.us
- Contact: 1-800-981-2491

Shire Plc (Carbatrol)
- Homepage: www.shire.com, www.takeda.com
- Contact: 1-888-227-3755

UCB Pharma Ltd. (Keppra, Keppra XR, Vimpat, Briviac)
- Homepage: www.ucb-usa.com, www.vimpat.com
- Contact: 1-844-599-2273

Meda Pharmaceuticals, Inc. (Felbatol)
- Homepage: http://www.medapharma.us, www.felbatol.com
- Contact: 1-732-564-2200

Bausch Health Companies, Inc. (Diastat, Mysoline)
- Homepage: www.bauschhealth.com, www.diastat.com
- Contact: 1-800-321-4576

Eisai Inc. (Fycompa, Banzel)
- Homepage: www.us.eisai.com, www.fycompa.com, www.banzel.com
- Contact: 1-201-692-1100

Sunovion Pharmaceuticals, Inc (Aptiom)
- Homepage: www.sunovian.us, www.aptiom.com
- Contact: 1-508-481-6700

Supernus Pharmaceuticals, Inc (Trokendi XR, Oxtellar XR)

- Homepage: www.supernus.com, www.trokendixr.com, www.oxtellarxr.com
- Contact: 1-866-398-0833

Aquestive Therapeutics (Sympazan Oral Film)

- Homepage: www.aquestive.com, www.sympazan.com
- Contact: 1-908 -941-1900

Greenwich Biosciences, Inc. (Epidiolex)

- Homepage: www.greenwichbiosciences.com
- Contact: 1-833-424-6724

Directory of Prescription Drug Patient Assistance Programs

For prescription drugs' financial assistance, you can contact the following patient assistance programs:

AbbVie Patient Assistance Foundation (Depacon, Depakote)

- Homepage: www.abbvie.com/patients/patient-assistance.html
- Phone: 1-800-222-6885
- Address: AbbVie Patient Assistance Foundation, PO Box 270, Somerville, NJ 08876

Teva Cares Foundation (Gabitril)

- Homepage: http://www.tevacares.org
- Phone: 1-877-237-4881
- Address: Teva Cares Foundation, PO Box 52028, Phoenix, AZ 85072

GSKForYou (Lamictal)

- Homepage: www.gskforyou.com
- Phone: 1-866-728-4368
- Address: GSK Patient Assistance Program, PO Box 220590, Charlotte, NC 28222-0590

Novartis Patient Assistance NOW (Tegretol, Tegretol XR Trileptal)
- Homepage: www.patientassistancenow.com
- Phone: 1-800-245-5356
- Address: PO Box 66556, St. Louis, MO 63166-6556

Johnson & Johnson Patient Assistance Foundation, Inc. (Topamax)
- Homepage: www.jjpaf.org
- Phone: 1-800-652-6227
- Address: Johnson & Johnson Patient Assistance Foundation, Inc., Patient Assistance Program, PO Box 42796, Cincinnati, OH 45242

Pfizer RxPathways (Cerebyx, Dilantin, Neurontin, Zarontin, Lyrica)
- Homepage: www.pfizerrxpathways.com
- Phone: 1-844-989-7284
- Address: Pfizer RxPathways, PO Box 66976, St. Louis, MO 63166-6976

Genentech Access Solutions (Klonopin)
- Homepage: www.genentech-access.com
- Phone: 1-866-422-2377
- Address: Genentech Access Solutions, 1 DNA Way Mail Stop #858a, South San Francisco, CA 94080-4990

Shire Cares (Carbatrol)
- Homepage www.shire.com/patients/patient-services/shire-cares
- Phone: 1-888-227-3755
- Address: PO Box 698, Somerville, NJ 08876

UCB, Inc. UCB Patient Assistance Program (Keppra, Keppra XR, Vimpat)
- Homepage: www.ucb.com/patients/programmes
- Phone: 1-877-785-8906
- Address: UCB, Inc., UCB Patient Assistance Program, 1330 Enclave Parkway, Suite 125, Houston, TX 77077

Bausch Health Patient Assistance Program (Diastat, Mysoline)

- Homepage:www.bauschhealthpap.com
- Phone: 1-833-862-8727
- Address: Bausch Health Patient Assistance Program, PO Box 6122, Lawrenceville, NJ 08648

Eisai Patient Assistance Program (Fycompa, Banzel)

- Homepage: www.eisaireimbursement.com
- Phone: 1-855-347-2448
- Address: 100 Tice Blvd., Woodcliff Lake, NJ 07677

Sunovion Support (Aptiom)

- Homepage: www.sunoviansupport.com
- Phone: 1-877-850-0819
- Address: Sunovian Support, PO Box 220285, Charlotte, NC 28222

Oxtellar XR $0 Co-Pay Savings Program (Oxtellar XR)

- Homepage: www.oxtellarxr.com/savings-resources
- Phone: 1-866-398-0833
- Address: Supernus Pharmaceuticals, Inc., 1550 East Gude Drive, Rockville, MD 20850

Trokendi XR Patient Savings and Support Program (Trokendi XR)

- Homepage: www.trokendixr.com/topiramate-cost
- Phone: 1-855-305-2066
- Address: Supernus Pharmaceuticals, Inc., 1550 East Gude Drive, Rockville, MD 20850

Sympazan Savings Program (Sympazan)

- Homepage: www.sympazanhcp.com/copay-and-access-support .html
- Phone: 1-833-278-3788
- Address: 30 Technology Drive, Warren, NJ 07059

Books

For additional information on epilepsy and seizure therapies, patients' anecdotes and resources for families of patients, the following books are available through popular book distributors. These can be found on Amazon.com:

- *Epilepsy Surgery: A Guide for Patients and Families*
  By: Ruben Kuzniecky, MD
  Approximately 30 percent of patients with epilepsy have intractable seizures. A portion of these patients can be cured with epilepsy surgery. This book is intended to help patients and families understand the process by which patients are selected for surgery and the types of surgery available to patients. The book lists the investigations, tests, procedures, and other critical information for patients. This book also helps prepare the patient for surgery and how to recover from epilepsy surgery.

- *Silently Seizing: Common, Unrecognized, and Frequently Missed Seizures and Their Potentially Damaging Impact on Individuals With Autism Spectrum Disorders*
  By: Caren Haines, RN, Nancy Minshew, MD
  Up to 50 percent of all children diagnosed with autism have undiagnosed seizure disorders, to a great extent because they are difficult to diagnose and due to a lack of awareness and understanding. Caren Haines, RN, with renowned behavioral child neurologist, Nancy Minshew, MD, is determined to change that. At age 2, author Caren Haines's son was diagnosed with autism. By the time he was 12, his diagnosis didn't account for his uncontrollable aggression, the acrid smells that lingered in his mind, and the odd voices that screamed at him from inside his head. By the time he was 18, his out-of-control behavior mirrored a mood disorder with psychotic features. *Silently Seizing* begins with a close-up look at this family's journey and examines a disorder that cannot always

be identified in a clinical setting. Intersecting at two medical sub-specialties—neurology and psychiatry—the child who has autism and partial seizures is at a serious disadvantage. By inadvertently allowing children's brains to "silently seize," we are robbing them of their ability to function normally. When treated early with antiseizure medications, many children show amazing gains in expressive language and comprehension. Many begin to speak and learn as many troubling behaviors begin to disappear. Even more important, many children lose their diagnosis of autism. Backed by up-to-the-minute research, this must-read book includes sections on what autism is, the seizure-autism connection, tips for diagnosing and treating seizures, as well as how to better understand children's behavior.

■ *Epilepsy: The Ultimate Teen Guide (It Happened to Me)*
By: Kathlyn Gay, Sean McGarrahan (Authors)
Teens can lead normal, active lives despite having epilepsy, and this book shows them how other teens are doing so. Through their stories, they offer advice on whether and how to tell friends, dates, teachers, or an employer about their condition. Important teen issues, such as driving, dating, sports, and college are addressed. How the Americans with Disabilities Act (ADA) applies to people with epilepsy is also reviewed.

■ *I Have Epilepsy. It Doesn't Have Me*
By: Jamie Bacigalupo, Judy Bacigalupo (Authors); Inga Shalvashvili (Illustrator)
Follow eight-year-old Jamie on her journey from being diagnosed with benign rolandic epilepsy at age five. Jamie persevered and overcame her epilepsy, and she went on to help other children by starting her own non-profit that provides gifts to children in over five states. Proceeds go to her non-profit to deliver to more children with epilepsy and/or asthma.

■ *Mommy, I Feel Funny! A Child's Experience with Epilepsy*
By: Danielle M. Rocheford (Author); Chris Herrick (Illustrator)
Based on a true story, *Mommy, I Feel Funny!* introduces the reader to Nel, a little girl diagnosed with epilepsy. The story takes you through the days following Nel's first seizure. Suddenly, Nel and her family are faced with thoughts, fears, and emotions that come with the discovery, understanding, and acceptance of epilepsy.

Paralleling medical terms with recognizable psychotic behaviors; Comprehending delusions and identifying hallucinations; Preparing for all aspects of brain surgery, including the steps before and the adjustments afterward; Finding hope and inspiration through reading the story of a man who fought seizures for 24 years and won.

■ *Epilepsy (What Do I Do Now?)*
By: Carl W. Bazil, Derek J. Chong, Daniel Friedman (Authors)
Patients with epilepsy pose many clinical challenges. Even experienced clinicians occasionally arrive at the point where diagnostic, work-up, treatment, or prognostic thinking becomes blocked. *Epilepsy* is the fifth volume in the *What Do I Do Now?* series, providing the clinician with the necessary tools to evaluate and treat an epilepsy patient. Applying a case-based approach of curbside consultation, the authors present 31 actual cases, providing key points to remember and recommendations for further reading at the end of each case, including EEGs and imaging where applicable. Concise and readable, *Epilepsy* is the perfect quick-reference guide for anyone working with epilepsy patients.

■ *Navigating Life with Epilepsy*
By: David C. Spencer, MD
Roughly 3 million people in the United States have already been diagnosed with epilepsy and another 200,000 new cases are diagnosed each year. Worldwide, approximately 1 percent of the global

population is diagnosed with epilepsy at some point in their lives. With the diagnosis come questions, concerns, and uncertainties from both the person diagnosed and their family. So, where to go? *Navigating Life with Epilepsy* provides accessible, comprehensive, and up-to-date information about epilepsy shared from the two decades of experience of epileptologist David Spencer, MD, FAAN. This book guides the reader through the initial diagnosis, offers explanations on current approaches to diagnostic testing, medications, and treatment options, as well as life management for the patient, their family, and their caregiver. Patient's stories are peppered throughout to illustrate that you are not alone: like you, they must navigate the myriad psychosocial challenges associated with epilepsy, including everyday concerns like driving, work, and relationships. *Navigating Life with Epilepsy* is a perfect resource for both patients with epilepsy and the family members and friends who care for them.

■ *Living Well with Epilepsy and Other Seizure Disorders: An Expert Explains What You Really Need to Know*
By: Carl W. Bazil, MD
Treatment options, lifestyle strategies, and emotional support for two million Americans.
Epilepsy, once mistakenly associated with demonic possession, has for centuries been a poorly understood illness. Today, although it affects nearly one out of every one hundred Americans, little comprehensive information can be found on bookshelves regarding this common and complex neurological disease. Until now!

Using his expertise in pharmacology and neuroscience, Dr. Carl Bazil demystifies epilepsy and other seizure disorders. He offers medical, practical, and emotional support to patients and their families. Dr. Bazil explains how and why seizures occur and thoroughly discusses treatment options, the pros and cons of surgery, experimental and alternative treatments, strategies for daily living, and much more.

Substantiated with case examples, this useful book provides a much-needed window into epilepsy, so patients can achieve the full life they deserve.

Home Safety Checklist

Kitchen, Cooking, Barbeque

- Do not start open fires, grills, and so forth. Ask someone to help you.
- Avoid boiling or frying in large pots and pans.
- Avoid a gas stove. Cook with an electric or microwave oven.
- Use rear burners when cooking.
- Avoid using an electric knife.
- Use oven mitts.
- Use a cart to wheel hot food from the stove to the table.
- Install heat control devices in the kitchen faucet to prevent scalding.
- Use plastic containers rather than glass.
- Consider placing security cameras in some rooms

Bathrooms

- Never lock bathroom doors.
- Take showers, not baths. If taking a bath, use only a few inches of water.
- Use a handheld shower head, and sit during showers.
- Shave with an electric shaver.
- Set the temperature of your water heather to warm.

General

- Do not hunt or handle guns, and so forth.
- Use an iron that shuts off automatically.
- Avoid using a curling iron or hot styling tools.
- Keep a protective screen in front of the fireplace.
- Avoid exposed heaters.
- Do not smoke cigarettes.
- Install smoke alarms.
- Choose a one-floor dwelling, if possible; limit use of stairs.
- Carpet all floors.
- Consider a home security system with a "panic button."
- Consider using seizure detection devices, such as watches, under-the-mattress alarms, or cameras.
- Keep phone numbers for hospital, doctor, and so forth, by your home phone and programmed into your mobile phone.
- Check in with a friend or family member at least once a day.
- Make sure a friend or family member has your doctor's phone number.
- Instruct friends and family on proper first aid for convulsions and when to call an ambulance.

First Aid for Seizures

Note: Most seizures are self-limited and require little intervention. Here are some practical guidelines.

Please note, these are general guidelines and should not be construed as medical advice. You should discuss them with your doctor or health care provider and act according to your own situation.

What should I do when someone is having a seizure? That question is asked over and over by families and friends of individuals of epilepsy, particularly concerning tonic-clonic seizure or convulsion. Witnessing a tonic-clonic seizure is an extremely frightening experience. When a seizure occurs, an observer can only do a few things to help. It's important that fear and frustration don't cause observers to respond in a way that may actually make things worse. The following are a few suggestions about what an observer should do during a seizure:

1. Time the seizure. This may be important in making a decision as to whether emergency help should be summoned.

2. Observe the seizure behavior carefully. This may help the doctor better understand the cause of the seizures and impact on the medication choice.

3. Protect the person having the seizure. Keep them from falling, hitting their head, or injuring themselves in some other way.

4. Do not put anything in the individual's mouth. During a seizure, the person having a seizure does not breathe well (and may at times appear blue around the lips). After the seizure is over, they will go back to breathing, but during the seizure, an observer can do nothing to help the person breathe. A person having a seizure cannot "swallow their tongue," so there's no need to try to put something into the individual's mouth.

5. Do not attempt cardiopulmonary resuscitation (CPR) unless the patient stops breathing. Call for emergency services if jerking movements last longer than 3 minutes.

6. When possible, roll the patient on their side. This may not be possible during the seizure itself, but it should be accomplished as soon as possible. While lying on their side, blood and saliva can more easily drain from the mouth, and it's easier for the individual to breathe. After the seizure, clear the airway of saliva, blood, or vomit, if possible.

7. Allow the person to wake up on their own. There is no need to stimulate or shake the individual who is sleeping after a seizure.

8. Do not restrain the individual, either during or after the seizure. Doing so may contribute to more agitation and aggressiveness.

You may need to intervene if the individual is going to do something dangerous (like walking out into traffic).

9. Stay with the individual after the seizure is over. Wait until the
    person is back to their normal level of alertness or until other
    help arrives.

10. Notify the individual's physician of the seizure. Tell the patient
    what happened, and do not allow them to drive.

For seizures that are not convulsive, the following is helpful:

1. Do not restrain the individual.
2. Protect the individual from wandering or walking into stairs,
    windows, and so forth, by gently guiding them into a safe area.
3. Do not try to reason with the individual after the seizure.
4. Stay with the individual until their confusion clears.
5. Notify the individual's family, friends, and physician of the
    seizure.
6. Do not allow the individual to drive that day.
7. Tell the individual what happened.

Glossary of Terms

Absence Seizures (childhood absence epilepsy; also known as petit mal, true petit mal, or pyknolepsy): A seizure disorder in children between 4 years old and adolescence. There is no warning of the attacks. Patients have a sudden change in consciousness, with staring and a blank facial expression, usually lasting less than 15 seconds. The EEG shows a typical pattern. Most patients outgrow the seizures by age 16. Seizures may be provoked by hyperventilation. The electroencephalogram reveals generalized 3-Hz spike and wave.

Atypical Absence Seizure: These seizures last longer than a typical absence seizure and more often have associated muscle tone changes. The EEG is faster or slower than the EEG seen in typical absence.

Agyria (lissencephaly): A type of cortical dysplasia with inadequate cortical sulcation and gyration. The cortex is smooth and thin, with most of the cortical neurons misplaced in a subcortical layer.

Aicardi Syndrome: This disorder affects only girls. Patients have mental retardation, infantile spasms, missing sections of the corpus callosum, and eye abnormalities. Patients often die early. Spinal bone abnormalities are common. This is a genetic disorder.

Ambulatory EEG: An ambulatory electroencephalogram (EEG) monitoring system that uses digital technology and can record EEG activity at home or any setting for up to 3 to 4 days.

Astatic Seizure: A seizure that result in a fall. A drop attack that may be due to a tonic, atonic, myoclonic, or partial onset seizure. Astatic seizures are usually seen in Lennox-Gastaut syndrome.

Atonic Seizure: A seizure that results in loss of muscle tone. The loss of tone may result in the patient falling to the ground. If less intense, the head may drop. Facial and dental injury is common.

Aura: Although an aura is often thought to be the warning of an impending seizure, it actually represents the beginning of a seizure. What the individual experiences depends on where the seizure starts. The most frequent auras are those seen in temporal lobe epilepsy patients. These auras are described as fear, impending doom, déjà vu, and so forth.

Automatisms: Abnormal involuntary or semi-purposeful movements that occur during or after an epileptic seizure, usually associated with memory loss. Patients may smack their lips, swallow, chew, rub their hands, walk, or perform more complex movements, such as undressing or saying things.

Benign Familial Neonatal Convulsions: Occurring primarily on days 2 and 3 after birth, these clonic seizures are inherited among family members. A minority of the children develop epilepsy.

Benign Rolandic Epilepsy: The most common epilepsy in children. Also known as *benign epilepsy with centrotemporal spikes*, the name refers to the electrical discharges seen on the EEG. Seizures begin between age 4 and 13 years in normal children. The seizures are characterized by speech arrest, salivation, and facial jerking. Convulsions also may occur. Most of the seizures occur during sleep or soon after waking up. Patients respond well to antiepileptic drugs, but many do not require medication. Benign rolandic epilepsy is age related, and seizures disappear by age 16.

Catamenial Epilepsy: Seizures somehow related to the time of menstruation. The seizures may take place any time before, during, or after the menstrual period. At least half the women with epilepsy have catamenial seizures.

Clonic Seizure: Repetitive jerking of muscles during a seizure. Most often, clonic seizures start in the upper or lower limb (hand, arm, face, and so forth). If the seizures follow a pattern of involvement of the hand to the face and the leg, they are called Jacksonian seizures.

Computerized Axial Tomography (CAT or CT scan): An imaging technique based on X-ray images taken in different planes by a movable gantry and reconstructed to provide views of the skull and brain. CAT scans are particularly useful when searching for blood or skull defects, but they may not detect small lesions causing seizures.

Convulsion: A generalized tonic-clonic seizure. A partial seizure may spread to become a convulsion, or a convulsion may begin globally without a focal onset.

Corpus Callosotomy: Splitting the fibers of the corpus callosum, which is the bridge of fibers that connects the right and left half of the brain. A type of epilepsy surgery particularly used for patients who have 'drop attacks' due to atonic seizures and who are at risk for injury. Many of these patients have Lennox-Gastaut syndrome. This surgery can greatly reduce drop attacks, but it does not improve partial seizures.

Dysplasia: Abnormal tissue or tissue in the wrong place; usually not tumor-related. Dysplasias constitute a large number of disorders often associated with childhood epilepsy.

Déjà Vu: A common aura. A sensation that a new experience has occurred before. A déjà vu sensation may occur as an aura prior to a complex partial or generalized seizure. Most common in temporal lobe epilepsy.

Depth Electrodes: Invasive electrodes used to determine the seizure focus when scalp electroencephalograms remain inconclusive. Typically, four to six electrodes are placed stereotactically into the brain under computed axial tomography or magnetic resonance imaging guidance through small holes drilled into the skull. These electrodes are associated with a small risk of hemorrhage and infection.

Electroencephalogram (EEG): Recording of brain electrical activity. The EEG was discovered by Dr. Hans Berger in 1929 and remains an essential component of epilepsy diagnosis and treatment. The EEG is usually recorded with scalp electrodes distributed in an array over the head. The electrical signal is filtered, amplified, and continuously recorded. Typically, 16 channels of electrical activity from different brain areas are displayed. Most EEG recordings take 30 minutes of continuous recording.

Epilepsia Partialis Continua: A form of continuous focal motor seizures, usually of the face or arms, lasting hours, days, or months. These represent simple partial seizures. Most common causes include Rasmussen's encephalitis and viral diseases.

Epilepsy with Grand Mal Seizures on Awakening: A genetic type of epilepsy with average age of onset at 16 to 17 years. Nearly all convulsions occur after awakening from sleep. Seizures respond well to antiepileptic medication, but often recur when drugs are stopped.

Epileptic Syndrome: A group of symptoms and signs, seizure types, cause, genetics, location, age of onset, precipitating factors, and other characteristics. Defining a patient within an epilepsy syndrome guides treatment and improves prognosis. Examples of epilepsy syndromes are benign rolandic epilepsy, childhood absence epilepsy, juvenile myoclonic epilepsy, and West syndrome.

Febrile Seizures: Seizures with fever that occur between the ages of 6 months and 5 years. Most occur during viral infections between 18 and 24 months of age. Very few of these children develop epilepsy. Children with one or two simple febrile seizures do not require chronic antiepileptic drug therapy. These seizures appear to be a benign response to fever that is age related and later outgrown. Children with many febrile seizures are more likely to require ongoing antiepileptic treatment.

Grand Mal Seizures: Convulsive seizures. Loosely translates from the French to "big bad" seizures. This term is not in use any longer.

Hemimegalencephaly: One side of the brain is larger than the other. It may be seen in rare developmental cerebral malformations. Usually associated with seizures, developmental delay, and mild weakness of the contralateral (opposite) side of the body.

Hemispherectomy: A type of epilepsy surgery. Removing or disconnecting either the entire or a part of one hemisphere. Many of these patients already have a severe dysfunction of that portion of the brain. Excellent seizure control after this operation is common.

Hertz: A unit of frequency (cycles per second) named after Dr. Heinrich Hertz, the discoverer of radio waves.

Heterotopia: A type of malformation of brain development. A cluster of neurons in an abnormal location resulting from abnormal migration. These misplaced neurons can be the source of epileptic seizures and other neurologic symptoms.

Hippocampal Sclerosis: Scar tissue in the hippocampus. A loss of neurons and scarring of the hippocampus is associated with temporal lobe epilepsy. It can appear on magnetic resonance imaging as atrophy and bright spots.

Hippocampus: A portion of the brain critical for memory function. The structure has the shape of a seahorse and it is often the location of seizures in temporal lobe epilepsy.

Hypsarrhythmia: A dramatic chaotic pattern on the EEG of patients with infantile spasms. Usually associated with poor response to antiepileptic drugs.

Ictal: "During a seizure." The period of clinical and electrical epileptic activity.

Infantile Spasms (West syndrome): Described in 1841, by Dr. William James West, on observing his own child. Seizures consist of flexor and/ or extensor spasms of the body, which tend to occur in clusters. Up to 60 percent of cases of infantile spasms are associated with strokes, malformations, and other brain lesions. Good outcome is seen in children who are normal when seizures begin and in whom no cause can be found for the spasms.

Interictal: The time between seizures or when patients are not having a seizure. Refers usually to the EEG.

Intractable Epilepsy: A changing definition. In general, seizures that persist despite appropriate treatment. Approximately 35 percent of patients have seizures that do not respond to adequate doses of appropriate antiepileptic drugs. Patients with intractable epilepsy are candidates for investigational drug trials, epilepsy surgery, and other treatments.

Jamais Vu: A type of aura. Is best described as a feeling that a familiar experience has never occurred before (opposite of déjà vu). Jamais vu and déjà vu are types of temporal lobe partial seizures.

Juvenile Myoclonic Epilepsy (Janz syndrome): A primary generalized epilepsy with onset between ages 12 and 18 years. Patients have brief jerks (myoclonic seizures) particularly when fatigued. These can occur in clusters and lead to convulsions. Continued treatment is required for most patients.

Ketogenic Diet: Special diet described in the beginning of the twentieth century to treat seizures. The ketogenic diet requires a high ratio of fat to carbohydrate and protein. Improvement in seizure control is seen particularly in children when the diet is rigorously followed.

Landau-Kleffner Syndrome: An epilepsy syndrome of unknown cause affecting children. It consists of progressive language problems and an epileptiform EEG. Seventy percent of patients have seizures. Severe behavior problems commonly occur. Outcome is variable, with some children making a complete recovery as adults, whereas others do not.

Lennox-Gastaut Syndrome: A childhood epileptic syndrome of intractable epilepsy, mental retardation, and slow spike-and-wave on EEG. Multiple seizure types occur, particularly atypical absence, tonic, and drop attacks. Seizures are extremely difficult to control. In addition to the seizures, most of these children have other neurologic abnormalities. The condition is likely genetic in at least 50 percent of patients.

Magnetic Resonance Imaging (MRI): Imaging technique developed in the late 1980s that uses powerful magnetic fields and computers to create images of the body based on the water content. It is the most accurate imaging technique to look at brain structure.

Mesial Temporal Sclerosis: *See Hippocampal Sclerosis.*

Monotherapy: The treatment of epilepsy using a single medication, rather than a combination. Monotherapy has fewer side effects, simpler dosing, and lower cost.

Myoclonus: Brief motor jerks that may represent epileptic seizures or nonepileptic etiologies. Usually affecting arms and hands. Myoclonus is often reported after awakening. Myoclonus is seen in juvenile myoclonic epilepsy.

Neuronal Migration Disorders: Brain malformations causing seizures. A number of conditions are classified as migration disorders.

Nonepileptic Seizures (Pseudoseizures, Psychogenic Seizures): These may be events such as tics or strokes that are mistaken as epileptic seizures. More commonly, staring spells, abnormal movements, or convulsions result from psychiatric problems, such as conversion disorder or panic attacks. Careful studies are often needed to make a correct diagnosis.

Partial Seizure (Focal Seizures): A seizure that begins in a specific area of the brain. Partial seizures are divided into "simple" and "complex" seizures. Partial seizures are the most common seizure type in adults.

Partial Complex Seizure: A seizure that causes alteration of consciousness. Partial complex seizures are sometimes called psychomotor seizures. Automatisms, such as lip smacking, chewing, and swallowing, are common. Most patients have no memory of the events.

Partial Simple Seizure: A seizure that does not cause alteration of consciousness. For example, a seizure that causes hand or arm movements. An epileptic aura, such as a smell, visions, or sound, is also a partial simple seizure.

Petit Mal Seizure: *See Absence Epilepsy.*

Polycystic Ovary Syndrome: A condition characterized by multiple cysts in the ovaries, increased body hair, acne, weight gain, loss of menstrual cycles, and hormonal disruptions. Polycystic ovary syndrome is seen in women with temporal lobe epilepsy and in those taking Depakote.

Polytherapy: The treatment of epilepsy using multiple medication combinations.

Positron Emission Tomography (PET): A computerized imaging technique that allows imaging of brain metabolism. Usually used prior to surgical interventions. May uncover areas that magnetic resonance imaging may not detect as abnormal.

Pseudoseizures: *See Nonepileptic Seizures.*

Psychomotor Epilepsy: *See Temporal Lobe Epilepsy.*

Pyknolepsy: An older term for childhood absence epilepsy.

Rasmussen's Encephalitis: Rare inflammatory disease in young patients affecting half of the brain and causing progressive weakness of one side, mental decline, and intractable seizures. Traditional treatment has been surgery, but immune therapy is also helpful.

Responsive Neural Stimulation (RNS): A battery-powered, programmable generator, connected to electrodes in the brain. It can detect seizures and electrical discharges, and then, via the same electrodes, it releases an electrical discharge to stop the seizure. It may help about half of the patients with seizure control.

Single Photon Emission Computed Tomography (SPECT): Nuclear medicine imaging technique. It may help determine the area of a seizure focus. The injection is given at the time of seizure. It is of use in surgical candidates prior to surgery.

Spike: A specific EEG abnormality associated with epileptic seizures.

Spike-Wave: A specific EEG abnormality associated with epileptic seizures.

Status Epilepticus: Recurrent seizures lasting without recovery for 30 minutes or more. Status epilepticus can be life-threatening and, thus, is a medical emergency.

Subclinical Seizures (Electrographic Seizures): Electrical seizures that do not have any outward signs. These seizures are visible on the EEG.

Subdural Electrodes: Electrodes used during epilepsy surgery. These electrodes are made of plastic and metal. They are placed on the surface of the brain by a neurosurgeon to record electrical activity and assist in the location of the seizure focus before surgery.

Temporal Lobectomy: Refers to *resection or removal of the temporal lobe or part of it. This is the most common operation for seizures.*

Tonic: The portion of a seizure during which stiffening of muscles occurs. It is part of a generalized tonic-clonic seizure.

Tuberous Sclerosis: A genetic condition characterized by skin lesions, seizures, and cognitive changes. Behavioral and learning problems are common. The diagnosis is essential for genetic counseling. Patients should have cardiac and renal ultrasounds, as well as an ophthalmologic exam to screen for extra-neurologic manifestations.

Vagal Nerve Stimulator (NeuroCybernetic Prosthesis): A battery-powered programmable generator, similar to a cardiac pacemaker, implanted in the neck. It sends repeated stimulation via an electrode attached to the left vagus nerve. It may help up to 25 percent of patients with seizure control.

Wada Test: Also known as Amytal procedure. Pioneered by Dr. Jun Wada, a Japanese neurosurgeon. This test evaluates how good memory is and locates on which side of the brain language is located. This test is done before surgical intervention in some patients.

West Syndrome: *See Infantile Spasms.*

Index

LaVergne, TN USA
13 October 2009
160677LV00003B/228/P